Lecture Notes on Cardiology

To the memory of Paul Wood

Lecture Notes on Cardiology

AUBREY LEATHAM FRCP, FACC (Hon)
Consultant Physician,
St George's and National Heart Hospitals;
formerly Dean, Institute of Cardiology,
London

CATHERINE BULL MB BChir, MRCP
Paediatric Cardiologist,
Senior Lecturer,
Institute of Child Health;
Honorary Consultant Cardiologist,
Hospital for Sick Children, London

MARK V. BRAIMBRIDGE MA, MB, BChir (Cantab) FRCS (Eng)
Cardiothoracic Surgeon
Department of Cardiovascular Research,
Rayne Institute,
St Thomas Hospital, London

With a chapter on Electrocardiography by
DEREK J. ROWLANDS BSc, MD, FACC, FESC, FRCP
Consultant Cardiologist,
Honorary Lecturer in Cardiology,
University of Manchester,

and a section on Echocardiography by
GRAHAM LEECH MA, CEng MIEE
Chief of the Non-Invasive Laboratory
St George's Hospital, London

THIRD EDITION

OXFORD

BLACKWELL SCIENTIFIC PUBLICATIONS

LONDON EDINBURGH BOSTON

MELBOURNE PARIS BERLIN VIENNA

© 1967, 1974, 1991 by
Blackwell Scientific Publications
Editorial Offices:
Osney Mead, Oxford OX2 0EL
25 John Street, London WC1N 2BL
23 Ainslie Place, Edinburgh EH3 6AJ
238 Main Street, Cambridge
    Massachusetts 02142, USA
54 University Street, Carlton
    Victoria 3053, Australia

Other Editorial Offices:
Librairie Arnette SA
2, rue Casimir-Delavigne
75006 Paris
France

Blackwell Wissenschafts-Verlag
Meinekestrasse 4
D-1000 Berlin 15
Germany

Blackwell MZV
Feldgasse 13
A-1238 Wien
Austria

First published 1967
Second edition 1974
Portuguese translation 1980
Reprinted 1975, 1977 (twice),
1980, 1982, 1983, 1984, 1985, 1986
Third edition 1991
Reprinted 1993
Four Dragons edition 1991
Reprinted 1993

Set by Times Graphics, Singapore
Printed and bound in Great Britain
at The Alden Press, Oxford

DISTRIBUTORS

UK
  Marston Book Services Ltd
  PO Box 87
  Oxford OX2 0DT
  (Orders: Tel: 0865 791155
          Fax: 0865 791927
          Telex: 837515)
USA
  Blackwell Scientific Publications, Inc.
  238 Main Street
  Cambridge, MA 02142
  (Orders: Tel: 800 759-6102
          617 876-7000)
Canada
  Times Mirror Professional Publishing, Ltd
  130 Flaska Drive
  Markham, Ontario L6G 1B8
  (Orders: Tel: 800 268-4178
          416 470-6739)
Australia
  Blackwell Scientific Publications Pty Ltd
  54 University Street
  Carlton, Victoria 3053
  (Orders: Tel: 03 347-5552)

British Library
Cataloguing in Publication Data

Lecture notes on Cardiology
  3rd ed.
  1. Medicine. Cardiology
  I. Leatham, Aubrey.   II. Bull,
  Catherine.   III. Braimbridge, Mark V.
  IV. Leech, Graham.
  616.12

  ISBN 0-632-01944-1 (BSP)
  ISBN 0-632-03076-3 (Four Dragons)

Contents

Introduction to the Third Edition

The first edition reflected the developments in clinical cardiology made by the late Paul Wood and his colleagues. Twenty-five years of technical advance in medical and surgical knowledge of the heart have since intervened but clinical cardiology is still fundamental to our approach to the patient and has become even more rewarding because of advances in fundamental knowledge. Indeed a careful history and clinical examination, followed, if necessary, by an exercise test and echocardiogram, available in most district hospitals, will give an exact diagnosis in the majority of cases.

The medical curriculum continues to become more crowded, making a 'Lecture Notes' approach to cardiology welcome. This edition has been completely rewritten, aiming to cover the needs of senior medical students, house officers and the many general physicians and general practitioners who welcome a concise and physiological account of the principles of modern cardiology. Echocardiography now has a central role in describing the anatomy and function of the heart, deserving a new section provided by Graham Leech. The sections on congenital heart disease and electrocardiography have been extensively rewritten, and great emphasis has been given to the illustrations, which are nearly all new.

Publisher's Note
Whilst the advice and information contained in this book are believed to be true and accurate at the date of going to press, neither the authors nor the publisher can accept any legal responsibility or liability for any errors or omissions that may be made.

Introduction to the First Edition

There is no lack of introductions to cardiology and little justification for another unless it is new in some respect other than the date on its cover. This book was designed as an extension of Blackwell's Lecture Notes series to provide an aid to the authors' undergraduate and postgraduate teaching, in which the students' preclinical physiological knowledge could be developed in a systematic and logical way towards the understanding of even the most complex cardiac lesions.

The main British contribution to the spectacular advances in cardiology in the last two decades has been this interpretation of each cardiac symptom and sign on a physiological basis. This advance was led by the late Dr Paul Wood and by Dr Aubrey Leatham.

The justification for placing another introduction to cardiology on the market is the commitment to this physiological approach in the presentation of cardiac disease, and also the continuation of this theme into the brief but comprehensive discussion of the surgical treatment available for each lesion.

The description of each cardiac condition is developed sequentially from its anatomy to the haemodynamic disturbances and thence to the physiological interpretation of the symptoms and physical signs. The prognosis and complications of the lesion lead rationally to description of medical treatment, indications for surgical treatment, the surgery available and its results.

It is immediately apparent that allocation of space has been heavily weighted in favour of congenital heart and acquired valve disease which lend themselves most favourably to physiological interpretation and surgical treatment. The main cardiac diseases in terms of incidence and community importance — coronary and hypertensive heart disease — are considered rather briefly, because there has been slower progress in their recognition and treatment in the last decade and because they are fully and satisfactorily covered in every textbook of medicine.

Surgical treatment also occupies a larger part of this book than most cardiological introductions. A physician has to know whether surgical treatment is possible for his cardiac patient, when it should be carried out, how his patient should be prepared for operation, what types of operation are available and what are the risks and complications of each. It is the general absence of such knowledge which has denied simple curative surgery to many patients in the last decade, and which has led to the emphasis and explanation of surgical treatment in an introduction to cardiology such as this which is designed for students who will become the general physicians and practitioners of the future.

Another function of an introduction to cardiology is the rationalization of description — aided by simple line diagrams — of the more complex cardiac lesions, which accounts for the space allotted to transposition of the great arteries, aneurysms of the thoracic aorta and others. The book has been aimed at those students who wish to widen their interest in cardiology beyond coronary and hypertensive heart disease, and the principle has therefore been adopted that almost *every* cardiac lesion merits inclusion, albeit briefly.

Dogmatism is inevitable in a Lecture Notes series because limited space precludes the development of conflicting theories and practice. The most widely accepted theory or practice has been outlined when alternatives exist. The results of surgery differ widely in varying centres and an attempt has been made to derive approximate mortality figures for each operation from current practice and the literature.

The pattern of description is standard throughout. The anatomy of the lesion is described, followed by its physiological disturbances. The symptoms and physical signs associated with each haemodynamic variation from normal are described. Prognosis is then outlined, followed by the types of treatment available and the benefits and risks of each. A balanced judgement on the diagnosis and treatment of any patient should then be possible.

J. S. Fleming
M. V. Braimbridge

Acknowledgements

We are immensely grateful to many of our colleagues for continuous help with the text, in particular to Mr Graham Leech for his section on echocardiography. A brief description of the principles of electrocardiography does not give enough information for the accurate reading of a standard 12 lead electrocardiogram: we therefore asked Dr Derek Rowlands, well known for the clarity of his teaching, to write a brief but comprehensive working basis for the subject. In order to be able to reproduce many illustrations from his magnificent ICI publication, *Understanding the Electrocardiogram*, we have placed this chapter at the end of the book, rather than in its logical position as an outpatient investigation in Chapter 2. We have also used his illustrations for Chapter 8. We are extremely grateful to Dr Roger Tittensor of ICI for providing these fine illustrations and also for his friendly co-operation and encouragement.

Professor Harold Lambert and Dr Susannah Eykyn helped us with the section on infective endocarditis and Sir Richard Bayliss with the chapter on systemic hypertension, and we are very grateful for their advice.

Our artists, Gillian Lee and Louise Perks, have laboured painstakingly to make our diagrams informative and it has been a pleasure to work with these two gifted people. The numerous printouts required to reduce the manuscript ruthlessly to essentials were patiently undertaken by Claire Millard at the Rayne Institute, St Thomas's Hospital.

The auscultatory diagrams are based on phonocardiograms and echophonocardiograms published in *Auscultation of the Heart and Phonocardiography* by Aubrey Leatham, Churchill Livingstone 1975.

List of Abbreviations

A	Aortic
AA	Aortic area
AF	Atrial fibrillation
AMV	Anterior mitral valve leaflet
Ao	Aorta
AP	Aortopulmonary
ASD	Atrial septal defect
AV	Atrioventricular
AVL	Aortic valve leaflet
BBB	Bundle branch block
BP	Blood pressure
CABG	Coronary artery bypass graft
CNS	Central nervous system
CPK	Serum creatine phosphokinase
CW	Chest wall
CW	Continuous wave
DC	Direct current
ECG	Electrocardiogram
Echo	Echocardiogram
EDM	Early diastolic murmur
Ej	Ejection sound
EjM	Ejection murmur
ESR	Erythrocyte sedimentation rate
F	Foot
HDL	High-density lipoprotein
HOCM	Hypertrophic obstructive cardiomyopathy
IABP	Intra-aortic balloon pump
IE	Infective endocarditis
ITU	Intensive therapy unit
IV	Intravenous
IVC	Inferior vena cava
IVS	Interventricular septum
JVP	Jugular venous pressure or pulse
LA	Left arm
LA	Left atrium
LAH	Left anterior hemiblock
LAH	Left atrial hypertrophy
LBBB	Left bundle branch block
LDH	Serum lactic dehydrogenase
LDL	Low density lipoproteins
LPH	Left posterior hemiblock
LSE	Left sternal edge
LV	Left ventricle
M	Mitral
MA	Mitral area
MDM	Mid-diastolic murmur
MI	Myocardial infarction
MV	Mitral valve
OS	Opening snap
P	Pulmonary
PA	Postero-anterior
PA	Pulmonary area
PA	Pulmonary artery
PDA	Persistent ductus arteriosus
PMV	Posterior mitral valve leaflet
PND	Paroxysmal nocturnal dyspnoea
PSM	Presystolic murmur
PTCA	Percutaneous transluminal coronary angioplasty
PVC	Premature ventricular contraction
PVE	Prosthetic valve endocarditis
PVR	Pulmonary vascular resistance
PW	Posterior wall
PW	Pulsed wave
RA	Right arm
RA	Right atrium
RAH	Right atrial hypertrophy
RBBB	Right bundle branch block
RV	Right ventricle
RVH	Right ventricular hypertrophy
SA	Sino-atrial
SAM	Systolic anterior motion
SGOT	Serum glutamic oxaloacetic transaminase
SVC	Superior vena cava
SVT	Supraventricular tachycardia
T	Tricuspid
TA	Tricuspid area
TG	Transposition of the great arteries
TPA	Tissue plasminogen activator
V	Voltage
VF	Ventricular fibrillation
VFM	Ventricular filling murmur
VSD	Ventricular septal defect
VT	Ventricular tachycardia
WPW	Wolff–Parkinson–White

Chapter 1
Clinical Diagnosis

An accurate diagnosis of cardiovascular disease, or of its absence, can usually be made at a single visit to an outpatient clinic by means of: history, physical examination, electrocardiogram (ECG) (often with exertion), echocardiogram (echo) and chest radiograph.

HISTORY

Careful evaluation of symptoms arising from the following haemodynamic disorders is the first and most important key to diagnosis:
- Raised pulmonary venous pressure
- Inadequate coronary blood flow
- Congestive (right heart) failure
- Low cardiac output
- Arrhythmia

Raised pulmonary venous pressure

Causes

1   Left ventricular (LV) failure.
2   Mitral stenosis (or other rare causes of obstruction at left atrial (LA) level, e.g. myxoma, cor triatriatum or obstructed total anomalous pulmonary venous drainage).

Symptoms

Dyspnoea

Definition

Dyspnoea is an inappropriate awareness of respiration and has many causes. The most frequent cause in heart disease is a high pulmonary venous pressure. Even severe oxygen desaturation in cyanotic congenital heart disease seldom causes dyspnoea at rest.

Mechanism

Rise in pressure in the LA and pulmonary veins is transmitted to the pulmonary capillaries. If it exceeds the oncotic pressure of the plasma proteins (normally 25 mmHg), it causes transudation of fluid from the capillaries into the interstitial tissues of the lungs, which become stiff. The work of inflating the lungs is increased and the greater muscular effort required gives the patient the sensation of dyspnoea. Usually the patient will then reduce his activities or change his posture to reduce the pressure below 25 mmHg. Frank pulmonary oedema represents the extreme situation when severe elevation of the pulmonary venous pressure keeps it continuously above 25 mmHg, which forces large amounts of fluid from the interstitial tissues into the alveoli.

Types of cardiac dyspnoea

Dyspnoea on exertion

On exertion the increased flow to the left side of the heart and the shortening of ventricular filling time from tachycardia temporarily raise the pulmonary venous pressure in the presence of mitral obstruction or impairment of LV filling.

It is conventional to use four grades to assess *severity* of dyspnoea on exertion (New York Heart Association):

1 Normal.
2 Moderate — walking on the level causes dyspnoea.
3 Severe — unable to continue walking even slowly on the level. All but the lightest housework has to be given up.
4 Gross — the slightest effort induces severe breathlessness. The patient is practically confined to bed by dyspnoea.

Poor effort tolerance may be concealed in a sedentary patient. It may be necessary for the physician to exercise the patient to check this.

Orthopnoea

Definition. Dyspnoea on lying flat which is relieved by sitting up.
Mechanism. Lying down increases the venous return to the right atrium (RA) and ventricle (RV) and thus the blood flow to the lungs. In the presence of mitral stenosis or LV failure, this results in an increase of LA and pulmonary venous pressure which, if 25 mmHg, causes interstitial oedema and dyspnoea. For orthopnoea to occur, the RA and RV must function normally and so this course of events does not occur with biventricular failure (e.g. acute myocarditis), tamponade or constrictive pericarditis.
Clinical presentation. The patient increases the number of pillows at night to avoid becoming dyspnoeic. Some patients, however, prop themselves up because they have been so instructed or for another reason, e.g. nasal catarrh or hiatus hernia: if they subsequently slip down without dyspnoea, they do not have orthopnoea.

Paroxysmal nocturnal dyspnoea

Definition. Acute dyspnoea, awakening the patient from sleep, forcing him to sit upright or stand out of bed for relief.
Mechanism. The blood volume is normally at its greatest at approximately 2 a.m. when the pulmonary venous pressure may build up to high levels. The reduced awareness during sleep allows the pressure to stay above 25 mmHg before dyspnoea awakens the patient.
Clinical presentation. The patient is awakened from sleep, dyspnoea lasts for 10–20 min and is not relieved by coughing. A dry cough and wheeze are commonly present during the attack.

Acute pulmonary oedema
Definition. Dyspnoea is severe at rest and is accompanied by cough and copious white or pink frothy sputum. There is cyanosis, perspiration, tachycardia, raised systemic blood pressure and widespread crepitations (fine crackles) over the lungs.
Mechanism. When levels of pressure of 30 mmHg are continuously exceeded in the pulmonary veins, in spite of the patient's sitting up at rest, the oncotic pressure of the plasma is overcome and fluid pours from the lung capillaries through the interstitial tissues into the alveoli in large quantities. Rupture of pulmonary capillaries from the high pressures makes the expectorated fluid pink.

The infant with raised pulmonary venous pressure
Causes. Pulmonary venous congestion may be due to LV failure in the face of excessive afterload (e.g. aortic stenosis or coarctation), to excessive preload (e.g. huge pulmonary venous return related to persistent ductus — PDA, or ventricular septal defect — VSD), or to obstruction to pulmonary venous return (e.g. cor triatriatum).
Clinical presentation. The child has a rapid respiratory rate at rest, breathing shallowly. The distress will be noticeably worse on feeding because the child is quickly exhausted by the effort of sucking and breathing at the same time. He becomes sweaty (sympathetic response to stress) and stops frequently, often not finishing the feed. Early introduction of solids to breathless babies is helpful as it takes less effort to ingest adequate calories. Pulmonary oedema occurs at lower atrial pressures in the very young, the physiological turnover of pulmonary transudate into, and lymphatic drainage out of, the alveoli being about five times greater in the neonate than the adult due to more permeable capillaries.

Differential diagnosis of cardiac dyspnoea
   1   *Respiratory dyspnoea* — usually a history of heavy smoking and recurrent bronchitis with infected sputum. Bronchospasm is suggested if dyspnoea varies from day to day and is sometimes absent. Attacks of asthma may resemble pulmonary oedema and indeed pulmonary oedema may produce bronchospasm, but in asthma there is more wheeze, less relief from the upright position and the attack is less circumscribed. Other respiratory causes are lymphangitis carcinomatosa, pneumothorax, pulmonary embolism.
   2   *Obesity* — interfering with diaphragmatic movement.
   3   *Anaemia* — which causes significant dyspnoea on exertion.
   4   *Anxiety* — Anxious patients often feel that they cannot fill their lungs with air and they may describe this as shortness of breath. Respiration is usually irregular and these feelings occur at rest when the patient's mind is unoccupied. Anxious *hyperventilation* causes a fall in $P\text{CO}_2$ with numbness of the arms, hands and lips, a feeling of unreality, even dimming of consciousness and, in extreme cases, tetany.

Other symptoms of raised pulmonary venous pressure

Cough

A raised pulmonary venous pressure may cause an irritating dry cough on exertion or at night, when it is relieved by sitting up or increasing the number of pillows. Rarely cough may be the first symptom, awakening the patient in an attack of pulmonary oedema.

Haemoptysis

Leakage of blood from engorged pulmonary veins may produce pink frothy sputum during an attack of acute pulmonary oedema. Rupture of a vein at abnormally high pressure may produce frank haemoptysis. More serious haemoptyses occur with severe pulmonary hypertension or pulmonary embolism.

Inadequate coronary blood flow causing myocardial ischaemia

Pathophysiology

The LV is more likely to become ischaemic than the RV because its coronary perfusion is confined to diastole (prevented in systole by the high intramural pressure), and its stroke work is greater (systemic arterial resistance is eight times that of the pulmonary). Ischaemia is exacerbated by elevation of systolic blood pressure (increased LV work) and by tachycardia (shortening the time available for coronary blood flow).

The causes of myocardial ischaemia are: coronary artery stenoses; LV hypertrophy in aortic stenosis, occasionally aortic regurgitation; and hypertrophic cardiomyopathy (often atypical pain).

Myocardial ischaemia, perhaps at metabolic level, also occurs in some cases of dilated cardiomyopathy. Anaemia by itself is rarely a cause of cardiac ischaemia but may be an exacerbating factor.

Symptoms

Angina pectoris on exertion

An uncomfortable sensation often described as tightness, less often as pain, most frequently in the sternal area and across the chest, typically radiating to one or both arms, lower jaw, or back. It may be confined to any one point in the area of cardiac distribution (e.g. the wrist, xiphisternum or jaw). (See p. 111.)

Dyspnoea

This is due to anoxic stiffening of the myocardium preventing ventricular filling, and thus raising LA and pulmonary venous pressures. Occasionally dyspnoea may be the only symptom of coronary disease. (See p. 117.)

Differential diagnosis of chest pain

1 *Cervical spondylosis or disc displacement* causing root irritation — the pain may be anywhere in the chest or arms, bears no relation to exertion, and usually

lasts for hours, though it may produce brief shooting pains.

2 *Colonic distension* — vague discomfort in the right or left chest, even the upper chest, and may cause brief stabs of pain.

3 *Anxious patients* greatly exaggerate symptoms from skeletal discomfort.

4 *Oesophageal pain* is central and substernal, may be difficult to differentiate from cardiac pain and may even be relieved by coronary dilators, but is not closely related to exertion.

Congestive (right heart) failure

Pathophysiology

Rise of RV end-diastolic pressure raises the RA and systemic venous pressures producing oedema (aggravated by hydrostatic pressure) and organ congestion. Low renal blood flow aggravates oedema by causing sodium retention.

Symptoms

Dependent oedema

Cause

The oedema fluid of congestive cardiac failure with a raised systemic venous pressure settles under the influence of gravity into the most dependent parts of the body. Pitting oedema of the feet and ankles occurs in the ambulant patient and a pad of oedema overlying the sacrum in the patient confined to bed. In severe failure the oedema may be widespread. Oedema is rarely seen in children.

Differential diagnosis of the cause of oedema
- Idiopathic — especially in premenstrual women after standing
- Deep vein thrombosis — often unilateral
- Low serum albumin from renal or hepatic abnormalities — not dependent, with the face, for instance, swollen
- Anaemia
- Obesity impeding venous return
- Lymphatic abnormalities — the oedema is firmer and less likely to pit on pressure

Hepatic pain

With exertion the venous pressure rises causing hepatic distension. This produces a dull ache in the right hypochondrium which has been termed hepatic angina. The relation to effort is less close than with angina and it is relieved by rest only slowly.

Low cardiac output

Symptoms

Fatigue

A low cardiac output has the effect of producing a constant feeling of fatigue, worse on exertion, related to poor blood supply to muscles and other organs.

However, the complaint of tiredness is so common in all types of illness, including psychological illness, that it cannot be regarded as reliable evidence of a low cardiac output. Indeed, the most common cause of fatigue in medical practice is boredom; another common cause is a β-blocking drug.

Effort syncope or dizziness

The vasodilatation of effort in the presence of a fixed low cardiac output (e.g. aortic stenosis, primary pulmonary hypertension) causes a marked fall in blood pressure and reduction in cerebral blood flow.

The infant with low cardiac output

A low cardiac output is reflected both by its direct consequences (hypotension, floppiness, low urine output) and by evidence of compensatory sympathetic overactivity (pallor, restlessness, sweating, cool peripheries).

Cardiac arrhythmia (See also Chapter 8.)

Symptoms

Palpitations

Palpitation is a commonly used term for any increased awareness of the heart beat. Occasional extrasystoles (premature ventricular contractions — PVCs) are described as the heart 'seeming to miss a beat'. The sudden onset of fast palpitations unrelated to exertion indicates an attack of paroxysmal tachycardia or of atrial fibrillation (AF).

Syncope

Cardiac syncope results from the sudden cessation of cerebral blood flow when there is an arrest of the cardiac pumping action. There is abrupt loss of consciousness with extreme pallor. The pupils dilate and *epileptiform convulsions* may occur. When efficient cardiac pumping action returns, there is abrupt restoration of consciousness, accompanied by a red flush of the skin as blood flows into vessels widely dilated by the accumulation of metabolites during the brief period of circulatory arrest.

Causes

1   Ventricular standstill or extreme bradycardia. The usual pathological finding is bilateral bundle branch disease.
2   Ventricular fibrillation (VF) or high rate ventricular tachycardia (VT), usually due to coronary or myocardial disease and occasionally secondary to bradycardia or standstill, metabolic or electrolyte abnormalities.
3   Other causes of loss of consciousness:
    (a) Effort syncope occurs only on effort due to low cardiac output.
    (b) Vasovagal attacks (faints) produce extreme pallor and, momentarily, complete cessation of all electrical activity of the heart. Start gradually, usually being precipitated by heat, standing or emotion and are associated with nausea, sweating and long lasting pallor. Recovery is rapid if the patient

is allowed to be recumbent. Liable to recur, particularly in patients with a naturally low blood pressure and during pregnancy. Often familial.

(c) Carotid sinus syncope (p. 157) — rare.

(d) Postural hypotension with loss or dimming of consciousness on standing.

(e) Epilepsy — prolonged or unilateral jerking movements during loss of consciousness. No pallor or disturbance of the pulse except for moderate sinus tachycardia. Incontinence, tongue biting or electroencephalograph (EEG) scans do not differentiate for certain from cardiac syncope.

(f) Symptoms from carotid (transient ischaemic attacks) and vertebrobasilar arterial disease seldom include loss of consciousness.

(g) Metabolic causes of loss of consciousness, e.g. hypoglycaemia, are seldom sudden.

(h) Pulmonary embolism (pp. 219–221)

(i) Transient mitral valve obstruction from myxoma or ball valve thrombus in the left atrium (very rare).

CLINICAL EXAMINATION

The examination of the cardiovascular system is carried out with the patient's head and back reclining so that the thorax is at an angle of 30–40° with the horizontal, with a pillow placed behind the neck so that the *sternomastoid muscles are relaxed*. The following features require particular attention: general appearance; the arterial pulse and blood pressure; the jugular venous pressure and wave form; the cardiac impulses; auscultation of the heart; the lungs; the liver; and oedema.

General appearance

Overall build

Chronic low cardiac output from heart failure may cause emaciation, and cyanotic congenital heart disease may cause stunted growth and poor development. Obesity aggravates the effect of cardiac disease.

Anatomical abnormalities

Genetic abnormalities

Many genetically determined disorders associated with cardiac disease are recognized from their effects on general body configuration. Some cardiac malformations are commonly associated with specific genetic defects:

Chromosome disorders

- Down's syndrome (trisomy 21) with atrioventricular septal defects
- Turner's syndrome (X0) with coarctation of the aorta
- Noonan's syndrome with pulmonary stenosis (phenotype of Turner's syndrome, normal genotype)

Dysmorphic syndromes

- Marfan's syndrome with aortic ectasia and dissecting aneurysm

- Hereditary haemorrhagic telangiectasia with pulmonary arteriovenous fistulae
- Neurofibromatosis with phaeochromocytoma
- Polydactyly with common atrium and atrial septal defect

Stigmas indicating maternal rubella infection

Mental deficiency, nerve deafness and cataract in a child suggest that the mother was infected during early pregnancy by rubella. The common associated cardiac lesions produced by the virus are: persistent ductus arteriosus; pulmonary valve stenosis; and pulmonary artery branch stenosis.

Thoracic deformity

Enlargement of the heart in early childhood may produce a permanent deformity of the overlying chest wall with the precordium bulging forward to the left of the sternum.

Pulmonary hypertension complicating a left to right intracardiac shunt in children may result in an abnormally rounded configuration of the upper part of the chest with indrawing of the lower chest.

Patients with floppy prolapsing mitral valves are often tall and thin with long arms, minor chest and spinal deformities and sometimes increased skin elasticity.

Malar flush

Patients with a chronic low cardiac output have a dusky mauve flush (peripheral cyanosis) of the cheeks associated with dilated capillaries in the dermis (telangiectasia). It is commonly seen in mitral stenosis complicated by pulmonary hypertension, and is hence termed a 'mitral facies'.

Cyanosis

Examination in daylight is essential. A blue discoloration of the skin caused by 5 g or more of reduced haemoglobin per 100 ml of blood in the capillaries. Cyanosis may be peripheral or central.

Peripheral cyanosis

A slow moving peripheral circulation allows prolonged contact between blood and tissues with greater oxygen extraction.

Physiological vasoconstriction resulting from cold, or compensation for a low cardiac output, is the usual cause of peripheral cyanosis, which is best seen in the lobes of the ears, the nose and the fingers.

Central cyanosis

Definition

Cyanosis caused by reduced oxygen saturation of the systemic arterial blood.

Clinical features

The following features accompany central cyanosis and distinguish it from peripheral cyanosis:

The warm mucous membranes are blue (tongue, inside of lips and conjunctivae).

Exercise immediately increases central, but not peripheral, cyanosis.
Polycythaemia with an abnormally high haemoglobin and haematocrit.
Finger clubbing (p. 9).
Arterial blood, obtained by needle puncture from a peripheral artery, is
desaturated — the absolute differentiating feature in doubtful cases.

Causes

1   *Cardiac shunt*. Venous blood enters the left heart without passing through
the lungs, i.e. right to left shunting of blood through an abnormal communication in the heart.
2   *Pulmonary shunt*. Inadequate oxygenation of the blood as it passes
unventilated alveoli. The breathing of oxygen increases oxygen tension in the
alveoli and compensates for poor lung function, lessening cyanosis due to lung
disease but having little effect on intracardiac shunts.

Differential cyanosis

Definition

Cyanosis more intense in the feet than in the hands when both are warm.

Cause

Oxygen content of the arterial blood in the legs is lower than in the arms because
of desaturated blood passing from the pulmonary artery through a PDA into the
descending aorta when high pulmonary vascular resistance raises pulmonary
artery pressure above systemic. The presence of differential cyanosis is diagnostic of this combination.

Clubbing of the fingers

Stages

1   Obliteration of the normal angle between the fingernail and skin on the
dorsum of the finger by an increase in the soft tissues underneath the nail bed.
2   The nail becomes curved longitudinally.
3   Swelling of soft tissues of the terminal phalanges gives a drumstick
appearance to the digits, nose and earlobes.

Causes

The exact stimulus producing finger clubbing is not known. In heart disease
finger clubbing is associated with cyanotic disease, infective endocarditis or left
atrial myxoma. It develops over the first year of life in those born with cyanotic
heart disease and resolves slowly if the defect is corrected.

THE ARTERIAL PULSE

The radial pulse is sufficiently obvious for analysis of *rate* and *rhythm*, palpating
both right and left simultaneously to check for discrepancies between the two
sides.

The carotid pulse is best for analysis of *amplitude* and *wave form*. The head is comfortably supported by a pillow and angled slightly backwards. The neck muscles must be relaxed. The left thumb (or finger) is pressed backwards to feel the patient's right carotid pulse against a transverse process. The right thumb (or finger) is used for the left side (but not simultaneously). Sometimes the carotid pulse is difficult to feel and the technique may not be successful in children. Palpation of the brachial artery against the lower end of the humerus with the arm straight or, better, higher up the humerus with the arm bent is then useful.

Rate (normally 55–90)

Abnormally fast
May represent:
1 Sinus tachycardia (sino-atrial node remains in control), e.g. excitement, fever, exertion, thyrotoxicosis, haemorrhage.
2 Arrhythmia (an ectopic focus has taken over pacemaking function from the sino-atrial node), e.g. atrial tachycardia, atrial flutter, AF, ventricular tachycardia.

Abnormally slow
May represent:
1 Sinus bradycardia (sino-atrial node remains in control), e.g. trained athletes, increased intracranial pressure, jaundice, sino-atrial disease.
2 AV dissociation. A regular pulse rate < 40 beats/min, except when asleep, usually indicates complete heart block.

Rhythm
The normal pulse is regular apart from a slight speeding up on inspiration and slowing on expiration (sinus arrhythmia) — most obvious in youth.

Complete irregularity indicates AF, but sinus rhythm with multiple extrasystoles (premature contractions) may simulate it. Auscultation is then superior for analysis of rhythm as premature beats without ejection still produce heart sounds. On exercise the irregularity of the pulse is accentuated in AF, whereas extrasystoles disappear except with severe myocardial disease, so that the pulse becomes regular in healthy subjects.

Amplitude
Judged by the movement of the palpating finger produced by the arrival of the pulse wave. A large amplitude pulse means that the pressure wave is large, i.e. there is a large difference between systolic and diastolic blood pressures.

Large amplitude pulse

Causes
• *Leakage of blood from the aorta or its large branches* — aortic valve regurgitation, PDA, arteriovenous fistula

- *Increased flow of blood from the aorta through dilated arterioles* — thyrotoxicosis and other high output states
- *Increased left ventricular stroke volume* — bradycardia, aortic regurgitation
- *Rigidity of the aorta* — atherosclerosis, almost the rule in the elderly.

Mechanism

The rapid escape of blood from the aorta in the first two groups lowers the pressure in the arterial system at the end of diastole while the large LV stroke volume ejected into the aorta causes a high systolic pressure.

The large stroke volume of bradycardia or aortic regurgitation gives an abnormally large pressure peak in the aorta. A normal stroke volume produces an abnormally large pressure rise when the aorta has lost its elasticity.

Small amplitude pulse

Causes

- Small LV stroke volume — shock, tachycardia, LV dysfunction, mitral stenosis
- Obstruction to LV ejection — aortic stenosis

Mechanism

In the low cardiac output states, the volume of blood ejected into the aorta with each beat is small.

Pulse varying in amplitude

Pulsus alternans (Fig. 1.1)

Description

The amplitude of a regular pulse wave is large and small alternately.

Significance

Pulsus alternans is evidence of LV failure, but the mechanism is still in dispute.

Pulsus paradoxus (Fig. 1.2)

Description

Marked (> 10 mm Hg) inspiratory diminution in amplitude of the arterial pulse (exaggeration of the normal). The 'paradox' is that the pulse disappears at the wrist when the heart sounds are still audible; a common error is to assume that the pulse is the opposite of normal, i.e. decreases on expiration.

Causes and mechanisms

1 *Asthma.* The powerful inspiratory effort to overcome airway obstruction increases the capacity of the lung vessels and reduces the flow of blood out of

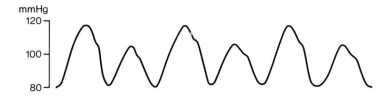

Fig. 1.1. Pulsus alternans — alternate large and small amplitude pulses.

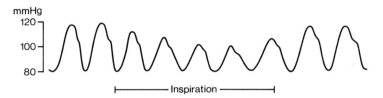

Fig. 1.2. Pulsus paradoxus — marked diminution of pulse amplitude during inspiration.

the lungs into the left heart. The systemic arterial pulse pressure is then diminished during inspiration.

2   *Tamponade.* When the diastolic volume of the heart is limited by a pericardial effusion or a rigid pericardium, the normal increase in filling of the right heart during inspiration decreases the space available for filling of the left heart. Thus LV stroke volume is reduced more during inspiration than normal. The degree of paradox can be measured with a sphygmomanometer.

Reduced amplitude of femoral pulses

Discrepancy of pulses between the upper and lower parts of the body indicates aortic obstruction, e.g. coarctation. Confirmed by comparing the systolic pressures at brachial and femoral level, remembering that the initial systolic peak is normally higher at femoral level owing to exaggeration of the initial pulse wave as it travels to the periphery. *Femoral pulse delay* is estimated by comparing radial and femoral pulses simultaneously.

Wave form (Fig. 1.3)

The wave form felt by the finger depends on the rate of change of pressure (dP/dt) rather than the recorded pressure wave. The initial pulse normally becomes sharper as it travels to the periphery. The normal brachial pulse has a smooth, fairly sharp upstroke, a momentarily sustained peak and a quick downstroke (Fig. 1.3a). The dicrotic notch, representing aortic valve closure, cannot be detected clinically, but the other features are readily analysed. Abnormalities of wave form are usually due to abnormalities of the aortic valve.

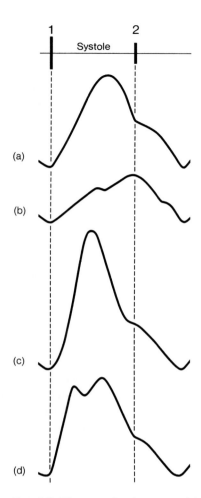

Fig. 1.3. The arterial pulse waves. (a) Normal. (b) Slow rising. (c) Sharp ('waterhammer'). (d) Bisferiens. 1 and 2 = first and second heart sounds.

Slow rising pulse (plateau pulse, anacrotic pulse)
(See Fig. 1.3b)

Description

Slow upstroke, particularly in the carotid or brachial pulse. The time taken to reach the peak is prolonged and the entire pulse wave is of small amplitude. These changes are less obvious in the peripheral pulses.

Cause

Aortic valve stenosis: the rate of ejection of blood into the aorta is decreased so that the duration of ejection is prolonged and the amplitude of the pulse diminished. Slow ejection from a poorly functioning LV may produce a similar pulse.

Sharp pulse (Waterhammer or collapsing pulse) (Fig. 1.3c)

Description

The upstroke is abrupt and steeper than normal, particularly at the periphery. The peak is reached early, is not sustained and the downstroke is also rapid. The amplitude is usually abnormally large. The examiner's finger appreciates the sharper than normal upstroke (rapid rate of rise) rather than the downstroke and experiences a sharp tap with each pulse beat.

Causes

The sharp upstroke represents the rapid ejection of a large stroke volume into an empty arterial system and the rapid downstroke indicates an abnormally fast escape of blood from the arteries during diastole. A waterhammer pulse is found in:

- Aortic valve regurgitation, persistent ductus arteriosus — (leak at aortic level)
- Systemic arteriovenous fistula — (leak at arterial level)
- Fever, thyrotoxicosis, anaemia, respiratory failure (due to generalised arteriolar dilatation).

Pulsus bisferiens (Fig. 1.3d)

Description

The initial upstroke is abrupt, the rate of rise of pressure then falls off but rises again to a second peak about the same height as the first before again falling off. The amplitude of the pulse wave is large and the palpating finger experiences two distinct impulses with each pulse beat, particularly at brachial level.

Cause

This wave form indicates combined regurgitation and stenosis of the aortic valve, both lesions being severe. The sharp upstroke represents the rapid ejection of a big stroke volume into an empty system, exaggerated as it travels to the periphery, and the second wave is due to prolongation of ejection from aortic stenosis.

THE BLOOD PRESSURE

The blood pressure depends primarily on the cardiac output and on the peripheral resistance (impedance), subsidiary factors being the elasticity of the aorta, the blood volume and blood viscosity.

Definition

- The *systolic* blood pressure is the peak pressure achieved during the ejection of blood from the ventricle into the arterial system.
- The *diastolic* blood pressure varies with the peripheral resistance (impedance). If there is a rapid escape of blood from the aorta, there will be a low pressure at the end of diastole. In the absence of anatomical leaks (aortic regurgitation, PDA, arteriovenous fistula), the peripheral resistance is governed by the small arteries and arterioles, vasodilatation lowering the diastolic pressure.

Measurement

Sphygmomanometer

An inflatable cuff firmly wound round the upper arm and connected to a mercury column is the most accurate way of measuring the blood pressure indirectly. The cuff used for adults should measure 12.5 cm in width. Narrower cuffs cause falsely high readings on large arms but are appropriate for children. Even a 12.5 cm cuff causes falsely high readings in grossly obese arms. The cuff should be inflated to 180 mm to avoid artifacts from 'silent periods' and on decompression the abrupt onset of the pulse sound is then an accurate measure of the *systolic pressure*.

The *diastolic pressure* lies somewhere between an abrupt muffling of sounds (so-called phase 4) and the total disappearance of sounds (phase 5) as used in the USA. Measurements are not accurate to more than the nearest 5 mmHg.

Direct intra-arterial measurement

A plastic cannula is inserted into a radial or femoral artery for continuous recordings, e.g. after cardiac surgery.

EXAMINATION OF THE FUNDI

Technique

A narrow beam of light from an ophthalmoscope illuminates the retina. The beam should be smaller than the pupil (which may have to be dilated) to avoid stray reflection. The patient sits on a high stool and fixes both eyes on one spot on a dark wall straight ahead. The operator uses his left eye for the patient's left and vice versa. Careful focussing is essential.

Hypertensive retinopathy

Haemorrhages and exudates, when due to hypertension, indicate that it is severe, and they are accompanied by marked irregularity of lumen of the arterioles. Papilloedema indicates the malignant phase.

Retinal arterioles

Hypertension is primarily due to constriction of small arteries and arterioles. The retinal arteriolar walls are invisible but irregular narrowing of the column of blood indicates that the lumen is irregular (Fig. 1.4) because of spasm or to thickening of the arteriolar wall, with the degree closely related to the diastolic pressure. Opacity of the wall and nipping and distortion at the arteriovenous crossings are also seen, but a mild degree may be present in the elderly without hypertension.

THE JUGULAR VENOUS PULSE AND PRESSURE (Figs 1.5–1.8)

Physiology

The RA pressure pulse is freely transmitted to the internal jugular veins of the neck, forming the jugular venous pulse (Figs 1.5–1.8). With the patient reclining

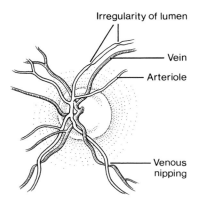

Fig. 1.4. Irregularity of lumen of a retinal arteriole and nipping of veins at arteriovenous crossings indicate sustained diastolic hypertension.

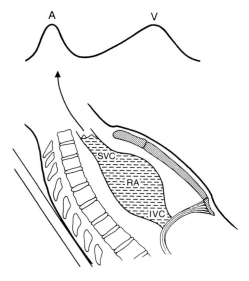

Fig. 1.5. Jugular venous pulse rising unimpended from RA to great veins just above level of the clavicle at 30–40°. SVC = superior vena cava; IVC = inferior vena cava.

at 30–40°, the waves can be seen just above the clavicles and about 1 cm vertically above the sternal angle (manubriosternal joint) (Fig. 1.8). They consist of the 'a' wave following atrial contraction; the 'x' descent of atrial relaxation; the small 'c' wave produced by the tricuspid valve bulging sharply into the atrium at the onset of systole or from the underlying carotid pulse; the 'v' wave is a passive rise of pressure from the continuing return of venous blood when the tricuspid valve is closed during ventricular systole; and the 'y' descent follows opening of the tricuspid valve in early diastole.

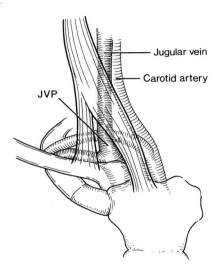

Fig. 1.6. Jugular venous pulse (JVP) best seen between the two heads of the relaxed sternomastoid muscle.

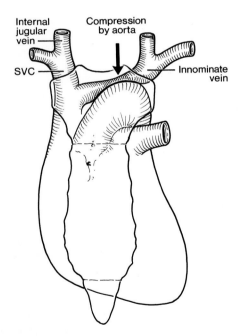

Fig. 1.7. Jugular venous pressure may appear elevated and damped on the left owing to compression of the innominate vein by the aortic arch. SVC = superior vena cava.

Clinical recognition

The neck is supported so that the sternomastoid muscles overlying the internal jugular veins are relaxed (Fig. 1.6). The pulse waves impart a gentle double

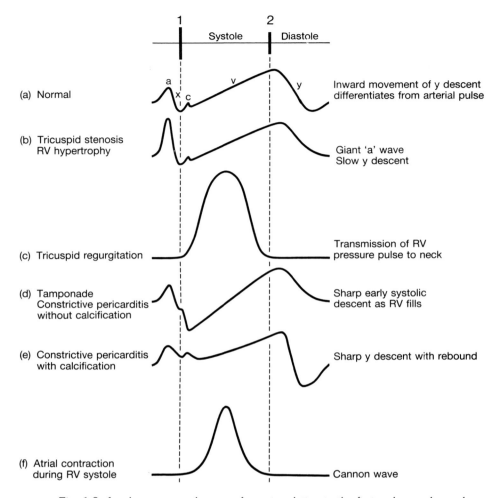

Fig. 1.8. Jugular venous pulse wave forms in relation to the first and second sounds.

undulation to the skin over the vein, unlike the sharp single outward movement from the nearby carotid pulse; the dominant movement of the venous pulse is inwards due to the 'y' descent, particularly when the pressure is elevated. This is useful for recognising venous waves elevated to the angle of the jaw because of severe right heart failure when pulsation may be reduced and the high venous pressure missed; the inward movement of the 'y' descent is in contrast to the sharp outward movement of the nearby carotid. In the normal pulse the 'a' wave usually becomes larger during inspiration because the increased flow into the RA causes more vigorous contraction.

These observations are best made on the right neck since the innominate (brachiocephalic) vein may be compressed by the arch of the aorta (Fig. 1.7) making the left-sided venous pressure appear to be abnormally high in some normal subjects. Inspiration lowers the mediastinum, allowing the pulse to fall to normal. In infants identification of the venous pulse is much more difficult and is therefore little used.

The mean pressure and the venous wave form are assessed.

Causes of a raised mean jugular venous pressure

1 High right ventricular filling pressure:

(a) RV failure

(b) High output states. A slight increase in RA filling pressure is required, even in normal hearts, for the RV to maintain a high cardiac output.

(c) Increased blood volume (overtransfusion, acute nephritis). Until the blood vessels dilate to accommodate the increased volume, there is an increased venous return and a raised RA pressure.

(d) Restriction of RV filling. Normal filling of the heart is impeded during diastole in tamponade, constrictive pericarditis and restrictive cardiomyopathy. An increase in ventricular diastolic pressure and in venous filling pressure is the result.

2 Obstruction to blood flow from RA to RV (tricuspid stenosis, right atrial myxoma). A high RA pressure serves to maintain blood flow across the obstructed region.

3 Superior vena caval obstruction e.g. bronchogenic carcinoma or retrosternal thyroid. The distended veins do not pulsate, which distinguishes this cause of an elevated venous pressure. Collateral venules may be seen on the chest wall.

4 Loss of negative intrathoracic pressure (emphysema, pleural effusion, pneumothorax). Any rise in pressure within the thorax is transmitted to the RA.

Clinical value of the venous pressure

• A *normal venous pressure* in an ambulant patient excludes right heart failure as the cause of oedema, which is commonly encountered in subjects without cardiovascular disease (unless diuretics have lowered the venous pressure before oedema has had time to disappear).

• A *raised venous pressure* is valuable in the recognition of right heart failure as symptoms may be minimal.

• An abnormally *low venous pressure* indicates over-diuresis or dehydration.

Abnormal venous pulse wave forms (Fig. 1.8)

• *The 'a' wave* is abnormally large if there is increased resistance to RA emptying from tricuspid stenosis or RV hypertrophy e.g. severe pulmonary stenosis (Fig. 1.8b). The 'a' waves are easily visible in the neck, are short and sharp and precede the carotid upstroke palpated on the other side of the neck. The 'a' wave is absent in AF.

• *Large systolic waves* occur with tricuspid regurgitation when the RV pressure pulse is transmitted to the RA (Fig. 1.8c). The wave may get larger when inspiration increases RV stroke volume.

• *Marked systolic descent.* Later than the normal 'x' descent, a negative wave may become large in tamponade, coinciding with filling of the RA as blood is ejected from the constricted pericardial cavity (Fig. 1.8d).

- *Rapid 'y' descent.* With elevated venous pressure from right heart failure, the 'y' descent is rapid.
- *Rapid 'y' descent and trough.* In constrictive pericarditis with a calcified pericardium the AV ring cannot move down (as it does in tamponade) when the stroke volume leaves the pericardial cavity (Fig. 1.8e). The atrial pressure does not then fall until the tricuspid valve opens when it falls rapidly; it quickly rises again as the constricted ventricle is rapidly filled, the so-called 'square root' venous pulse.
- *A slow 'y' descent* is seen with tricuspid stenosis and RV hypertrophy from slow emptying of the right atrium (Fig. 1.8b).
- *The 'c' and 'v' waves.* In AF, where there is no 'a' wave, there are still two positive waves in the venous pulse, the 'c' and the 'v' waves, so that recognition of AF is difficult from visualising the venous pulse alone. The 'c' wave, however, coincides with the carotid pulse whereas an 'a' wave precedes it.

The venous pulse in arrhythmia

Large abrupt waves, termed 'cannon waves', are caused by atrial contraction during ventricular systole when the tricuspid valve is closed (Fig. 1.8f). These occur with ventricular ectopics, distinguishing them from AF. Periodic cannon waves, with a regular, slow pulse, indicate atrioventricular dissociation. Regular cannon waves with each beat indicate nodal rhythm.

THE CARDIAC IMPULSES

The precordium is palpated for:

The position of the apex beat.
An abnormal left ventricular impulse at the apex.
An abnormal right ventricular impulse at the parasternal region.
Abnormal impulses at both apex and parasternal areas.
Other abnormal movement.
Palpable heart sounds.
Palpable murmurs (thrills).

Position of the apex beat

This is the lowest and outermost point at which the finger is lifted, and was formerly used to assess heart size. The apex beat, however, may be displaced by scoliosis or thoracic deformity or disease and the apical impulse is often impalpable in adults; in an infant, check that it is not in the right chest (dextrocardia). The quality of the cardiac impulse at the apex is more important than its position. Heart size should be assessed by echo or chest radiography.

An abnormal left ventricular impulse at the apex

A ventricle reacts to increased stroke volume with a *hyperkinetic* contraction, which can be detected by the finger as a sharp outward movement before hypertrophy appears on the ECG or echo, particularly in mitral and aortic regurgitation. This can be mimicked by catecholamine stimulation resulting from anxiety.

A *sustained* outward movement at the apex indicates LV hypertrophy. In order to detect these abnormalities, the patient is turned almost on to the left side, but even then a thick chest wall or hyperinflation may conceal any abnormality.

Abnormal right ventricular impulses at the left sternal edge

These may be analysed in the same way. No movement normally can be felt, except in thin, excited children. In atrial septal defect with left to right shunt, the *hyperkinetic* dilated RV may extend to the apex. A *sustained* lift indicates RV hypertrophy.

Abnormal impulses at both apical and parasternal areas

The right hand detects an abnormal lift at the apex, and the left hand a similar lift parasternally with the two separated by an inward movement. This indicates hypertrophy of both RV and LV.

Other abnormal movement

Systolic expansion of the *left atrium* from moderate or severe mitral regurgitation thrusts the RV forwards, causing a sharp outward movement in the left parasternal region which is indistinguishable from a hyperkinetic RV.

With an anterior *ventricular aneurysm*, the systolic anterior movement may be palpated internal to the apex.

Palpable heart sounds

A very loud sound may be palpable. The loud first sound (M_1) of mitral stenosis can usually be felt, as can the loud pulmonary component of the second sound (P_2) in severe pulmonary hypertension. Loud ventricular filling sounds (third and fourth) may also be palpated.

Palpable murmurs

Any loud murmur may be palpated as a thrill: its longer duration differentiates it from a palpable sound.

AUSCULTATION

Stethoscope

The chest piece should have a *rigid* diaphragm and a bell. High frequency sounds and murmurs are heard better with the diaphragm, e.g. splitting of sounds, opening snap, aortic diastolic murmur. The bell, applied lightly to the chest, transmits low frequency sounds better, e.g. ventricular filling sounds, mitral diastolic murmur. Ideally it should be large but adjustable in diameter to fit between the ribs in thin subjects. The stethoscope should have good fitting ear pieces and double tubing, and the patient should be in a comfortable reclining position, tipped partly to the left for auscultation at the apex.

Frequency

The human hearing mechanism is very sensitive to high frequency sounds and murmurs and insensitive to low frequencies. For example, third and fourth sounds are not heard by medical students until their attention has been 'tuned in' to the low frequencies.

Systole

Differentiation of systole from diastole is easy at normal heart rates as systole is the shorter. It is more difficult with tachycardia, when a thumb on the carotid upstroke will identify the first sound which just precedes it.

Concentration on the *first sound* usually reveals splitting, which may be close (normal), or wide, raising the possibility of bundle branch block or an additional ejection sound; differentiation between them is best achieved with the rigid diaphragm over the apex (mitral area) for an ejection sound and at the lower left sternal edge (tricuspid area) for a split first sound (which is accompanied by wide splitting of the second sound).

Concentration on *systole* may reveal a murmur, its site of maximal intensity, and, more important, its 'shape' and timing, particularly whether it reaches the second heart sound or not. The frequency and quality of systolic murmurs are not of great diagnostic value except that, in general, large pressure gradients generate high-velocity jets which tend to be of high frequency or pitch. Thus the systolic murmur of mitral regurgitation is of high frequency and best heard with the diaphragm, while a physiological right ventricular outflow murmur is of low frequency and best heard with the bell.

Diastole

Appreciation of splitting of the *second heart sound* into its aortic and pulmonary components is the key to auscultation of the heart and requires the use of the rigid diaphragm in the pulmonary area during continuing slow and quiet respiration. Once both components have been recognized and their intensity compared, it is easy to detect a slightly later, but similar quality, opening snap of the mitral valve.

The diaphragm is used at the left sternal edge to detect high-frequency aortic *early diastolic murmurs* (easily missed). For the remainder of diastole the bell is used at the mitral and tricuspid areas for low-frequency *third and fourth (atrial) sounds*, and mitral and tricuspid *ventricular filling murmurs*.

Effect of respiration and pharmacological agents

Inspiration increases right heart flow and thus accentuates right heart sounds and murmurs; later, during expiration, the increased flow reaches the left heart. Thus left heart murmurs are accentuated during *expiration*, but the effect of respiration on the left heart is less pronounced. Respiration should not be halted (except for hearing aortic diastolic murmurs) as this diminishes the flow of blood through the heart.

The intensity of murmurs is also influenced by *pharmacological agents*, amyl nitrite and other vasodilators dropping systolic pressure and lessening the intensity of a mitral regurgitant murmur. Phenylephrine increases peripheral vascular resistance and therefore the intensity of an aortic diastolic murmur. The use of such agents is seldom necessary if the timing of the murmurs is correctly related to the heart sounds.

Sites for auscultation (Fig. 1.9)

The site of maximum intensity of a sound or murmur is useful but does not always decide its origin, e.g. the murmur of aortic stenosis is frequently loudest at the apex. The direction of selective spread (e.g. axilla in mitral regurgitation) and the effect of respiration are also useful factors to take into account.

Mitral valve sounds and murmurs

These are loudest at the apex (MA), with the patient turned on the left side.

Tricuspid valve sounds and murmurs

These are localized to the lower left sternal edge (TA), but spread to the apex if the RV is dilated and the LV rotated posteriorly, e.g. atrial septal defect (ASD).

Aortic valve sounds and murmurs

- *Ejection* murmurs are loudest in the aortic area (AA, second right interspace) and at the cardiac apex. They are often transmitted to the carotid arteries in the neck, but a short murmur confined to the neck may be heard in young normal subjects with a big stroke volume; in older subjects it suggests carotid stenosis.
- *Regurgitant* early diastolic murmurs are usually loudest in the third and fourth left intercostal spaces at the left sternal edge with the patient leaning forward in expiration. With aortic dilatation, however, the murmur is usually maximal in the aortic area.

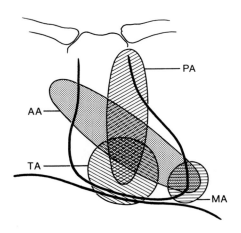

Fig. 1.9. Sites for auscultation. MA = mitral area; TA = tricuspid area; AA = aortic; and PA = pulmonary area.

Pulmonary valve sounds and murmurs

Loudest in the pulmonary area (PA, third left interspace) but often heard lower.

Murmurs over the back

The systolic murmurs of peripheral pulmonary stenosis and coarctation of the aorta are heard maximally over the back. A continuous murmur suggests a communication between the descending aorta and pulmonary circulation.

The cardiac cycle

A proper understanding of heart sounds and murmurs can only be achieved by understanding the phases of the cardiac cycle and appreciating that there is slight asynchrony between the two sides of the heart.

The sino-atrial (SA) node is in the RA which contracts first, followed by the LA. *Atrial systole* lasts 0.1 s, preceding ventricular systole. The LV contracts before the RV because the left side of the septum is depolarized by the left bundle branches before the right. The mitral valve closes before the tricuspid and the pressure in the LV rises with the aortic valve closed, the *isovolumic contraction* phase. The aortic valve then opens and blood is ejected into the aorta, the *ejection* phase. At the end of systole, usually lasting 0.3 s, the aortic valve closes. The LV pressure falls to atrial level, the *isovolumic relaxation phase* lasting 0.1 s. The mitral valve opens initiating the *rapid filling phase*. The ventricle then fills slowly with a further abrupt increase following atrial contraction. RV systolic events are similar but start earlier (low PA pressure) and finish later.

THE HEART SOUNDS

The total vibrations caused by ventricular contraction and relaxation are shown in Fig. 1.10 and are divisible into two major groups depending on their mechanism, i.e. *valve*, or *ventricular filling*. In addition the slight asynchrony between the two sides of the heart doubles the number of sounds making a total of 12 which may be grouped in the following way:

Valve sounds

First sounds   — closing of mitral and tricuspid valves.
Ejection sounds — opening of aortic and pulmonary valves.
Second sounds — closing of aortic and pulmonary valves.
Opening snaps — opening of mitral and tricuspid valves.

The valve sounds are of high frequency and have been shown by echophono-cardiography to coincide with the final halt of opening and closing valves. Only the closing sounds are normally audible.

Ventricular filling sounds

Rapid filling (third) — LV and RV.
Atrial (fourth)   — RV and LV.

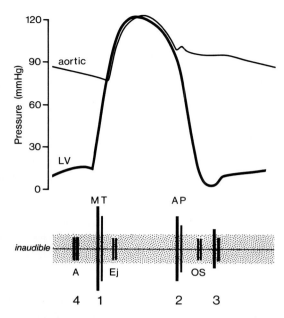

Fig. 1.10. The heart sounds and their relation to the LV and aortic pressure pulses (RV pulse occurs 10–20 ms later). Left sided events precede right except for RA contraction (sinus node in RA) and RV ejection (low pressure in PA). 4 and A = atrial sounds (right and left); 1 = first sound — mitral (M) and tricuspid (T) components; Ej = ejection sounds (pulmonary and aortic); 2 = second sound — aortic (A) and pulmonary (P) components; OS = opening snaps of mitral and tricuspid valves; 3 = third sounds (left and right). Only those sounds spreading beyond the shaded area are audible in a normal subject.

The ventricular filling sounds are of very low frequency and therefore difficult to hear. The third sound is audible in children normally and diminishes in intensity with increasing age, becoming inaudible (but recordable) in normal subjects in middle age with increasing ventricular stiffness.

Valve sounds

First sounds

Description

The loudest sound in the cardiac cycle is caused by the abrupt halt of the closing movement of the mitral valve (M_1) followed by the softer tricuspid (T_1), initiated by contraction of the LV followed by the RV. This produces close splitting of the first sound (Fig. 1.11a). Abnormally wide splitting is heard when tricuspid closure is delayed as in right bundle branch block, pacing from an electrode on the LV, or with LV ectopics (Fig. 1.11b).

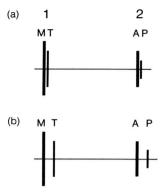

Fig. 1.11. First heart sounds. (a) Physiological splitting of first sound. (b) Wide splitting of first (and second) sounds. (Right bundle branch block, pacing from LV, LV ectopic.) M and T = mitral and tricuspid components of first sound. A and P = aortic and pulmonary components of second sound.

Intensity of the first sound

Varies and is closely related to the timing of the final halt of the closing atrioventricular (AV) valves (mainly mitral) in relation to the ventricular pressure pulse (Fig. 1.12). This timing depends on the position of the leaflets at the start of ventricular contraction. Early closure during the initial slow rise of LV pressure is soft while late closure on the steep part of the LV pressure pulse is loud.

Causes of soft first sound

1   Early AV valve closure (leaflets semi-closed at end of diastole):
    (a) Low flow at the end of diastole

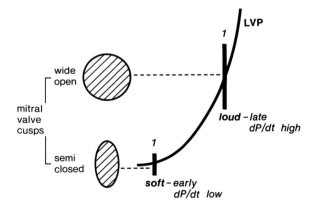

Fig. 1.12. Variations in intensity of first sound depend on the position of the cusps of the AV valves (mainly mitral) at the start of contraction. A wide open valve takes longer to reach its final closure point (causing the sound) which therefore occurs on a later and steeper part of the LVP — LV (pressure) pulse — with greater velocity. A semi-closed valve reaches its final closure point early when pressure change is slower.

(b) P–R interval > 0.2 s. Atrial contraction causes eddies which not only open the valve but, circulating behind the valve curtain, also semi-close it before ventricular contraction if there is sufficient time (Fig. 1.13).

2 Rigid calcified valve.

3 Poorly contracting LV (seldom useful in diagnosis).

Causes of loud first sound (leaflets wide open at end of diastole)
Late AV valve closure
(a) High flow at the end of diastole (mitral stenosis, short diastole from tachycardia, left to right shunts).
(b) P–R interval < 0.2 s. Atrial contraction has opened the valve and the eddies have not had time to close it before ventricular contraction.

Varying intensity of first sound

1 Varying duration diastole.

2 Complete atrioventricular dissociation (regular rhythm—p. 161).

Ejection sounds — opening of aortic and pulmonary valves (Fig. 1.14)
High pitched, often 'clicky', in early systole and best heard with a rigid diaphragm chest piece.

Aortic ejection sound (click)
In early systole soon after the first sound (often best appreciated at the apex). Caused by the abrupt halt of the fused aortic cusps carried sharply upwards in systole when they fail to fold back on to the aortic wall. Causes are:

1 Bicuspid aortic valve. Does not open fully.

2 Aortic stenosis with mobile valve. An aortic ejection sound indicates that the stenosis is at valve level. With calcification the sound disappears. It is also absent in subvalvar and supravalvar stenosis.

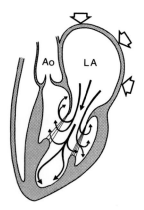

Fig. 1.13. Re-opening and closing of mitral valve following LA contraction (broad arrows). Ao = aorta.

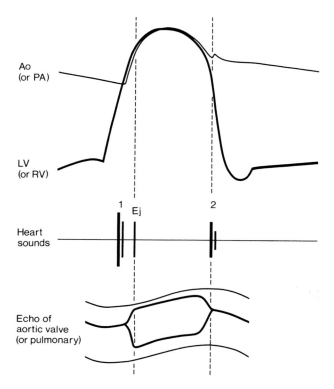

Fig. 1.14. Ejection sounds (Ej) occur on the upstroke of the aortic or pulmonary pressure pulse and coincide with the final halt of the opening aortic (or pulmonary) valve on the echo.

Pulmonary ejection sound (click)

Coincides with the final halt of the upward movement of the pulmonary valve in early systole. Causes are:

1 Pulmonary valve stenosis. Soon after tricuspid closure (shortened isovolumic contraction time of RV) and recognized by its disappearance on inspiration when the increase in the 'a' wave from powerful atrial contraction opens the pulmonary valve *before* ventricular contraction.

2 Pulmonary hypertension. With a dilated main PA. The ejection sound is later because of the prolonged isovolumic phase of the RV and it does not disappear on inspiration as the 'a' wave cannot exceed the elevated pulmonary diastolic pressure. The exact mechanism is obscure.

Other systolic clicks

Occur in mid or late systole in patients with floppy prolapsing mitral valves (p. 91). May occur alone or precede a late systolic murmur indicating slight mitral regurgitation (Fig. 4.17).

Second sounds (Fig. 1.15)

The second heart sounds are caused by closure of the aortic (A_2) and pulmonary (P_2) valves as ventricular pressures fall below those in the aorta and pulmonary artery.

On inspiration the two sounds separate (Fig. 1.15a), mainly because of delay of P_2 resulting from the increase in stroke volume of the RV from its extrathoracic venous reservoir; inspiratory splitting of the second sound is audible in the pulmonary area, but P_2 is relatively soft, is not transmitted to the mitral area, and may be inaudible in older subjects with thick chest walls and hyperinflation. A_2 is louder, even in the pulmonary area, and at the apex it alone forms the second sound.

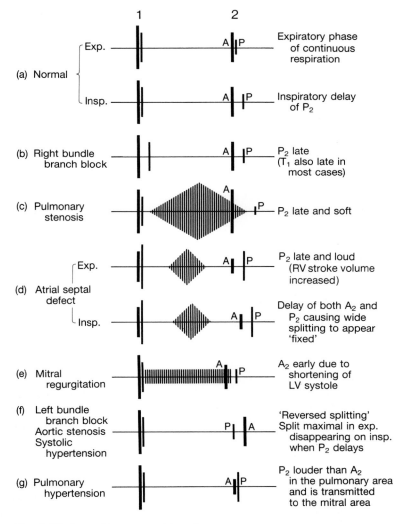

Fig. 1.15. Second heart sound in pulmonary area.

In the expiratory phase of continuous respiration in normal subjects reclining at 30–40° to reduce venous return, there is near fusion of A_2 and P_2 as LV and RV systoles terminate simultaneously (Fig. 1.15a).

Abnormally wide splitting of the second sound (Fig. 1.15).
The second sound is widely split if P_2 is delayed or if A_2 is early.
Delay of P_2:
1   Right bundle branch block (RBBB) — electrical delay in activation of the RV (Fig. 1.11b & 1.15b).
2   Pulmonary stenosis — P_2 is soft and its delay is related to the severity of the stenosis (Fig. 1.15c).
3   Atrial septal defect with left to right shunt — the increased stroke volume of the RV causes delay of P_2. The wide splitting is 'fixed' when the defect is large because inspiratory inflow from a common atrial reservoir causes simultaneous increase in stroke volume of both ventricles with delay of both A_2 and P_2 (Fig. 1.15d).
4   Right ventricular failure causing prolonged RV contraction.

Early A_2
Mitral regurgitation — shortening of LV systole because of diminished resistance to LV ejection (Fig. 1.15e).

'Reversed' splitting (P_2 before A_2)
On expiration the second sound is split if A_2 is delayed beyond P_2: on inspiration the split disappears with the normal inspiratory delay of P_2.
1   Left bundle branch block (electrical delay) (Fig. 1.15f).
2   Severe aortic stenosis, systolic hypertension: large PDA (LV overload prolonging contraction).

Loud second heart sound
1 A_2. Systemic hypertension: dilated proximal aorta.
2 P_2 (Fig. 1.15g). Pulmonary hypertension (also in ASD without pulmonary hypertension because of the sharp rise and fall of PA pressure). P_2 is louder than A_2 in the pulmonary area and is transmitted to the mitral area (where splitting is not normally heard). Concentration is required to hear the soft A_2 preceding the loud P_2. Fusion of A_2 and P_2 only occurs with a single ventricle or large VSD with high pulmonary vascular resistance equalling systemic (Figs 9.7 and 10.4).

Opening snaps (Fig. 1.16)
Opening of mitral and tricuspid valves. Opening snaps occur in diastole at the final halt of a rapidly opening AV valve at the end of isovolumic relaxation (normally 0.1 s after A_2). The higher the atrial pressure, the shorter the isovolumic relaxation phase and the earlier is the opening snap. Loud snaps indicate that there is a large area of cusp fusion (big 'sail area'). Recognition of a snap and differentiation from P_2 is achieved by hearing A_2, P_2 and the opening snap in rapid succession during inspiration.

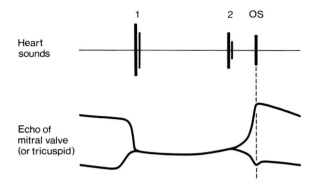

Fig. 1.16. Opening snaps of the mitral (or tricuspid) valve coinciding with the final halt of the opening valve on the echo.

Mitral opening snap
    1   Mitral stenosis with a mobile valve. Maximal internal to the apex.
    2   Rapid mitral flow, e.g. left to right shunting VSD or PDA, or severe mitral regurgitation. Snap is soft.

Tricuspid opening snap
    1   Tricuspid valve abnormalities — rheumatic stenosis; Ebstein's anomaly.
    2   Increased tricuspid flow — left to right shunting ASD.

Ventricular filling sounds (Fig. 1.17)
    These sounds of rapid ventricular filling are much lower in frequency than the valve sounds. Best heard with the bell chest-piece gently applied to the chest and may be described as a dull thud becoming palpable when loud. Caused by the final halt of the ventricular wall 0.15 s after A_2 following rapid diastolic filling.

Rapid filling (third) heart sounds

LV third sound
    Maximal at the apex with the patient inclined to the left.
    1   Normal in children and in thin young adults — rarely physiological over the age of 40 because the ventricle becomes less compliant with increasing age.
    2   Raised LA pressure — LV failure or severe mitral regurgitation. May also occur with normal LA pressure following a large anterior infarct (ventricle flapping).

RV third sound
    Maximal at the lower left sternal edge on inspiration and never normal.
    1   Right heart failure.
    2   Tricuspid regurgitation.
    3   RV preload (volume overload) — from ASD.

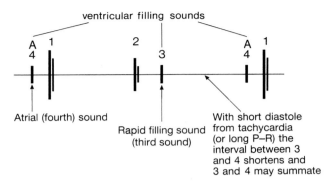

Fig. 1.17. Ventricular filling sounds.

Early third sound

In *constrictive pericarditis* with elevated atrial pressures, filling is rapid and halted early by the constricted pericardium producing an early (0.1 s after A_2), high energy and higher frequency sound.

Atrial (fourth) heart sounds

Never audible in normal subjects (but can be recorded). Caused by powerful atrial contraction filling an abnormally stiff ventricle. Atrial sounds are difficult to differentiate from splitting of the first sound when the first component (mitral) is of low frequency — a phonocardiogram is then required.

LA (fourth) sound (maximal at the apex)

1 LV hypertrophy (e.g. hypertension, aortic stenosis).
2 Fibrotic LV (e.g. old infarction).
3 Hypertrophic cardiomyopathy (loudest of the atrial sounds).

RA (fourth) sound (maximal at the lower left sternal edge and on inspiration)

RV hypertrophy.

Summation of atrial and third sounds (Fig. 1.17)

Occurs with tachycardia or a long P–R interval and may have no abnormal significance.

HEART MURMURS (Fig. 1.18)

Murmurs are caused by turbulence of blood flowing through valves or ventricular outflow tracts. They are classified by their relation to the heart sounds and phases of the cardiac cycle:

• *Systolic*
   Midsystolic (ejection)
   Pansystolic (regurgitant)

- *Diastolic*
    Early diastolic (regurgitant)
    Mid or delayed diastolic (ventricular filling)
    Atrial systolic (presystolic — ventricular filling)
- *Continuous*
- *Pericardial friction rub.*

The site of maximum intensity is useful (*see* Fig. 1.9) but may be misleading (e.g. aortic ejection murmurs are often maximal at the apex). Large pressure gradients generate high velocity and high frequency murmurs and small pressure gradients low velocity and low frequency murmurs. The intensity is conveniently graded into four grades: 1/4 (= soft); 2/4 (= moderate); 3/4 (= loud); and 4/4 (= very loud). Loud murmurs are palpated as thrills.

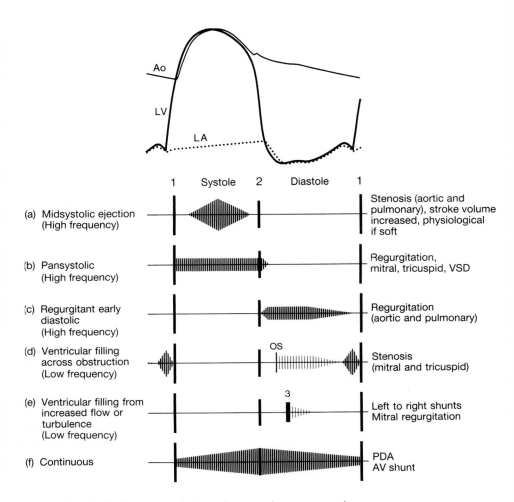

Fig. 1.18. Murmurs and their relation to the pressure pulses.

Systolic murmurs

Midsystolic (ejection) murmurs (Fig. 1.18a)
   Occur during ejection of blood through the ventricular outflow tracts into the great arteries. Their intensity varies with stroke volume and is reduced with premature beats and low cardiac output. They begin with the ejection sound, if present, and cease before the relevant valve closure sound (A_2 or P_2).

LV ejection murmurs (Fig. 1.18a)
   Maximal at the aortic area, lower left sternal edge and apex. (See Fig. 1.9.) Causes are:
   1 Aortic valvar, subvalvar or supravalvar stenosis. Murmur is loud (3–4/4), carotid pulse slow-rising and LV hypertrophied. The murmur is softer with reduced stroke volume from LV failure, or if transmission is impaired by a thick chest wall or hyperinflated lungs.
   2 Hypertrophic obstructive cardiomyopathy (idiopathic hypertrophic subaortic stenosis, p. 130). Intensity 2–3/4. Carotid pulse sharp and LV greatly hyper-trophied with loud atrial sound.
   3 Increased stroke volume (1–3/4). Aortic regurgitation; bradycardia; anaemia; high output states.
   4 Aortic cusp sclerosis (1–2/4). Increased rigidity of cusps without haemody-namic obstruction is common in the elderly. Murmur seldom loud. Carotid pulse normal and LV not hypertrophied (unless from another cause, e.g. hypertension).
   5 Bicuspid aortic valve with no obstruction. A bicuspid valve cannot open com-pletely during ejection. Aortic ejection sound with soft murmur (1/4).
   6 Coarctation of aorta (2/4). A coarctation murmur (p. 241) can, when audible anteriorly, be confused with an ejection murmur.

RV ejection murmurs (Fig. 1.18a)
   Maximal in the pulmonary area and below it, and louder on inspiration. Causes are:
   1 Physiological murmurs over the RV outflow tract in normal thin children and young adults. Moderately loud (2/4) with a flat-fronted chest or sternal depression (RV outflow tract pressed against the sternum) or with bradycardia increasing stroke volume.
   ASD and pulmonary stenosis are excluded if the second heart sounds become single in expiration — the subject should be reclining at 30–40° with respiration slow and deep.
   2 Pulmonary stenosis (3–4/4). Valvar stenosis – associated ejection sound; infundibular stenosis – no ejection sound. P_2 is soft and late, corresponding to the degree of obstruction (Fig. 1.15c).
   3 Increased stroke volume (2/4). ASD (Fig. 1.15d), VSD, pulmonary regur-gitation.

Pansystolic ('holosystolic', 'regurgitant') murmurs (Fig. 1.18b)
   These murmurs reach and engulf their second heart sound — e.g. A_2 in mitral regurgitation — because the pressure gradient between ventricle and atrium (or

LV and RV) continues through isovolumic relaxation. The murmur is high pitched ('blowing') and is loud because the large pressure gradient gives a high velocity jet, even when it is of little haemodynamic significance. Causes are:

1 Mitral regurgitation. Maximal at the apex and often in late systole, transmitted to the axilla. Trivial regurgitation may be confined to late systole. If the chordae to the posterior (mural) cusp rupture, the hood of the cusp directs the regurgitant jet upwards and centrally (Fig. 4.18), causing confusion with an aortic ejection murmur unless the shape of the murmur is noted.

2 Ventricular septal defect with left to right shunt. Maximal at the lower left sternal edge and may be loud when the defect is small (Maladie de Roger).

3 Tricuspid regurgitation. Maximal at fourth left interspace with inspiratory augmentation and a systolic wave in the jugular venous pulse.

Diastolic murmurs

Early diastolic (regurgitant) murmurs (Fig. 1.18c)

Immediately follow aortic or pulmonary closure when the valve is regurgitant; continue throughout diastole, unless the regurgitation is trivial, because of the pressure gradient between great artery and ventricle.

Aortic regurgitation

High pitched because of the large pressure gradient, best heard with a rigid diaphragm chest-piece. Usually maximal near the fourth left interspace below the aortic valve, but higher and to the right of the sternum if the aorta is dilated. The murmur is best heard with the patient sitting forward in held expiration (the noise of respiration has the same frequency). An aortic ejection sound indicates that it is associated with a bicuspid aortic valve.

Pulmonary regurgitation

Usually secondary to a dilated valve ring from pulmonary hypertension or following pulmonary valve surgery. With pulmonary hypertension the diastolic pressure gradient causes a high velocity regurgitant jet and a high-pitched early diastolic murmur indistinguishable from that of aortic regurgitation, except that it is usually maximal about the third left space rather than the fourth. Differentiated from aortic regurgitation by finding evidence of pulmonary hypertension (RV hypertrophy and an enlarged main pulmonary artery on X-ray), with no waterhammer pulse or LV hypertrophy, and by its being louder on inspiration.

Mid (delayed) diastolic (ventricular filling) murmurs (Figs 1.18d & e).

Low-frequency rumbles (low-velocity flow, best heard with the bell chest-piece gently applied), starting appreciably after the second sound in the rapid filling phase after isovolumic relaxation. Respiration should not be halted as this diminishes flow. Causes are:

Obstruction (Fig. 1.18d)

1 Mitral stenosis — murmur maximal exactly at apex with patient inclined to left. Begins after the opening snap; is long if the stenosis is severe, short if mild (no gradient in late diastole).

2   Tricuspid stenosis — murmur maximal at lower left sternal edge and increased by inspiration.

Flow murmurs (Fig. 1.18e)

Murmurs of high flow across the AV valves are short and soft and follow the third sound 0.15 s after A_2. The sudden inflow of a large volume of blood from the atrium rapidly distends the ventricle and causes the third sound. The cusps of the AV valve are pulled together at this moment and produce a short period of relative stenosis, over which blood continues to flow rapidly, causing the murmur.

1   Mitral flow murmurs — maximal at the apex.

   (a) Mitral regurgitation — the regurgitant volume augmenting ventricular filling.

   (b) Left to right shunts (PDA; VSD) — increased flow across the mitral valve.

2   Tricuspid flow murmurs — maximal at the left sternal edge and on inspiration. Left to right shunts — ASD, anomalous pulmonary venous return (increased flow across the tricuspid valve).

Turbulence — murmurs soft and short

1   Mitral vegetations from acute rheumatic valvulitis (Carey Coombs murmur)

2   Anterior mitral cusp prolapse into LV inflow caused by jet from aortic regurgitation (Austin Flint murmur). See Fig. 4.9.

3   Tricuspid — Ebstein's anomaly (p. 192).

Atrial systolic (presystolic) murmurs (Fig. 1.18d)

Brief ventricular filling murmurs caused by atrial contraction immediately preceding the first sound; higher pitched than the other ventricular filling murmurs because of a bigger pressure gradient. Necessarily disappear with the onset of AF.

Continuous murmurs (Fig. 1.18f)

Due to a communication in the circulation with a continuous pressure gradient throughout the cardiac cycle (leaking from aorta or pulmonary artery or their branches). Usually maximal in late systole which differentiates it from an ejection murmur accompanied by an early diastolic murmur. Causes of a continuous murmur are:

1   Aorta to pulmonary artery communication. PDA murmur maximal below the left clavicle. A congenital aortopulmonary communication (AP window) may be too large to produce turbulence and a murmur but there is an ejection murmur from the increased stroke volume of the LV.

2   Systemic arteriovenous communication. May be congenital, e.g. aortic sinus of Valsalva aneurysm rupturing into the right heart; or traumatic, e.g. knife wound.

3   Pulmonary arteriovenous communications. Produce central cyanosis and

clubbing. A murmur is rarely heard over the fistula because the pressure gradient is small.

4 Aortopulmonary collaterals. In pulmonary atresia with ventricular septal defect (usually loudest at the back).

5 Pulmonary artery branch stenosis.

6 Venous hum. Frequently heard over the neck and under the clavicles of children, a continuous murmur which varies with the position of the neck and *invariably disappears when the child is horizontal.*

Pericardial friction rubs

Pericarditis without appreciable effusion causes a 'murmur', usually of a quality different from an intracardiac murmur, and sounding closer to the stethoscope. It coincides with heart movement in midsystole and during ventricular filling (rapid filling phase in middiastole and in atrial systole). All three components are louder during inspiration when increased flow of blood into the heart increases the friction. They may also be louder with increased pressure on the stethoscope.

EXAMINATION OF THE LUNGS

Pleural effusions

A small pleural effusion is not uncommon in heart failure. Large pleural effusions complicating heart disease usually indicate an underlying pulmonary infarct.

Crackles at the lung bases

Crepitations or fine crackles are due to fluid in the respiratory bronchioles, frequently from a pulmonary venous pressure constantly raised above the oncotic pressure of the plasma proteins forcing fluid onwards from the interstitial space into the alveoli (pulmonary oedema) and respiratory bronchioles.

Basal crackles (crepitations) in pulmonary oedema occur late in inspiration because of the late inspiratory opening of airways narrowed by cuffs of peribronchial oedema. The sounds are profuse, high-pitched, inaudible at the mouth and silenced by bending forwards. The basal crackles of chronic bronchitis occur early in inspiration, are scanty, low-pitched, transmitted to the mouth and unaffected by posture (because of fluid in larger, central airways).

THE LIVER

The patient is examined supine and relaxed. Palpation starts low in the abdomen and lateral to the rectus muscle. As the patient inspires, the liver edge is felt and when enlarged may be percussed. If the stethoscope is placed on the liver below the xiphisternum, the sound of a scratching finger terminates at the lower edge of the liver.

Enlargement

An enlarged, tender liver edge below the costal margin is evidence of a raised systemic venous pressure, particularly useful in infants when the jugular venous pressure cannot be easily determined in a short neck. If the patient has cardiac cirrhosis, the liver may not be enlarged, even with a high venous pressure.

Systolic pulsation

The systolic pressure wave of tricuspid regurgitation is transmitted to the liver causing expansile systolic pulsation.

OEDEMA

Dependent oedema (See pp. 5 and 137.)

1   Site (p. 5.) The added hydrostatic pressure causes ankle oedema in ambulant patients and sacral oedema in those confined to bed.
2   Differential diagnosis (p. 5.)

Ascites

Persistent high venous pressure produces ascites, diagnosed by shifting dullness on percussion of the abdomen in two positions.

Chapter 2
Non-invasive Investigations

ELECTROCARDIOGRAPHY

Electrocardiography is the graphic recording of the electrical activity of the heart which immediately precedes and causes muscular contraction (depolarization); it is followed by a recovery phase (repolarization). Originally devised and much used for studying abnormalities of rhythm, its greatest use now is for the detection of myocardial ischaemia and infarction and other myocardial abnormalities.

Although a normal electrocardiogram (ECG) is frequent in patients with coronary disease, no cardiac examination is complete without one. Although interpretation is based to some extent on theoretical knowledge, it is largely the result of pattern reading requiring visualisation of multiple leads and therefore requiring many examples. This is out of keeping with the rest of the book and so Dr. Derek Rowlands has written a special chapter on electrocardiography (see Chapter 14).

EXERCISE TESTING WITH THE ELECTROCARDIOGRAM

Testing the performance of the heart on exertion is useful for objective assessment of the patient's symptoms in every type of heart disease but its greatest value is in diagnosis in patients with chest pain when the history is not clear, and particularly for assessing the severity of ischaemic heart disease.

Methods available

Exact measurements can only be made with a treadmill or a bicycle ergometer but any type of exercise may be used, such as mounting and dismounting steps, a brisk walk or climbing stairs. The first two methods enable the ECG to be monitored during the measured exercise as a precaution. The most widely used method is the treadmill with the Bruce protocol, incorporating up to five stages of exertion depending on the speed and elevation of the treadmill. A calibrated bicycle ergometer is more accurate but requires the ability to cycle.

Procedure

A 'control' ECG is taken at rest immediately before exercise to identify any recent acute change. The test is graded to suit the patient's physical fitness and is terminated when a given heart rate is reached, depending on the patient's age (obtained from tables — roughly 220 minus the patient's age). It is terminated with the onset of pain, marked S–T depression, arrhythmia, dyspnoea, or particularly with generalized weakness accompanied by a fall in blood pressure. Muscle fatigue, particularly in the legs, is the commonest cause of termination of the test in healthy subjects. At the end of the exercise the patient lies down to avoid a vasovagal attack and to improve the clarity of the postexercise ECG.

Assessment

Attention is directed to blood pressure, symptoms, and the ECG, in that order of importance.

Blood pressure

A fall during exertion is a sign of serious ischaemic or myocardial disease.

Symptoms

The onset of chest pain and its type are noted in relation to the degree of exercise. Dyspnoea may be an 'ischaemic variant' or the dominant symptom if the myocardium is affected.

ECG changes (Fig. 2.1)

A steady baseline and freedom from interference are essential for the interpretation of S–T changes, best done on the ECG immediately after exertion. Severe ischaemia requiring angioplasty or surgery almost invariably produces marked S–T depression (> 2 mm) at low levels of exercise. Localization of the artery affected is seldom possible since S–T depression usually represents ischaemia of the endocardium, which is the most vulnerable part of the myocardium.

S–T depression

This is the only certain evidence of cardiac ischaemia and has to be looked at critically. With tachycardia, diastole is short and there is no zero baseline between the end of the T wave and the next P wave. The P–R interval, if long enough, has then to be used as the baseline for measurement of S–T depression.

Physiological S–T depression

With or without tachycardia, is up-sloping and is due to negative atrial repolarization. See Chapter 14, p. 2 and Figs 14.3 and 14.4.

Ischaemic S–T depression

This is horizontal or down-sloping (Fig. 2.1). It may be exactly mimicked by digitalis (Fig. 14.36), producing horizontal S–T depression at rest, increased by exertion. Digitalis must therefore be stopped 3 weeks before the test. Left ventricular (LV) hypertrophy may also produce horizontal S–T depression (Fig. 14.18). T wave changes with or after exercise do not necessarily indicate cardiac ischaemia.

Mild S–T depression, increased by exertion, is not uncommon in women without coronary disease.

Arrhythmia

Ventricular ectopics of no clinical importance disappear with exertion but may reappear immediately after exertion in the early resting phase. Runs of ventricular ectopics or ventricular tachycardia induced by exercise are usually evidence of ischaemia or myocardial disease.

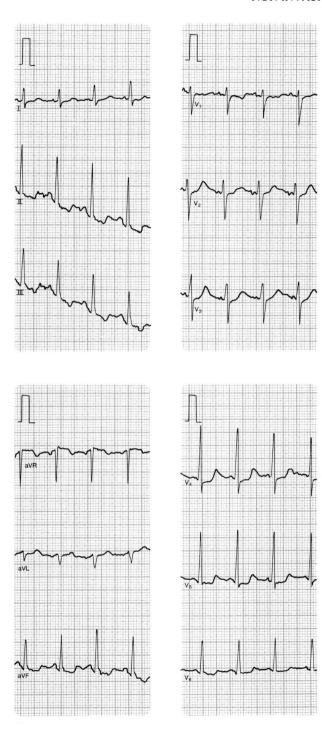

Fig. 2.1. Positive exercise test. The immediate postexercise heart rate is only 115/min. The patient was unable to complete the exercise programme because of the development of anginal pain. There is 2 mm S–T depression clearly seen in V_4 and V_5. There is lesser S–T depression in V_6 and aVF. Assessment of S–T changes in II and III is not possible because of the sloping S–T segment. At coronary angiography the patient had a localised 90% occlusion of the proximal part of the anterior descending branch of the left coronary artery.

Precautions

Careful history-taking before an exercise test is essential; it is unwise and unnecessary to exercise a patient with severe angina of effort, or recent angina, infarction or ECG change. While it is safe to exercise a patient who regularly undertakes more exercise than is required for the test, an exercise test in a sedentary patient requires the presence of a doctor trained in resuscitation with the immediate availability of a direct current (DC) defibrillator. With these precautions the risk of an exercise test is negligible and it is the most widely used test for the assessment of the severity of ischaemic heart disease.

ECHOCARDIOGRAPHY

Basic concepts of cardiac imaging

Echocardiography is a 'non-invasive' procedure which is harmless and uses echoes from sound waves to map the heart and study its function. To study the heart it is necessary both to visualize structures and to observe their functional dynamics. For these reasons still 'pictures' are of little use and methods have been devised to record patterns of cardiac structures.

Equipment

Ultrasound waves are generated by electrical excitation of a piezo-electric crystal, which vibrates and sets in motion a short burst or 'pulse' of waves lasting a few microseconds. The waves can be focussed into a 'beam' and aimed selectively at particular regions of the heart. To provide detailed images, a small wavelength is required, necessitating a high frequency (from 2 MHz for large adults to 7 MHz for neonates). The same crystal is used to detect the arrival of returning echoes and convert them back to electrical signals.

Technique

The major problem of echocardiography is the restricted access to the heart afforded by the lungs and rib cage, which form impenetrable barriers to ultrasound in the adult subject. This limits the quality of most studies and, in cases of obstructive airways disease or chest wall deformity, can make it impossible to obtain useful information. Normally small 'windows' can be located in the third and fourth intercostal spaces (termed *left parasternal*), just below the xiphoid process of the sternum (*subcostal*) and, with the subject turned to the left and exhaling, from the point where the apical impulse can be palpated (*apical*). By positioning the transducer successively over these areas and angling and rotating it to align the image scan plane, a series of standard views is obtained. The aortic arch can be imaged from a suprasternal position. Transoesophageal echo improves access further.

Display and recording

When an ultrasound pulse travels into the thorax and through the heart, it encounters interfaces between different types of tissues: — muscle, blood, etc. (Fig. 2.2). In crossing each interface, some of the energy is reflected and, provided that the angle of incidence is close to 90°, the reflections return to the transducer as echoes. The resulting electrical signals are amplified and used to

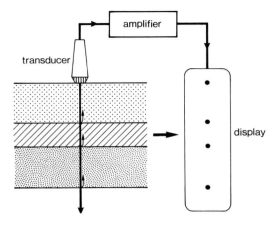

Fig. 2.2. Echoes generated at tissue interfaces are processed electronically to form a display showing the distance of each interface from the ultrasound transducer.

increase the brightness of the light spot on a cathode-ray tube which travels from top to bottom of the display, starting at the moment the ultrasound pulse is generated. The velocity of the ultrasound pulse is approximately constant (about 1550 m/s) so the time delay between arrival of echoes from the various interfaces is proportional to the distances between them and this in turn is indicated by the positions of the bright spots on the display. Once the echo from the furthermost structure of interest has returned, a second ultrasound pulse is transmitted and the process is repeated. In practice, several thousand pulses per second can be transmitted.

The echocardiographic examination

Two-dimensional images

Technique
To generate cross-sectional images, the machine scans the ultrasound beam rapidly across the heart (typically 25 times per second). This can be done by rocking the transducer crystal or spinning it on a wheel or by dividing the crystal into a number of small segments and exciting these electrically in a varying, but precisely controlled, sequence which alters the direction of pulse propagation without moving the transducer. The operator aims the transducer so as to image particular sections of the heart. Echo signals are displayed with the direction of the scan on the cathode-ray tube synchronized to that of the ultrasound beam. This builds up a tomographic image of the heart which shows both the anatomy of the selected anatomical section and its motion (Fig. 2.3). The cross-sectional ('two-dimensional') images are viewed on a video monitor and can be recorded on videotape. Individual frames from the videotape can be photographed, but this loses the motion information.

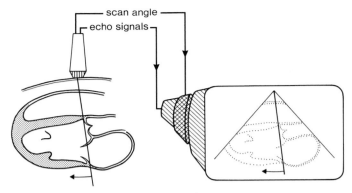

Fig. 2.3. Diagram showing how a cross-sectional ('two-dimensional') image is formed using a mechanical scanning system.

Nomenclature of views (Fig. 2.4)

1 *Left parasternal position.* Long-axis and short-axis planes can be obtained. Tilting the plane of the short-axis scan produces a series of sections from the LV apex to the atria and great arteries.

2 *Apical approach.* Also gives a long-axis view, but with the apical region in the foreground, and shows the four-chamber plane.

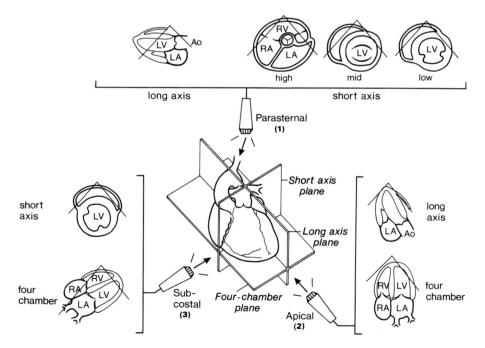

Fig. 2.4. Diagram showing the standard two-dimensional echocardiographic images and their terminology. **1** = left parasternal position; **2** = apical approach; **3** = subcostal approach.

3 *Subcostal approach.* For short-axis and four-chamber views in children to image systemic and pulmonary venous returns and the atrial septum.
4 *Transoesophageal approach.* For aorta and LA.

M-mode echocardiograms

Technique

To document in detail the motion patterns of individual cardiac structures such as valves, a technique called *M-mode* is used. The echo signals from one particular beam direction are recorded as columns of dots on a roll of photosensitive paper which is pulled past the cathode-ray tube display at constant speed. Stationary structures thus generate straight lines along the paper and movements such as those of heart valves are indicated by continuous undulating lines (Fig. 2.5). By convention, the position of the transducer is at the top of the paper, with increasing distance from it indicated by vertical displacement of the echo trace. Time calibration is provided by lines on the paper edges at 0.04 s intervals and it is normal to add an ECG trace as an aid to identifying the phases of the cardiac cycle.

Recording

M-mode recordings are obtained from the left parasternal position to document motion patterns of the aorta, aortic valve and left atrium; mitral valve; and right and left ventricles (Fig. 2.6).

Calibration of M-mode recordings is provided by columns of dots on the recordings, the separation of the dots being equivalent to 1 cm of body tissue. It

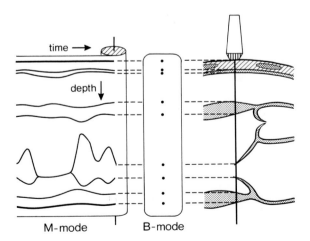

Fig. 2.5. Diagram showing how echo signals from the heart are converted into a M-mode recording. The returning echoes are registered as a column of dots on the display tube (B-mode) and the moving recording paper turns this into the M-mode.

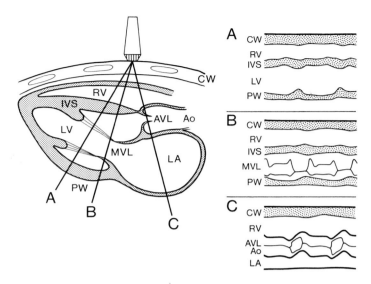

Fig. 2.6. Derivation of M-mode recordings of the major structures of the left heart. CW = chest wall; RV = right ventricle: IVS = interventricular septum; LV = left ventricle; PW = posterior wall; MVL = mitral valve leaflet; LA = left atrium; Ao = aorta; AVL = aortic valve leaflets.

is thus possible to obtain the dimensions of the major cardiac structures at any desired point in the cardiac cycle and with an accuracy of ±2–3 mm. Normal adult values for echo dimensions are listed in Table 2.1.

Comparison of end-diastolic and end-systolic values then allows parameters of cardiac function to be derived, e.g. percentage systolic reduction in LV cavity size (*shortening fraction*).

Table 2.1. Normal adult measurements of M-mode echocardiograms

Measurement	Normal Adult Range (± 2 x SD)
Aortic root diameter	2.0–3.7 cm
Left atrium (end systole)	1.9–3.8 cm
Excursion of anterior mitral valve leaflet	1.5–2.5 cm
Right ventricle (end diastole)	1.0–2.3 cm
Interventricular septum	
End diastole	0.7–1.1 cm
End systole	0.9–1.4 cm
Systolic thickening	30–50%
Left ventricle cavity	
End diastole	3.5–5.5 cm
End systole	2.5–4.1 cm
Systolic dimension reduction	20–40%
Posterior left ventricular wall	
End diastole	0.7–1.1 cm
End systole	0.9–1.4 cm
Systolic thickening	60–75%

Doppler echocardiography

Basic concepts

Echocardiographic imaging uses the relatively strong spectral echoes generated at tissue interfaces. Using high amplification, it is possible to detect weak echoes from much smaller structures, including those from red blood cells. If the blood is moving relative to the direction of the ultrasound beam, the frequency of the returning waves will be changed according to the Doppler equation and, for a given ultrasound frequency, the Doppler frequency shift is directly proportional to the blood velocity. A direct relationship exists between peak flow velocity and pressure gradient across a restrictive lesion such as a stenotic heart valve and is given by the Bernoulli equation (Fig. 2.7):

$$P_1 - P_2 = 1/2.\rho.(V_2^2 - V_1^2).$$

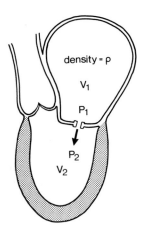

Fig. 2.7. Derivation of the pressure gradient across a stenotic mitral valve from the blood velocity across it using Bernoulli's equation.

For most practical purposes, this can be approximated as:

$$P_1 - P_2 = 4.V_2^2,$$

where the pressure gradient $(P_1 - P_2)$ is measured in mmHg and the velocity (V_2) is in metres/second. It is necessary to establish the peak jet velocity accurately and to align the ultrasound beam with it, otherwise falsely low readings will be obtained. Since velocity values are squared in the Bernoulli equation, such errors can lead to serious under-estimation of pressure gradients.

In order to obtain undistorted velocity data, a continuous train of ultrasound waves (continuous wave — CW) has to be used. This precludes obtaining any information about the depth at which a jet is located and it is not possible to generate a simultaneous image.

It is possible to extract some Doppler information from the short pulses used for imaging and thus to provide spatial location of velocities. This is called pulsed wave (PW) Doppler. Pulsed wave Doppler is useful for showing the location of abnormal flow, e.g. across the interventricular septum in a child with a ventricular septal defect (VSD), but the gaps between pulses generally prevent quantification of high velocities. It is also possible to miss a lesion if every possible location is not checked. Real-time colour flow imaging analyses velocities from a matrix of cells covering the entire two-dimensional image and displays velocity data as a colour overlay on a moving two-dimensional image. This provides a graphic illustration of abnormal flow jets, which appear as brightly coloured 'candle flames'.

Applications of echocardiographic imaging and Doppler

There are five ways in which ultrasound data are used:
1 Two-dimensional images to demonstrate cardiac anatomy.
2 M-mode recordings to provide dimensions and detailed motion patterns.
3 Continuous wave Doppler to give quantitative velocities for calculation of pressure gradients.
4 Pulsed wave Doppler for location of individual jets.
5 Colour-flow mapping for qualitative display of all velocity data.
Together they are vital adjuncts to the history and clinical examination in the majority of cardiac disorders and have superseded radiology for examining intracardiac structures.

Valve stenosis

The presence of calcium in a valve generates intense echoes and reverberations from these show as multiple parallel lines on M-mode recordings. The degree of calcification is more accurately assessed, however, by the X-ray image amplifier. In mitral stenosis M-mode recordings show thickening of cusps, reduced movement, abnormal motion and the orifice area can be measured from 2-D views. The small, distorted orifice in severe aortic stenosis precludes direct measurement, but M-mode recordings show the degree of hypertrophy, and the reduced diastolic filling rate.

Continuous wave Doppler velocities allow true peak and mean pressure gradients to be calculated for all stenotic lesions.

Valve regurgitation

Continuous wave Doppler is extremely sensitive in detecting valve regurgitation and PW Doppler allows precise localization of the site of the lesion but quantification of regurgitation is difficult. Pulsed wave and colour-flow Doppler can be used to map penetration of a regurgitant jet into the receiving chamber and the overall intensity of the jet on CW Doppler gives some idea of the total regurgitant flow, since the signal is comprised of the sum of the echoes from all the red cells in the path of the ultrasound beam. For mitral and aortic regurgitation, an indication of the degree of volume overload can be obtained from the LV end-diastolic dimension.

Examination of the valve usually indicates the aetiology (e.g. vegetations following endocarditis, prolapse or annular dilatation).

Aortic aneurysms and dissection

The proximal ascending aorta, the top of the aortic arch (using a suprasternal transducer position) and a short section of the descending aorta as it passes behind the left atrium can be seen in most patients. The diameter of the aorta can be measured; the presence of a reflecting structure moving within the aortic lumen suggests an intimal flap associated with dissection. Transoesophageal echo is the most accurate technique for this purpose.

Prosthetic heart valves

Each type of heart valve prosthesis has characteristic echocardiographic features. Irregularity of movement which is due to wear or formation of pannus around the orifice can be shown on M-mode recordings. The presence of stenosis or regurgitation can be indicated by CW Doppler and the location of regurgitant jets, especially paravalvar leaks caused by breakdown of the suturing, located by colour-flow mapping or PW Doppler. LV function can be studied by two-dimensional or M-mode recordings.

The heart muscle and heart failure

Dilated cardiomyopathy is characterized by a large, thin-walled and poorly contracting LV, while in hypertrophic cardiomyopathy the LV is small, with a grossly thickened, immobile septum.

Restrictive cardiomyopathies usually have large atria; M-mode recordings of the LV in diastole show early expansion, followed by sudden cessation of filling.

The end-systolic dimension is increased with poor ventricular function from any cause affecting the LV. The RV is more difficult to assess.

Pericardial effusion

Fluid in the pericardial cavity is indicated by an echo-free region next to the myocardium, separating it from the intense echo of the pericardium (Fig. 2.8).

Masses within the heart

Echocardiography is a sensitive method for detecting abnormal masses within the heart. Although their location, shape and size may give clues as to their pathogenesis, echocardiography cannot be used for tissue characterization.

Ischaemic heart disease

Echocardiography is useful to assess abnormal wall motion where the ECG is invalidated, e.g. by bundle branch block, or inaccurate, e.g. in differentiating inferior and posterior infarctions. It is excellent for detecting complications such as mitral papillary muscle rupture, ventricular septal defect and tamponade.

In the postinfarction period, it is valuable for diagnosis of LV aneurysm, thrombus in the left ventricle, pericardial effusion (Dressler's syndrome) and chronic myocardial failure.

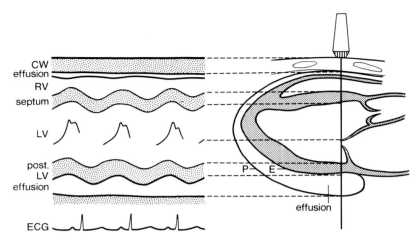

Fig. 2.8. M-mode pericardial effusion. P = pericardium; E = epicardium. Other abbreviations as in Fig. 2.6.

Congenital heart disease

Echocardiography has replaced cardiac catheterization and angiography for diagnosis in children. The examination is relatively easier than in an adult because the ribs and lungs do not offer resistance to the passage of ultrasound.

In skilled hands, echocardiography and Doppler can diagnose almost all congenital heart disease correctly, not only after birth but *in utero* by 22 weeks' gestation.

PHONOCARDIOGRAPHY

Modern auscultation is based on the graphic recording of heart sounds and murmurs. Accurate timing of sounds is achieved by simultaneous carotid pulse recordings giving the onset of aortic ejection and valve closure and by simultaneous echocardiography showing the movements of valves without phase shift.

Apparatus

The minimum requirements are two sound recordings (from different areas), a carotid pulse and an ECG taken simultaneously on a recorder with a good high-frequency response. Each amplifier should have three filter positions — low frequency to show filling sounds and murmurs, medium frequency, and high frequency for systolic murmurs, early diastolic murmurs and valve sounds.

Indications for phonocardiography

For identification of sounds and murmurs

Sounds

Atrial sounds

Differentiation from the first component (M_1) of a split first sound may be difficult clinically if M_1 is soft and of low frequency due to a long P–R interval: on the phono the atrial sound precedes QRS.

Ejection sounds

Aortic. Differentiated from the second component of a split first sound (T_1) by its occurrence during the upstroke of the aortic pressure pulse (coincident with the beginning of the upstroke of the indirect carotid pulse). A simultaneous echo shows synchronicity between an aortic ejection sound and the final halt of the outward movement of the aortic cusps while a delayed tricuspid component of the first sound (T_1) coincides with the final halt of the closing tricuspid valve.

Pulmonary. Pulmonary ejection sounds are confusingly near to T_1, but they disappear during inspiration when augmentation of the 'a' wave pushes up the pulmonary valve in presystole.

Second sound

Wide splitting. Found with atrial septal defect (ASD) or single atrium ('fixed' split), right bundle branch block and pulmonary stenosis (see Chapter 1, p. 30 and Fig. 1.15).

Single second sound. P_2 cannot be recorded when severe pulmonary stenosis is accompanied by a right to left shunt diminishing pulmonary blood flow (Fallot's tetralogy). A_2 and P_2 are fused in Eisenmenger's complex with a VSD (p. 218). A_2 is absent in severe calcific aortic stenosis.

Reversed splitting of the second sound (P_2 preceding A_2). Left bundle branch block, hypertension or severe aortic stenosis. A_2 is identified by occurring 0.02 s after the dicrotic notch of the indirect carotid pulse.

Amplitude of second sound. In pulmonary hypertension and in ASD the second component (P_2) is greater than the first (A_2) in the pulmonary area and is transmitted to the apex. A_2 is loud in systemic hypertension (high pressure) and Fallot's tetralogy (anteriorly displaced aorta).

Opening snaps. These resemble the second component of a split second sound in quality but are identified by recording all three sounds $(A_2, P_2,$ opening snap) during inspiration — or by synchrony of the sound with the final halt of the opening valve on the echo.

Murmurs

Systolic

Aortic ejection murmurs are often loud at the apex and phonocardiography may be needed to exclude a pansystolic murmur from mitral regurgitation. An ejection murmur always stops before A_2. In hypertrophic obstructive cardiomyopathy the ejection murmur peaks late but its termination before A_2 is shown on the phono.

Diastolic

An aortic regurgitant murmur seldom requires a phono because the human hearing mechanism is highly sensitive at high frequencies and can discriminate between murmur and background noise. At low frequencies a sound recording is superior to the ear and may pick up inaudible mid-diastolic murmurs, third and fourth sounds.

For teaching

Auscultation followed by analysis of the phonocardiogram and re-auscultation is the ideal method for teaching students.

CARDIAC RADIOLOGY

Cardiac silhouette

A radiological silhouette is produced by the X-rays making a tangent between a structure of one density and another of different density, in this case water density (heart, great vessels) and air (lungs).

The radiological density of water is similar whether it is in a pleural effusion, heart, blood vessel or mediastinal structure.

Postero-anterior radiograph (PA view, 1.5 m distance, Fig. 2.9)

Cardiothoracic ratio

The normal transverse diameter of the heart should not exceed 155 mm and should be well within 50% of the widest internal diameter of the chest. May be artificially small if the diaphragm is low.

Individual silhouettes

The right heart (cavae, atrium, ventricle and pulmonary artery) lies anteriorly: the left heart (pulmonary veins, atrium, ventricle and aorta) lies posteriorly. Little of the left heart therefore reaches the postero-anterior cardiac silhouette.

Eleven silhouettes need to be recognized: eight from the cardiac chambers and three in the lungs. Normally there are five cardiac silhouettes visible, two on the right and three on the left, and two pulmonary silhouettes (arteries and veins).

Right heart border

On the right, from above downwards, the normal silhouettes are the superior vena cava and the right atrium. Another silhouette appears at the lower end of the superior vena cava and upper end of the right atrium if there is dilatation of the ascending aorta.

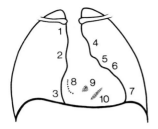

Fig. 2.9. Anterior chest X-ray: cardiac contours (exaggerated to indicate site). 1 = superior vena cava; 2 = ascending aorta; 3 = right atrial border; 4 = aortic knuckle; 5 = main pulmonary artery; 6 = left atrial appendage — only visible when enlarged; 7 = left ventricle; 8 = margin of left atrium lying behind the right atrium; 9 = position of aortic valve calcium; and 10 = position of mitral valve calcium.

Left heart border

Normally on the left there are three silhouettes: the aortic knuckle, the main pulmonary artery and the ventricular mass. The term 'ventricular mass' is used because either ventricle may occupy the lower part of the left silhouette when either dilates. The abnormal silhouette that may appear on the left border is that of the left atrial appendage below the pulmonary artery and above the ventricular mass.

There is normally no silhouette formed by the left atrium itself because it is entirely related to water density tissue in the mediastinum. Dilatation of the left atrium occurs towards the right when it may project into that pleura and give rise to a silhouette inside or outside the right atrial silhouette, best seen on a penetrated PA radiograph.

Lung markings

The relevant lung markings are those of pulmonary arteries, pulmonary veins and pulmonary lymph. The pulmonary arteries tend to form a horizontal Y with upper and lower lobe vessels: the pulmonary veins enter the left atrium horizontally and are rarely individually visible but form a hazy outline to the lower hila of the lungs when they are dilated.

Oligaemia of the lung fields occurs in pulmonary stenosis and atresia: plethora in left to right shunts. Diversion of blood flow to the upper lobes occurs in conditions with a raised left atrial pressure. Reactive pulmonary arteriolar constriction is greater in the lower lobes where hydrostatic pressure is added to the pulmonary venous pressure. Pulmonary lymphatics run in the interlobular septa and when the mean left atrial pressure is raised, the dilated lymphatics and septal oedema form horizontal lines at the costophrenic angles, first described by Kerley and known as Kerley's 'B' lines.

Frank pulmonary oedema shows patchy, semiconfluent, ill-defined, mainly parahilar shadowing.

Anteroposterior radiograph

Patient in bed. Heart size assessment is inaccurate as the heart is nearer to the X-ray plate than in PA view and the diaphragm is raised, the two causing the appearance of spurious cardiac enlargement.

Lateral chest radiograph

Particularly valuable to show calcification of valves or pericardium. The only silhouette normally seen on the lateral chest radiograph is the posterior border of the left ventricle protruding into the left pleura. Dilatation of the right ventricle can sometimes be seen filling the space between the heart shadow and the sternum. A barium swallow will show posterior displacement of the oesophagus by a dilated left atrium.

Enlargement of a cardiac silhouette

Enlargement of a cardiac silhouette occurs because of dilatation only: hypertrophy of a ventricle is rarely enough to exceed the variations caused by respiration and systole/diastole. Echo is superior for chamber size.

Causes of dilatation

Dilatation of atria and great vessels (aorta, pulmonary vessels and venae cavae) is caused by both a *raised pressure* (e.g. pulmonary hypertension, mitral stenosis) or an *increased flow* (e.g. left to right shunt). Dilatation of ventricles only occurs with a raised volume overload (preload, e.g. aortic regurgitation): pressure overload (after-load, e.g. aortic stenosis) causes hypertrophy, not dilatation, and rarely therefore appears on the radiograph. When the ventricle with aortic stenosis fails, however, it will then dilate. A vessel also dilates because of turbulence immediately distal to stenosis (e.g. *poststenotic dilatation* of aorta and PA because of aortic and pulmonary valve stenosis).

Differential radiological diagnosis

Diagnosis of the causative lesion can often be suggested by the appearance of the chest radiograph, e.g. *aortic stenosis* has a normal silhouette except for poststenotic dilatation of the ascending aorta: *aortic regurgitation* has a dilated ventricular mass; *mitral stenosis* has a dilated left atrium and appendage, upper lobe diversion and Kerley's lines but a normal ventricular mass; *mitral regurgitation* has the same but with a dilated ventricular mass; *pulmonary hypertension* has a dilated pulmonary artery and right atrium but a normal ventricular mass, unless heart failure, pulmonary regurgitation, or a previous left to right shunt has caused ventricular dilatation; *pulmonary valve stenosis* has a poststenotic dilated pulmonary artery, a normal ventricular mass and a dilated right atrium; in *infundibular* pulmonary stenosis, the pulmonary artery is normal; and 'uncoiling' of the ascending aorta and aortic knuckle is suggestive of *hypertension* and may be confused with an aneurysm.

Calcification

Cardiac calcification may be seen in valves (Fig. 2.9), pericardium, coronary arteries, aorta and left atrium.

Valve calcification

Knowledge of valve calcification is important clinically because it tends to abolish valve sounds (ejection clicks, opening snaps and second sounds).

Aortic valve calcification is seen in the centre of the heart on a penetrated lateral film. On the image amplifier the degree of calcification can be graded and is a measure of severity of stenosis when caused by a bicuspid valve. *Mitral valve* calcification is inferior and posterior to this. When confined to the annulus, it has little effect on function.

Pericardial calcification

Surrounds the cardiac silhouette and is best seen on a lateral view. It is associated with constrictive pericarditis.

Coronary artery calcification

This is rarely seen on a routine radiograph, because of cardiac movement, but is clearly seen on screening.

Other calcification

The aortic wall may be calcified in the elderly and in syphilitic aortitis and there may be calcification of thrombus lining the left atrium in mitral valve disease.

Other radiological techniques

CT scanning

Normal computerized tomography (CT) scanning is rarely used in cardiac diagnosis because of the movement of the heart but may identify aortic aneurysms from other lesions of the mediastinum.

Rapid CT scanning, gated to the ECG, can, however, produce images as precise as two-dimensional echocardiography in elucidating intracardiac pathology.

MAGNETIC RESONANCE IMAGING

Magnetic resonance is a physical property exhibited by certain elements with an odd number of protons in their nuclei (e.g. hydrogen and phosphorus). When placed in a magnetic field and excited by a pulse of radio waves at an appropriate frequency, these nuclei emit a radio signal which can be detected by a suitable receiver. The signals detected during magnetic resonance imaging are relayed to a computer which constructs an image based on the amplitude of signal emitted point for point over a 'slice' through the patient. The amplitude of the signal depends largely on the abundance of hydrogen nuclei and so the image reflects proton density through the chosen tomographic slice.

Advantages

Any plane can be chosen. Offers high soft tissue contrast and high resolution. Flowing blood is clearly distinguished from stationary structures, without the use of contrast media.

Disadvantages

'Gating' to the ECG is required to compensate for movement of the heart and acquisition times for the image are long. The technique has applications in the assessment of ventricular function, imaging of aorta, pulmonary arteries and pericardium and applications in flow visualization. The technique has not yet displaced other non-invasive imaging methods, e.g. two-dimensional echocardiography or CT scanning.

NUCLEAR CARDIOLOGY

Nuclear cardiology involves the use of radiopharmaceuticals to obtain information about the myocardium and cardiac chambers.

Advantages

It is non-invasive and provides functional information. It can be used during exercise and rest.

Disadvantages

Spatial resolution is poor so that anatomy is not easily demonstrated.

Technique

Radiopharmaceuticals

The most commonly used are:
1   Technetium 99m in tagged red cells (for ventricular function) or as pyrophosphate (in acute infarction).
2   Thallium 201 whose myocardial distribution is proportional to blood flow (for myocardial perfusion).

Gamma-camera and online computer

A γ-camera alone can be used for thallium imaging but an online computer is necessary for ventricular function.

Radionuclide ventriculography

Technetium 99m labelled erythrocytes are used on a first pass study to show blood pools in the cardiac chambers or as an equilibrium study after activity is evenly dispersed throughout the blood. A left anterior oblique view with craniocaudal tilt separates ventricles and atria. The number of counts give different colours. Ventriculography is used to assess the following:

Ejection fraction

This technique is independent of ventricular geometry, unlike echo- or angiocardiography. Valuable in left ventricular failure and to show right ventricular ejection fraction in congenital and pulmonary disease.

Regional ventricular function

Dyskinetic and akinetic areas in coronary artery disease are shown by the extent and timing of motion of each ventricle, e.g. ventricular aneurysms and infarcts show a low amplitude (hypokinesia) and delayed contraction.

Valve regurgitation

Calculated from the ratio of RV and LV volumes.

Intracardiac shunting

In a left to right shunt there is a normal peak as the bolus passes through the lungs plus an earlier than usual second peak. The shunt can be quantified.

Stress imaging

Stress is produced by: dynamic exercise on a bicycle with the upper body immobilised or supine; isometric exercise squeezing a bulb; cold pressor test, immersing the hand in cold water; and intravenous dipyridamole (vasodilator).

Distinction of ischaemia from infarction

New wall motion abnormalities appear with thallium 201 imaging in ischaemic ventricles under stress compared with resting views, distinguishing ischaemia from infarction in which there is no change.

Acute infarction imaging

Technetium 99m pyrophosphate shows areas of acute infarction as a 'hot spot'. It is maximal on the second day but little is left by the fifth day, so only a narrow time window is available. Large old infarcts, e.g. ventricular aneurysms, also take up technetium 99m and need to be distinguished from acute infarcts.

Chapter 3
Invasive Investigations

CARDIAC CATHETERIZATION AND ANGIOGRAPHY

Objectives

1 *Pressure measurements* can be made within the cardiac chambers and great vessels. (Fig. 3.1).

2 *Samples of blood* may be obtained from the cardiac chambers and great vessels and analysed for their percentage oxygen saturation.

3 *Radio-opaque contrast medium* can be injected directly into any cardiac chamber or vessel. Cine angiograms can then delineate a cardiac or extra cardiac lesion as the contrast passes through the heart.

Techniques

Studies require an image intensifier and cine-angiography equipment, fluid-filled catheters and transducers for pressure measurements and an oximeter if oxygen saturations are to be measured.

Studies are usually performed under sedation and local anaesthetic, though some children need general anaesthesia. Catheters are introduced percutaneously by the Seldinger technique (Fig. 3.2) or directly into the vessel dissected out through a small incision.

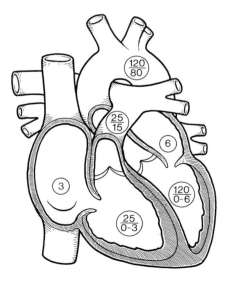

Fig. 3.1. Normal intracardiac pressures.

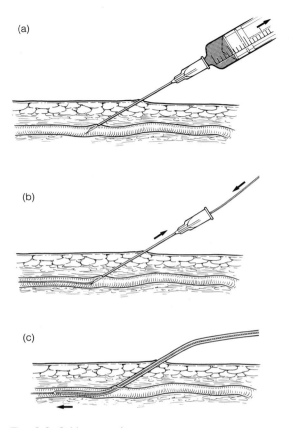

Fig. 3.2. Seldinger technique.

Right heart catheterization

The cardiac catheter is introduced through the femoral vein (or a vein in the arm). Under radiographic control, it can be directed into right atrium, right ventricle and pulmonary artery. Pushed out into a small branch pulmonary artery, it 'wedges' and records a pressure tracing which closely corresponds to the pressure in the pulmonary veins and left atrium.

Left heart catheterization

Retrograde approach

The catheter is introduced from the femoral or brachial artery and can be directed through the aortic valve and into the left ventricle.

Across the atrial septum

If, as in many children, the foramen ovale is patent, the left atrium and left ventricle can be entered with a catheter introduced from the femoral vein. In adults with an intact atrial septum, the atrial septum can be punctured by a needle and a catheter passed over it into the left atrium.

Derived data

Valve stenosis

An abnormally high pressure is found proximal to a narrow valve, a low pressure may be found distal to it. The gradient across the valve is one index of the severity of the obstruction but flow must be taken into account. Equations relating pressure gradient, flow and heart rate can be used to estimate valve orifice areas — Gorlin equations.

Shunt calculations

In congenital heart disease, blood samples are taken in the cavae, pulmonary veins, atria, ventricles, aorta and pulmonary artery. There is a rise in oxygen saturation of samples taken from a chamber into which a left to right shunt occurs and the bigger the 'step up' in saturations the bigger the shunt. Conversely desaturated blood reaching the left side of the heart documents a right to left shunt.

The size of the overall shunt is usually expressed as the *pulmonary : systemic flow ratio* which can be quantitated:

$$\frac{\text{Pulmonary flow}}{\text{Systemic flow}} = \frac{\text{Systemic artery } O_2 \text{ sat.} - \text{Systemic venous } O_2 \text{ sat.}}{\text{Pulmonary artery } O_2 \text{ sat.} - \text{Pulmonary venous } O_2 \text{ sat.}}$$

If the actual pulmonary flow can be measured or derived from the oxygen consumption (Fick principle), the pulmonary vascular resistance can then be calculated:

Pulmonary vascular resistance (normally 1 Wood unit)

$$= \frac{\text{Mean pulmonary artery pressure} - \text{Mean left atrial pressure}}{\text{Pulmonary flow}}$$

Angiography

Radio-opaque contrast medium, usually iodine based, is injected under pressure into a ventricle or major artery over the course of one to three cardiac cycles. Cine cameras record images at 60 frames per second, often in two planes simultaneously. Views are selected to delineate the structures of interest.

Specially shaped catheters may be used to deliver contrast selectively into particular vessels, e.g. the left and right coronary arteries.

In some systems in which the image is digitized, computer aided systems can be used to enhance the image (digital subtraction angiography).

General indications for invasive investigations

To establish a precise diagnosis

Part of an assessment prior to operation. Detailed angiography may be needed, e.g. coronary angiography prior to coronary artery bypass grafting.

Estimation of the severity of a lesion

1 *Valve stenosis.* Withdrawal gradient or simultaneous pressures across the valve, together with estimate of flow.

2 *Valve regurgitation.* Pressure tracings can give an indication of the severity of valvar regurgitation, e.g. in the severe mitral regurgitation with a small LA, the left atrial pressure tracing shows a prominent systolic wave. Angiography also demonstrates the severity of valvar regurgitation which is graded according to the amount of contrast refluxing backwards across the affected valve.

3 *Size of shunt.* Step up or down in oxygen saturations documents size of intra- or extracardiac shunt.

Delineation of additional lesions

Suspected additional lesions must be confirmed or excluded before surgery for congenital heart disease.

Assessment of results of surgery

Particularly for congenital heart disease.

Interventional catheterization

Specially designed catheters can be used to treat or palliate some congenital and acquired heart diseases:

1 *Coronary angioplasty.* A flexible wire is guided past an atheromatous lesion and a balloon is inflated to compress the plaque and improve coronary flow. Case selection is important as the coronary lesion must be proximal and collateral coronary flow adequate.

2 *Balloon valvotomy* of stenotic pulmonary, aortic and mitral valves. Case selection is very important as the procedure should split fused commissures without rendering the valve grossly incompetent.

3 *Balloon atrial septostomy.* A Fogarty catheter is guided from the right atrium, across the atrial septum, inflated in the left atrium and pulled back sharply to tear the atrial septum. This is part of the early palliation of transposition of the great arteries and mitral atresia.

4 *Blade septectomy.* If the atrial septum is too thick to tear, a catheter with a retractable blade may be used to cut the atrial septum.

5 *Embolization.* Any vessel that can be selectively cannulated can be occluded. Wire coils, detachable balloons and 'umbrella devices' have been used. Some fistulae and abnormal pulmonary vessels are managed in this way but occlusion of persistent ductus is still experimental.

Complications of cardiac catheterization

1 *Atrial and ventricular arrhythmias.*

2 *Systemic embolism* during left heart catheterization.

3 *Haemodynamic changes* related to contrast medium — patients with high pulmonary vascular resistance or low cardiac output particularly precarious.
4 *Puncture of the heart* producing tamponade.
5 *Intramyocardial injection* of contrast medium.
6 *Damage to an artery* through which a catheter is introduced.

The electrocardiogram and intravascular pressures are continuously monitored and anaesthetic and resuscitation equipment must be available.

Swan–Ganz catheterization

Even when radiological facilities are not available, right heart pressures can be measured. A light flexible catheter with a balloon on the end is introduced into a vein and the balloon inflated with air or carbon dioxide. (Fig. 3.3) The balloon 'floats' through the right heart and into the pulmonary artery with the blood flow and registers pulmonary arterial pressure. It eventually wedges in a small pulmonary artery and registers a pressure similar to left atrial pressure. This technique is sometimes used intra-operatively and in coronary care units to monitor left atrial pressure.

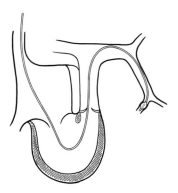

Fig. 3.3. Swan–Ganz catheterization.

MYOCARDIAL BIOPSY

Myocardial biopsy is usually performed by passing a flexible bioptome transvenously into the right ventricle. Left ventricular biopsies can be obtained by a transseptal approach. Biopsies can also be taken at surgery with a Tru-Cut needle or from an excised papillary muscle at mitral valve replacement.

Uses

Diagnostic

1 *Myocardial disease*, e.g. amyloidosis.
2 *Evidence of rejection* following cardiac transplantation. Serial biopsies of the right ventricle are routine postoperative management following cardiac transplantation.

Myocardial deterioration during surgical ischaemia

Adenosine triphosphate (ATP) or creatine phosphate levels or change in birefringence in response to ATP and calcium show deterioration due to ischaemia.

Complications

Perforation of the ventricle (rare).

Chapter 4
Valve Disease and its Complications

Abnormalities of heart valves are due to congenital, rheumatic, connective tissue or degenerative disease, and range from minor distortion to severe stenosis, regurgitation or both.

Complications are arrhythmia (p. 101), thromboembolism (p. 102), infective endocarditis (p. 103) and ventricular failure (Chapter 6).

AETIOLOGY

1. Congenital heart disease
(See Chapter 9.) The most common congenital anomaly (1% of the population) is a bicuspid aortic valve, which has a risk of infective endocarditis and may later cause aortic stenosis resulting from calcium deposition.

2. Acute rheumatic fever
Still the commonest cause of valve disease but has almost disappeared in countries with high standards of nutrition and hygiene.

Pathogenesis
Endothelial surfaces under stress, particularly the joints, develop an allergic response weeks after general infection with a haemolytic streptococcus (Lancefield Group A). The immunological trigger lies in the protective coat of the coccus and affects children between the ages of 5 and 20 years, younger in areas of poverty, and produces nodules which may disappear or leave behind scarring with giant cell Aschoff nodules.

About half the children develop acute non-bacterial vegetations on the mitral, less often on the aortic, and occasionally on the tricuspid valves, the relative frequency of involvement seeming to be related to the pressure sustained by the valve. In florid cases the myocardium and pericardium are also affected. Occasionally the immunological trigger causes chorea (p. 65).

Mitral valve disease, most commonly stenosis, develops over the next 10 years (more rapidly in areas of low standards of living), and may be associated with aortic regurgitation and stenosis. Isolated aortic valve disease is rare but isolated mitral regurgitation occurs. The joints always return to normal.

Clinical presentation

Symptoms
Two to three weeks after a haemolytic streptococcal pharyngitis or scarlet fever, joint pains develop which typically flit between large joints, but occasionally affect only one. Erythrocyte sedimentation rate (ESR) and antistreptolysin titres are high.

Clinical examination

General

Fever, with painful, swollen joints; erythema marginatum — red areas with definite margins; and nodules on pressure points, e.g. elbows. Manifestations other than fever may be minimal.

Cardiovascular system

- Sinus tachycardia
- Raised jugular venous pulse (JVP) from heart failure — now rare
- Auscultation. Soft, short ventricular filling murmur (Carey Coombs murmur from vegetations on the mitral valve) and sometimes a soft early diastolic murmur (aortic regurgitation). Ejection murmurs may be physiological because of high flow from fever, or may be due to aortic valvulitis. An apical pansystolic murmur indicates mitral regurgitation

The diagnosis is often missed (50% of patients with rheumatic mitral stenosis give no history of acute rheumatic fever or chorea).

Complications

1 *Pericarditis* — with a friction rub and later effusion in severe cases.
2 *Heart failure* — rheumatic myocarditis or severe valve lesions.
3 *Central nervous system* — resulting from the immunological reaction to the haemolytic streptococcus. Chorea (involuntary movements) may be the main manifestation.

Electrocardiography

Prolonged P–R interval (usually slight — serial measurements required).

Echocardiography

May show vegetations or pericardial effusion. Serial measurement of left ventricle (LV) size assesses progress in severe cases.

Prognosis

If no murmurs develop, the heart has escaped. A mitral mid-diastolic murmur may be transient. An aortic early diastolic murmur is usually permanent.

Treatment of acute rheumatic fever

Rest in bed but not immobilization. Penicillin to eradicate the streptococcus. Large doses of aspirin or steroids improve the clinical picture but do not diminish the valvulitis.

- *Recurrent attacks* occur particularly in the first year
- *Prophylaxis* is effective as the streptococcus does not become resistant to penicillin. Oral penicillin 125 mg b.d. monthly, long-acting penicillin parenterally, or a sulphonamide, e.g. sulphadimidine 0.5 g b.d. are given for 5 years after an attack or until the age of 20

3. Disorders of connective tissue

Marfan's syndrome

An inherited disorder of connective tissue (Chapter 12). Aorta almost invariably affected, with dissection the usual cause of death. Aortic regurgitation is due to dilatation of aortic ring or secondary to dissection. Associated mitral regurgitation is due to prolapsed cusps.

Dissection of aorta (of ascending aorta — type A).

This causes aortic regurgitation, the initial tear allowing one aortic cusp to prolapse. Most commonly an isolated abnormality of the aorta and not associated with Marfan's syndrome.

Prolapse of redundant mitral cusps (floppy valve)

This is a common (5% of the population over the age of 50) disorder of collagen affecting only the mitral cusps and chordae (most highly stressed collagen in the body). May be inherited. Stature often tall and thin with chest deformity and big arm span and abnormal collagen may be detected in the skin. Ballooning and prolapse of mitral cusps may cause mitral regurgitation which is usually slight unless there is chordal rupture (Fig. 4.18), or infective endocarditis (p. 103).

Isolated dilatation of the aortic root

This is now the commonest cause of aortic regurgitation in Europeans (p. 76).

4. Degenerative disease of valves

In old age, deposition of calcium in the hinge areas of the aortic cusps (so-called aortic sclerosis) causes rigidity and turbulence and an ejection murmur. This may progress to 'senile' calcific aortic stenosis.

Calcification of the mitral annulus is not uncommon in the elderly but seldom interferes with haemodynamics.

AORTIC STENOSIS

Types of aortic stenosis

Obstruction in the LV outflow occurs at three levels (Fig. 4.1a):

1   *Valve stenosis* — congenital or acquired — calcium deposition common.
2   *Sub-valve stenosis* — congenital (Fig. 4.1b), or hypertrophic obstructive cardiomyopathy (Chapter 6), when septal hypertrophy causes LV outflow obstruction.
3   *Supravalvar aortic stenosis* — congenital (Fig. 4.1c) and frequently associated with mental retardation and a peculiar facies.

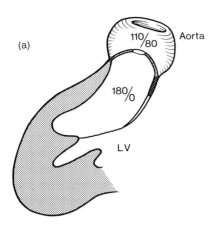

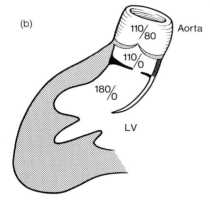

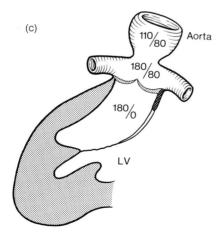

Fig. 4.1. Types of aortic stenosis: (a) Valvar. (b) Subvalvar diaphragm. (c) Supravalvar.

1. Aortic valve stenosis

Aetiology and pathology

Bicuspid valve

The commonest cause of aortic stenosis is calcification of a congenitally bicuspid valve. By itself a bicuspid valve has no effect on function and is only diagnosed by an aortic ejection sound and a soft ejection murmur (Fig. 4.2a).

True congenital stenosis

Manifest from birth. A small hole in a domed valve.

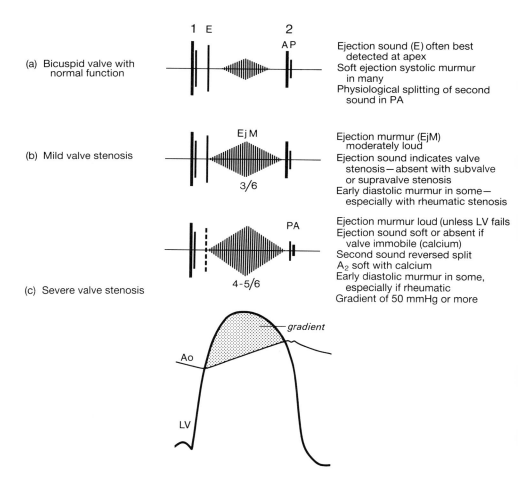

(a) Bicuspid valve with normal function

Ejection sound (E) often best detected at apex
Soft ejection systolic murmur in many
Physiological splitting of second sound in PA

(b) Mild valve stenosis

Ejection murmur (EjM) moderately loud
Ejection sound indicates valve stenosis—absent with subvalve or supravalve stenosis
Early diastolic murmur in some— especially with rheumatic stenosis

(c) Severe valve stenosis

Ejection murmur loud (unless LV fails)
Ejection sound soft or absent if valve immobile (calcium)
Second sound reversed split
A_2 soft with calcium
Early diastolic murmur in some, especially if rheumatic
Gradient of 50 mmHg or more

Fig. 4.2. Aortic valve abnormalities — auscultatory findings. A = aortic; P = pulmonary; Ao = aorta; EjM = ejection murmur.

Senile aortic stenosis (aortic cusp sclerosis)

Calcium deposition spreads from the hinge areas of three otherwise normal cusps causing stenosis in the elderly.

Rheumatic

Rheumatic fusion of the valve commissures with thickening of cusps associated usually with aortic regurgitation and mitral valve involvement.

Haemodynamics

Reduction in valve aperture causes no haemodynamic abnormality until it is one-quarter of normal.

1 *Systolic gradient across the valve.* The pressure during systole is higher in the LV than in the aorta (Fig. 4.1a).

2 *Left ventricular hypertrophy.* Increased LV work results in LV hypertrophy. LV dilatation does not occur until the ventricle fails or if aortic regurgitation is also present.

3 *Poststenotic dilatation.* Localized dilatation occurs distal to the obstruction because of the lateral force on the aortic wall exerted by the turbulence of the jet of blood.

Clinical presentation

Symptoms

Symptoms may be *absent* in sedentary persons even with severe stenosis, particularly in the older age groups (5% of sudden, unexpected deaths are due to calcific aortic stenosis).

Dyspnoea

This is due to the raised filling pressure of the hypertrophied LV raising the left atrial (LA) pressure. Usually mild in early stages ('a' wave only).

Angina of effort

Coronary blood flow is inadequate for a hypertrophied myocardium. Angina at rest is rare unless there is coincidental coronary disease (about 25% of the older age groups).

Syncope or dizziness

This may occur with exertion (low cardiac output and peripheral vasodilatation). Syncope may also occur without exertion due to arrhythmia.

Clinical examination

The patient is well, unless suffering from infective endocarditis or heart failure.

Pulse

Rhythm. Usually sinus — atrial fibrillation (AF) suggests a rheumatic aetiology with co-existing mitral stenosis.

Amplitude. Reduced (low cardiac output).

Wave form. Slow upstroke (carotid or brachial pulse (see Fig. 1.3b;): in peripheral pulses this may be lost).
Blood pressure. Normal except terminally.

Jugular venous pressure

Usually normal unless LV failure has caused pulmonary hypertension and right ventricular (RV) failure. Sometimes a dominant 'a' wave in the venous pulse (mechanism unknown).

Cardiac impulses

LV hypertrophy can usually be detected, except in obese patients, by inclining the patient to the left.

Auscultation (Fig. 4.2b & c)

Ejection murmur: loud, in the aortic area, at the apex and in the neck. In the elderly the murmur may be maximal at the apex (close apposition of the LV to the chest wall).
Ejection sound (click): usually best appreciated at the apex; absent with severe valve calcification.

Electrocardiography

LV hypertrophy (Fig. 14.18) with occasional unexplained exceptions, particularly in children.

Chest radiography

Calcium deposition on a lateral chest X-ray is related to severity of obstruction in a bicuspid valve. Accurate grading of calcification, however, needs an image intensifier. On the PA chest X-ray, *poststenotic dilatation of the ascending aorta* with a normal-sized LV until the onset of LV failure or coincident regurgitation.

Echocardiography and Doppler scanning (Fig. 4.3)

Calcification is difficult to quantitate, may be seen in older age groups without significant obstruction and may be absent in rheumatic stenosis. Thick LV free wall and septum (> 1 cm). The LV cavity is not dilated unless there is associated aortic regurgitation or failure. The gradient may be assessed by Doppler ultrasound (p. 47).

Cardiac catheterization and angiocardiography

The *pressure gradient* across the aortic valve is measured by withdrawing a catheter from LV into the aorta (Fig. 4.1) or by using a double lumen catheter for simultaneous recording. From simultaneously measured valve gradient and stroke volume, the *Gorlin valve* area (p. 60) may be calculated. A Gorlin area of 0.5 cm^2 indicates *severe stenosis*. Echocardiographic assessment of aortic stenosis is so accurate that measurement of the gradient is seldom necessary, but a *coronary arteriogram* is required if valve replacement is proposed: 25% of patients over 50 will have significant coronary disease.

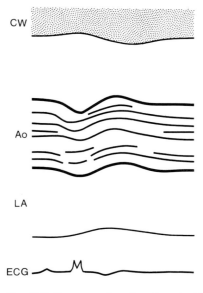

CW

Ao

LA

ECG

Fig. 4.3. Severe aortic valve stenosis. M-mode echo showing heavy linear echoes from the calcium in the valve (compare Fig. 2.6). CW = chest wall; Ao = aorta.

Associated lesions

In rheumatic aortic stenosis, mitral stenosis may be missed because the hypertrophied LV reduces the rate of LV filling so that the velocity of flow is insufficient to produce an opening snap or diastolic murmur. Suggested by long-standing dyspnoea, atrial fibrillation or a loud first sound.

Differential diagnosis

Aortic cusp sclerosis

Soft ejection murmur but with a normal carotid pulse and no LV hypertrophy unless systemic hypertension is present.

Ejection murmurs in normal children

It is common to hear a short, low frequency, soft or moderately loud, mid-systolic murmur over the RV outflow tract (pulmonary area and lower left sternal edge) in thin children and young adults. A murmur maximal at the apex and preceded by an ejection sound suggests a bicuspid aortic valve.

Mitral regurgitation

Both murmurs may be maximal at the apex with A_2 inaudible from calcification or drowned by the pansystolic murmur. A phonocardiogram shows the pansystolic murmur running through A_2. A sharp upstroke on the pulse is characteristic of mitral regurgitation.

Assessment of severity

Symptoms
Dyspnoea, particularly paroxysmal nocturnal dyspnoea, exertional angina and syncope suggest severe stenosis unless there is associated coronary or myocardial disease.

Wave form of the pulse
A normal sharp upstroke on the carotid or brachial pulse excludes significant stenosis except in children. No conclusion can be reached if the pulse is small as it may be difficult to palpate for anatomical reasons or due to a low output state.

LV hypertrophy
LV hypertrophy indicates significant stenosis, unless hypertension is also present.

Calcium
Marked calcification in a congenital bicuspid or sclerotic valve indicates severity, but rheumatic valves may be severely stenosed without calcification.

Complications of aortic stenosis
- *Left ventricular failure.*
- *Sudden death* (from arrhythmia)
- *Systemic embolism* from a calcified valve blocking small arteries, e.g. retinal
- *Infective endocarditis* difficult to diagnose in the elderly when fever may be minimal but unexplained anaemia and clubbing are suggestive
- *Atrioventricular (AV) block.* Calcium spreading into the septum

Prognosis
Symptoms appear late and carry a poor prognosis. Survival following LV failure seldom exceeds 2 years and sudden death is not infrequent.

Surgery
The aim is to replace a severely stenosed valve before symptoms appear because a damaged LV never completely recovers. On the other hand, it is never too late to replace the valve.

Indications for surgery
1 Symptoms, e.g. dyspnoea, angina, dizziness, syncope.
2 In an asymptomatic patient, significant peak gradient, e.g. > 40 mmHg or reduction of Gorlin valve area, e.g. < 0.5 cm^2.
3 Before irrevocable damage to the ventricle, e.g. deteriorating ECG or LV dilatation on chest X-ray.

Operation
1 Infancy — balloon angioplasty.

2   Childhood — for congenital stenosis, open aortic valvotomy on cardiopulmonary bypass (Fig. 4.4).
3   Adult — aortic valve replacement. For choice of valve, see Figs. 4.5a, b & c, and pp. 262–263.

Complications of valve replacement
- *Hospital mortality* 2–4%, higher with LV failure
- *Infective endocarditis* 2–3%
- *Valve thrombosis and embolism* (prostheses 3%, xenograft 1%)
- *Paraprosthetic leak* 1–3% (higher with heavy calcification and active endocarditis)
- *AV dissociation*

2. Subvalvar aortic stenosis (Fig. 4.1b)
Subvalvar stenosis is due to (i) a fibrous or fibromuscular diaphragm immediately below the valve; (ii) to diffuse narrowing; or (iii) to hypertrophic obstructive cardiomyopathy.

Fibromuscular congenital stenosis
The anatomy varies from a localized subaortic diaphragm to a longer fibromuscular narrowing. The ejection murmur is present with no ejection sound. Stenosis is frequently mild with the murmur noticed at routine examination. The aortic valve is often regurgitant from interference with its function by the jet from the subaortic stenosis.

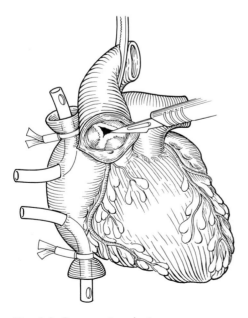

Fig. 4.4. Open aortic valvotomy.

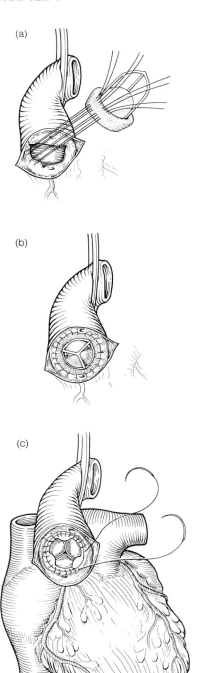

Fig. 4.5 (a) A Starr-Edwards ball valve being inserted with interrupted sutures.
(b) Ball valve *in situ*. (c) Aortic xenograft.

The diagnosis of the subaortic site of obstruction is suggested by the absence of an ejection sound without calcification to explain this and is made by echocardiography or cardiac catheterization (Fig. 4.1) and angiocardiography. Significant stenosis is treated by open resection through the aortic valve including both diaphragm and muscular component.

Hypertrophic obstructive cardiomyopathy (idiopathic hypertrophic subaortic stenosis)

Left ventricular outflow obstruction occurs in some cases of hypertrophic cardiomyopathy (see Chapter 6) with obstruction occurring only in mid-systole when the mitral valve is pulled towards the hypertrophied septum.

The pulse is sharp and the LV severely hypertrophied (loud atrial (fourth) sound and abnormal ECG).

No ejection sound and an ejection murmur later in systole than in valve stenosis but finishing before A_2. No diastolic murmur. The diagnosis is established by echocardiography (p. 49).

Surgical relief of the obstruction is seldom indicated as the obstruction is part of a generalized disease of the heart muscle, but if symptoms are severe, a gutter can be cut through the septum on cardiopulmonary bypass (Fig. 6.6) or, rarely, the mitral valve may be replaced.

3. **Supravalvar aortic stenosis** (Fig. 4.1c)

A rare congenital abnormality, often associated with an abnormal facies similar to that in infantile hypercalcaemia. The obstruction varies from a narrow ring above the aortic valve to an hour-glass deformity. The murmur is similar to valve stenosis but with no ejection sound.

Diagnosis is by echocardiography. The LV outflow tract and aortic valve are normal. Cardiac catheterization and angiography delineate the stenosis. Surgery is advised for severe stenosis which is relieved by one or more patches across the narrowed area. (Fig. 4.6)

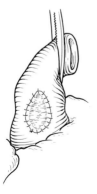

Fig. 4.6. Supravalvar aortic stenosis patched.

AORTIC REGURGITATION

Aortic regurgitation may be classified as being due to cusp abnormality or to aortic ring dilatation.

Aetiology and pathology

1. Cusp abnormality

Rheumatic valvulitis

Vegetations appear on the aortic cusps during acute rheumatic fever and are followed by fibrotic shrinkage, causing aortic regurgitation.

Congenital

In many cases the valve is bicuspid as well as deficient. A ventricular septal defect may allow prolapse of the associated cusp through it.

Infective endocarditis

Usually on an abnormal valve but occasionally a normal valve is the site of infection
- In older age with degenerative changes
- In drug addicts
- With virulent organisms, e.g. staphylococcus

2. Aortic root dilatation

Isolated dilatation (Fig. 4.7)

In Europe the commonest cause of aortic regurgitation. The cusps fail to meet centrally (Fig. 4.8).

Dissection of ascending aorta Type A (p. 252)

The intimal tear allows prolapse of an aortic cusp.

Secondary dilatation

Marfan's syndrome (cystic medionecrosis causes dilatation of the ascending aorta as well as the ring), syphilis (where the cusps may be abnormal as well), ankylosing spondylitis, Reiter's syndrome. Hypertension, particularly if untreated, may cause root dilatation.

Haemodynamics

Regurgitant jet in diastole (early diastolic murmur — Fig. 4.9)

The LV fills with regurgitant blood in addition to that received from the LA and dilates and hypertrophies to accommodate its increased preload.

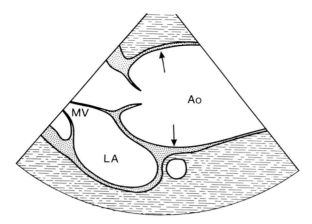

Fig. 4.7. Two-dimensional echo (parasternal long axis view) showing gross dilatation of aortic root, causing aortic regurgitation. MV = mitral valve; Ao = aorta.

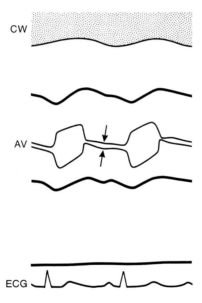

Fig. 4.8. M-mode echo showing aortic root dilated in relation to the valve. The double diastolic closure line (arrow) suggests defect in closure causing regurgitation. CW = chest wall; AV = aortic valve.

Increased stroke volume in systole (ejection murmur)

Only a proportion is effective forward flow to the periphery, the remainder returning to the ventricle during diastole. The duration of systole is normal with the increased stroke volume ejected more rapidly, causing a fast rate of rise of arterial pressure (dP/dt) and often an ejection murmur.

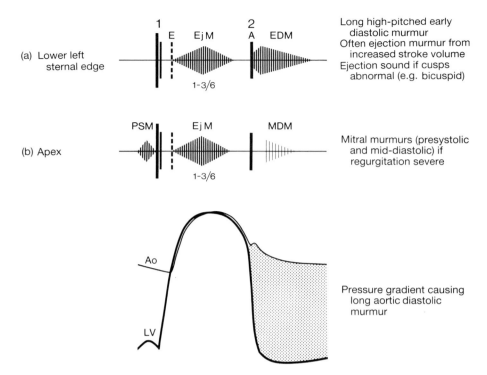

(a) Lower left
    sternal edge

Long high-pitched early
  diastolic murmur
Often ejection murmur from
  increased stroke volume
Ejection sound if cusps
  abnormal (e.g. bicuspid)

(b) Apex

Mitral murmurs (presystolic
  and mid-diastolic) if
  regurgitation severe

Pressure gradient causing
long aortic diastolic
murmur

Fig. 4.9. Aortic regurgitation — auscultatory findings. EjM = ejection murmur;
E = ejection sound; EDM = early diastolic murmur; PSM = presystolic murmur;
MDM = mid-diastolic murmur; Ao = aorta.

Clinical presentation

Symptoms

Usually symptomless because the LV accommodates the gradually increasing
stroke volume — dyspnoea occurs late when the LV fails. Acute LV failure,
however, occurs at the onset of sudden, severe regurgitation, e.g. infective
endocarditis, when the LV has no time to adapt to the increased work load.

Angina pectoris may occur and is often atypical, except in syphilitic
regurgitation where there may be associated narrowing of the coronary ostia.

Clinical examination

In mild cases the only sign is a soft early diastolic murmur.

Pulse

1 *Sinus rhythm* (atrial fibrillation suggests rheumatic aetiology with involvement of the mitral valve).

2 *Large amplitude.* High systolic, low diastolic blood pressure.

3 *Waterhammer character.* Rapid rise of pressure wave to a poorly sustained peak (ejection of a large stroke volume into a relatively empty arterial tree) with rapid fall.
4 Abrupt distension and collapse of carotid arteries (Corrigan's sign).
5 Capillary pulsation in nail beds and pulsation of retinal arterioles in the optic fundi (arterial pulsation transmitted to the arterioles and capillaries).

Blood pressure
Increased systolic, low diastolic pressures.

Jugular venous pressure
Normal until the onset of cardiac failure.

Cardiac impulses
The apex beat is displaced and the apical impulse is abrupt and of large amplitude (hypertrophied and dilated LV with a large stroke volume).

Auscultation (Fig. 4.9)
1 *Early diastolic murmur.* Blowing high pitched, beginning immediately after A_2, loudest at the third and fourth left intercostal spaces but also heard in the aortic area and at the apex.
2 *Ejection murmur* (large volume flow during systole). Loudest in the aortic area and propagated into the carotid arteries and may be preceded by an ejection sound if the cusps are abnormal.
3 *Austin Flint murmur.* Low-pitched rumbling presystolic and mid-diastolic murmurs at the apex in severe cases. The regurgitant aortic jet pushes the anterior leaflet of the mitral valve backwards (Fig. 4.10) into the inflow in diastole, causing it to vibrate as with mitral stenosis (Fig. 4.11).

Electrocardiography
Left ventricular hypertrophy (p. 286 and Fig. 14.18).

Chest radiography
Increased transverse diameter of the heart (dilated LV). Dilatation of ascending aorta (increased blood flow to and fro between LV and aorta).

Echocardiography

Mitral valve flutter
In diastole the regurgitant jet strikes the anterior cusp of the mitral valve (Fig. 4.11) causing vibrations. Premature closure of the mitral valve — in severe cases, the mitral valve is closed by the aortic regurgitation rather than LV contraction.

Dilated left ventricle
Left ventricular systolic and diastolic dimensions are increased.

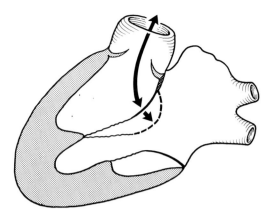

Fig. 4.10. Haemodynamics of aortic regurgitation.

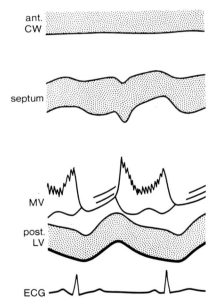

Fig. 4.11. M-mode echo of mitral valve showing fluttering of anterior cusp struck by regurgitant jet from aortic valve. CW = chest wall; MV = mitral valve.

Dilated ring

A dilated aortic root (Fig. 4.7) and failure of the cusps to meet (Fig. 4.8) can be diagnosed and associated mitral valve disease excluded (p. 87).

Cardiac catheterization and angiocardiography

An aortogram shows the anatomy of the aortic root and roughly assesses the severity of the regurgitation. The ventriculogram assesses LV dilatation and contractility. A coronary arteriogram is performed in patients over the age of 40 requiring surgery.

Variations in presentation with different aetiologies

Rheumatic aortic regurgitation

Rheumatic fibrosis tends to cause stenosis in addition, particularly in middle age. Progression is slow with, almost invariably, coincidental mitral valve disease which may be difficult to diagnose as the regurgitant jet damps out the opening snap and causes Austin Flint murmurs. A soft ejection sound may be present.

Congenital

Usually identified by the loud ejection sound of the associated bicuspid valve or the pansystolic murmur of the ventricular septal defect (VSD). The ascending aorta may be dilated.

Infective endocarditis

May cause acute regurgitation and LV failure: signs of endocarditis (p. 103).

Isolated aortic root dilatation

Progresses more rapidly than rheumatic valvulitis. No ejection sound. Root dilatation diagnosed on echo.

Dissection of the ascending aorta

Usually presents as an emergency with the sudden onset of chest pain and collapse. Regurgitation is seldom severe.

Prognosis

Usually well tolerated unless acute (infective endocarditis), or severe. Asymptomatic patients with the triad of low diastolic pressure, LV hypertrophy on the ECG and marked dilatation on the chest X-ray and echo (> 5 cm in systole) are likely to deteriorate with irreversible damage to the LV.

Assessment of severity

Exertional dyspnoea, and particularly paroxysmal nocturnal dyspnoea, indicate severe regurgitation, as does *angina* in the absence of coincidental coronary disease. The heart murmurs are of little value in assessing severity except that a soft early diastolic murmur usually indicates that regurgitation is minimal. The degree of sharpness of the *arterial pulse*, the *diastolic blood pressure*, the amount of *LV hypertrophy* and the *LV cavity size* on echo assess severity. *Premature closure of the mitral valve* on echo always indicates severe regurgitation.

Treatment

Medical

None, except for avoidance of severe physical activity and prophylaxis against infective endocarditis, until LV failure supervenes.

Surgical

Indications

Symptoms

In an asymptomatic patient, a combination of low diastolic blood pressure, LV hypertrophy on ECG, ventricular dilatation on chest X-ray and echocardiogram.

Operation

1 *Reposition cusp* when due to prolapsed cusp through VSD, or to dissection of the ascending aorta.

2 *Aortic valve replacement* for all other patients (Figs. 4.5a, b & c). For choice of valve, see p. 262–263.

Complications of surgery

As in aortic stenosis (p. 73).

MITRAL STENOSIS

Aetiology

Rheumatic (99% of cases)

Mitral stenosis is the most common valve lesion caused by rheumatic fever, and is four times as frequent in females as in males.

Fifty per cent of patients with mitral stenosis have no history of rheumatic fever or chorea — either the acute illness was mild and escaped notice or it has subsequently been forgotten.

Congenital

Rare, seldom occurs alone.

Pathology

Rheumatic mitral stenosis

1 Commissures adherent, leaving small, oval, central orifice.

2 Cusps thickened and fibrous.

3 Chordae tendineae thickened and shortened.

Progressive fibrotic thickening and rigidity of the cusps lead to critical stenosis (valve area $< 1.5 \, cm^2$) by the age of 30–40 years, occurring much earlier (15–20 years) in India and the Middle East.

Congenital mitral stenosis

Diaphragm with a hole in it, to which anomalous chordae tendineae are attached. Never isolated.

Haemodynamics

Raised LA pressure

No effect until valve area is less than one-quarter of normal ($1–1.5 \, cm^2$) when it causes a rise of LA pressure and a diastolic gradient across the valve. When

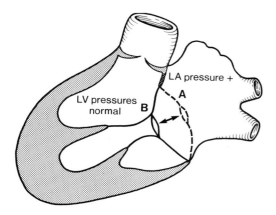

Fig. 4.12. Mitral stenosis. Mechanism of loud first sound and opening snap. The fused cusps of the mitral valve act as a diaphragm with a small central orifice. Their final halt at **A** with their delayed, high velocity closure causes the loud first sound; their final halt in the LV at **B** early in diastole causes the opening snap.

pulmonary venous pressure exceeds the oncotic pressure of the plasma proteins (30 mmHg), exudation of fluid causes interstitial, then pulmonary oedema. There is a corresponding rise in PA pressure.

Pulmonary hypertension and low cardiac output

A chronically raised LA pressure may cause, by an unknown mechanism, an excessive rise of pulmonary vascular resistance from intimal thickening and medial hypertrophy, especially if LA is small and indistensible. The cardiac output falls, particularly when dilatation of the RV and tricuspid ring causes tricuspid regurgitation.

Clinical presentation

There are two types of clinical presentation in mitral stenosis:

1 *The younger patient with a normal pulmonary arterial resistance* presents primarily with a raised LA pressure (dyspnoea, pulmonary oedema).

2 *The older patient with pulmonary hypertension* presents primarily with a low cardiac output and right heart failure (fatigue, mitral facies, raised JVP, RV hypertrophy). Dyspnoea is less prominent and such patients may present in the chest clinic with a diagnosis of cor pulmonale (p. 223) if the valve is immobile with opening snap and murmur difficult to hear.

Symptoms

1. Normal pulmonary vascular resistance

Dyspnoea

Gradual elevation of LA pressure causes increasing exertional dyspnoea, orthopnoea and paroxysmal nocturnal dyspnoea and finally pulmonary oedema. Aggravated by the increased blood volume of pregnancy or the tachycardia of atrial fibrillation (AF).

Palpitations
> The rising LA pressure dilates the left atrium and atrial ectopics and brief runs of atrial tachycardia progress to chronic AF.

2. Raised pulmonary vascular resistance
> Fatigue (low cardiac output).
> Hepatic pain, ascites, dependent oedema (RV failure).

Clinical examination
> The two clinical presentations of mitral stenosis again apply.

1. Normal pulmonary vascular resistance

Pulse
> Small (reduced cardiac output) and may be irregular (AF).

Jugular venous pressure
> Normal.

Cardiac impulses

> *Palpable mitral first sound ('tapping' impulse).* The loud first sound is palpated as an abrupt shock preceding the ventricular impulse at a normally positioned apex beat.

Auscultation (Figs 4.12 and 4.13)

> *First heart sound.* Loud, unless fibrosis and calcification of the valve reduce its mobility. Valve closure is late because of the high LA pressure and therefore occurs on a later, steeper part of the LV pressure pulse, with consequent greater velocity of closure in a valve held open by the end-diastolic gradient and flow.

> *Opening snap (OS).* A high-pitched early diastolic sound, maximal internal to the apex owing to the final halt of the fused cusps moving rapidly into the LV. The higher the LA pressure, the earlier the OS (e.g. 0.06 s after A_2 = high pressure; 0.1 s = almost normal pressure). May be mistaken for P_2 which it resembles in quality, but in the pulmonary area A_2, P_2 and the opening snap are all heard separately during inspiration. The opening snap is the best physical sign of mitral stenosis and also indicates that the valve is mobile. It softens or disappears with a rigid, calcified valve.

Diastolic murmurs

> *Presystolic murmur.* In sinus rhythm the obstruction to ventricular filling causes a brief murmur following LA contraction in presystole.

Mid-diastolic murmur. A longer, low-frequency, rumbling murmur, best heard with a bell stethoscope exactly at the apex. The tighter the stenosis, the longer the gradient between LA and LV persists and the longer the murmur. Loud murmurs may be palpable (thrill).

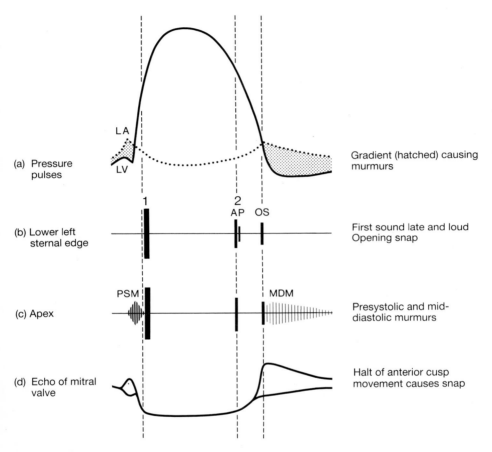

Fig. 4.13. Mitral stenosis — auscultatory findings. A = aortic; P = pulmonary; OS = opening snap; MDM = mid-diastolic murmur; PSM = presystolic murmur.

Lung bases

Fine crackles (crepitations): raised LA pressure with respiratory bronchiolar fluid.

2. Raised pulmonary vascular resistance

Malar flush and loss of weight

Chronic low cardiac output.

Pulse
> Very small; low cardiac output. Usually AF but may be sinus rhythm if LA small before onset of failure.

Jugular venous pressure
> May be raised, with a systolic wave of tricuspid regurgitation.

Cardiac impulses
> Right ventricular hypertrophy (RV afterload); palpable P_2 (pulmonary hypertension).

Auscultation
> Mitral sounds and murmurs are difficult to hear because of low flow but a soft opening snap is usually audible. Loud P_2 (pulmonary hypertension). Tricuspid pansystolic murmur (tricuspid regurgitation).

Liver
> Enlarged and may be pulsatile (raised RA pressure and tricuspid regurgitation).

Ascites (raised RA pressure)

Dependent oedema (raised RA pressure)

Electrocardiography
- Often normal
- LA hypertrophy (P mitrale, Fig. 14.21) — increased voltage of the later part of the P wave evident as a large, second hump on a bifid P in leads 2, 3 and aVF, and a negative second half of the P in V1 (biphasic)
- Atrial fibrillation. Invariable with a large LA and middle age
- Right ventricular hypertrophy. A dominant or a secondary R in V1 and V2 indicates pulmonary hypertension (Fig. 14.20).

Chest radiography

Cardiothoracic ratio
> The heart size is normal (small LV) but pulmonary hypertension causes RV failure and tricuspid regurgitation (dilated RA and pulmonary artery).

Dilated left atrium
> Left atrial appendage dilatation appears on the left border below the pulmonary artery. A large LA is visible on the right border.

Pulmonary vessels
> Increased flow through upper lobes as pulmonary vascular changes begin in lower lobes (hydrostatic pressure increases pulmonary venous pressure in lower lobes). With pulmonary hypertension PA and branches dilate.

Kerley's lines

Interlobular oedema and dilated lymphatics cause horizontal line shadows at the costophrenic angles, indicating high LA and pulmonary venous pressure.

Echocardiography (Fig. 4.14)

Orifice remains open throughout diastole. Anterior cusp thickened. Posterior cusp tethered to the anterior cusp, moving with it anteriorly instead of in the opposite direction in diastole. Immobility and calcification are noted. The LA is dilated: the LV normal size.

The rate of LV filling is slow unless there is additional aortic regurgitation. Two-dimensional echocardiography shows the mitral orifice size. Doppler scanning assesses jet velocity and therefore gradient, and demonstrates any associated mitral regurgitation but not its degree.

Cardiac catheterization and angiocardiography

Mitral valve gradient

LA pressure at rest and on exertion can be estimated indirectly by wedging a catheter in a PA, measuring retrograde transmission of pressure pulses from the pulmonary veins and LA or directly by transeptal catheterization of the LA.

The *end-diastolic gradient* between LA and LV is a measure of the severity of the stenosis but is exaggerated by a short diastole (adjust for heart rate). From simultaneous cardiac output measurement, a formula calculates the *Gorlin valve area*. A ventriculogram shows associated mitral regurgitation.

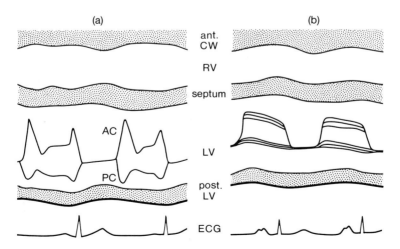

Fig. 4.14. M-mode echoes of mitral cusp movements. Normal (a) and mitral stenosis (b) showing in (a) normal separation of anterior and posterior cusps: in (b) thickening and adhesion causing both cusps to move anteriorly and stay open throughout diastole. CW = chest wall; AC = anterior cusp; PC = posterior cusp.

Pulmonary arterial resistance (p. 60)

Mean pulmonary arterial wedge pressure, less mean LA pressure divided by cardiac output allows calculation of the pulmonary arterial resistance.

Assessment of severity

Symptoms

Severe exertional dyspnoea, and particularly paroxysmal nocturnal dyspnoea, indicate critical mitral stenosis but can occur with mild stenosis in the presence of tachycardia (e.g. onset of AF).

Right ventricular hypertrophy

Clinically or on the ECG always associated with severe stenosis.

Auscultation

Close opening snap (short isovolumic relaxation phase from high LAP).
Long mid-diastolic murmur.
Abnormally loud P_2.
All these indicate severe stenosis.

Chest radiography

Pulmonary venous congestion, upper lobe diversion and Kerley's lines indicate severe stenosis.

Echocardiography

A mitral valve area of < 1.5 cm^2 is critical stenosis. Usually accurately assessed on the two-dimensional picture, except with very small orifices when Doppler scan measurements of jet velocity are a measure of the gradient and valve orifice.

Cardiac catheterization

An end-diastolic gradient of 10 mmHg without tachycardia, and a Gorlin valve area of < 1.5 cm^2, indicate critical stenosis.

Associated valve lesions

Mitral regurgitation (p. 91), aortic stenosis and regurgitation (pp. 64, 76), tricuspid stenosis and regurgitation (pp. 98, 99) may all co-exist with rheumatic mitral stenosis.

Complications of mitral stenosis

Atrial fibrillation

The consequence of age and increasing LA pressure and size. At its onset the ventricular rate is fast, resulting in short diastoles raising LA pressure with risk of pulmonary oedema and low cardiac output.

Thrombo-embolism

From the LA or appendage with AF, particularly at onset (rare in sinus rhythm). May occur in the elderly even with mild stenosis.

Pulmonary hypertension (p. 83)

Infective endocarditis
Rare in pure mitral stenosis.

Differential diagnosis

'Lone' atrial fibrillation
Mitral stenosis has to be excluded (echocardiography useful).

Primary pulmonary hypertension
'Silent' mitral stenosis should always be considered as a possible cause.

Left to right shunts
In atrial septal defect the dilated RV may reach the axilla causing apical short ventricular filling murmurs because of high flow through the tricuspid valve (p. 171). Ventricular septal defect and patent ductus may cause mitral flow murmurs (pp. 176, 183).

Austin Flint murmur (see Fig. 4.9)
In pure aortic regurgitation the Austin Flint murmur (p. 79) may be indistinguishable from that of mitral stenosis — differentiated by echo.

Left atrial myxoma
Often misdiagnosed as mitral stenosis because the tumour may lie in the mitral orifice and cause delayed mitral closure and a loud first heart sound, a systolic murmur of mitral regurgitation, a soft opening snap described as 'tumour plop', and often a soft mitral diastolic murmur. Variable with posture. Embolism is frequent and myxoma should be considered in a patient with systemic embolism in sinus rhythm. The diagnosis is made by echocardiography or histology of an embolus.

Prognosis
The course of mitral stenosis is long with many surviving to the age of 60, or even into old age in mild cases. The most serious of the complications (p. 102) is thrombo-embolism. The course may be accelerated by further attacks of rheumatic fever in populations with low standards of living.

Treatment

Prevention of recurrent rheumatic fever
Penicillin or sulphonamides are given for 5 years after the last attack of rheumatic fever or until the age of 20 (p. 65).

Anticoagulation
Highly successful in preventing thrombo-embolism. Start before the onset of AF; imminence is indicated by an age of over 40, a history of paroxysmal

palpitations, atrial ectopics on ECG or an LA dimension on echo above 4 cm. Attempts to maintain sinus rhythm with drugs such as quinidine are seldom worthwhile.

Control of tachycardia (AF)
Digoxin, if necessary aided by a β-blocker or by verapamil.

Diuretics
Lessen pulmonary venous pressure.

Surgery

Indications
1   Symptoms (dyspnoea) despite control of AF. Operate early before AF becomes permanent.
2   Signs of critical stenosis with calculated valve area (echo, Gorlin) < 1.5 cm^2.

Technique
1   Mobile valve in less developed countries and during pregnancy. Closed mitral valvotomy, inserting dilator through a beating LV via left thoracotomy (Fig. 4.15).
2   Mobile valve, method of choice. Open mitral valvotomy with separation of fused papillary muscles and chordae, mobilization of posterior leaflet by division of secondary chordae and correction of any resulting mitral regurgitation by inserting a valvoplasty ring (p. 97).
3   Rigid, calcified valve. Mitral valve replacement (for severe symptoms) (Fig. 4.16).

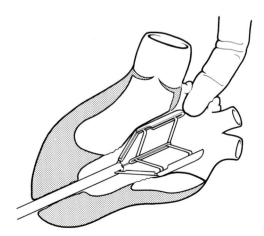

Fig. 4.15. Closed mitral valvotomy.

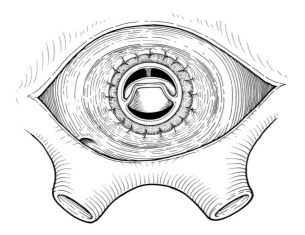

Fig. 4.16. Mitral disc valve *in situ*.

Results

1 Closed mitral valvotomy — mortality 2%, perioperative embolism 2%, restenosis 2% per year.

2 Open mitral valvotomy — mortality 2%, less risk of embolism, better long term function.

3 Mitral valve replacement — mortality 5%, higher if tricuspid valve also involved. Thrombosis and embolism 5%.

MITRAL REGURGITATION

Aetiology and pathology

Mitral regurgitation may be primary (due to valve disease) or secondary to left ventricular dilatation.

1. Primary mitral regurgitation

Redundant cusp mitral leaflet prolapse ('floppy' mitral valve).

Commonest cause of mitral regurgitation in Europe and North America. The association of chest pain (skeletal, exacerbated by anxiety), ventricular ectopics, a late systolic murmur and click and valve prolapse on the angio or echo have been described as Barlow's syndrome.

Rheumatic mitral regurgitation

Frequently associated with stenosis and aortic valve disease. Chordal rupture does not occur. Cusps are fibrotic and shrink: chordal shortening restricts posterior cusp movement.

Ischaemic heart disease

A mild degree of mitral regurgitation (late systolic murmur) frequently follows inferior infarction, but is relatively unimportant unless there is papillary muscle rupture.

Localized cardiomyopathy affecting a papillary muscle (p. 119).

Rare cause of primary mitral regurgitation.

2. Secondary mitral regurgitation

Regurgitation secondary to a dilated LV (cardiomyopathy, ischaemic fibrosis, acute myocarditis) is seldom severe. May be difficult to differentiate from end-stage primary regurgitation.

Haemodynamics

Forward output is diminished because of loss of stroke volume into the LA. Left atrial pressure is only elevated in systole so that the mean LA pressure does not rise greatly and orthopnoea is absent until LV failure supervenes — usually late because of reduced LV afterload.

Clinical presentation

Symptoms

No cardiac symptoms with mild regurgitation except for ventricular ectopics in patients with prolapsing valves. *Dyspnoea on exertion, orthopnoea and paroxysmal nocturnal dyspnoea* are absent until LV failure supervenes. Associated exertional angina makes coronary disease likely to be the cause of the mitral regurgitation. Non-specific chest pains are frequent in patients with prolapsing valves but are usually skeletal in origin and are exaggerated by anxiety (often from unwise medical management).

Clinical examination

Arterial pulse

Sinus rhythm unless the mitral regurgitation is severe enough to cause LA enlargement and AF. Upstroke sharp but ill-sustained.

Jugular venous pressure

Normal unless severe regurgitation results in a raised pulmonary arterial resistance and RV failure (less common than in mitral stenosis because mean LA pressure is lower).

Cardiac impulses

The apical LV impulse is hyperkinetic, often detectable when there is no abnormality of the electrocardiogram or echo. In the parasternal region, systolic expansion of the LA causes a heave indistinguishable from that of RV hypertrophy.

Auscultation (Fig. 4.17)

Apical *pansystolic murmur* of high frequency ('blowing'). Always reaches and may drown A_2 and continues after it (continuation of pressure gradient between LV and LA up to opening snap). In mild cases the murmur may be confined to late systole, or have a late systolic crescendo. The murmur radiates to the axilla, except with ruptured posterior chordae when the posterior leaflet 'hood' directs the jet forwards to the parasternal region (Fig. 4.18).

A *third sound* and *short mid-diastolic flow murmur* (volume overloaded ventricle with increased diastolic flow) occur with severe regurgitation (regurgitant volume returning to ventricles).

Electrocardiography

Except for AF, the ECG is often normal. LV not greatly hypertrophied (preload only).

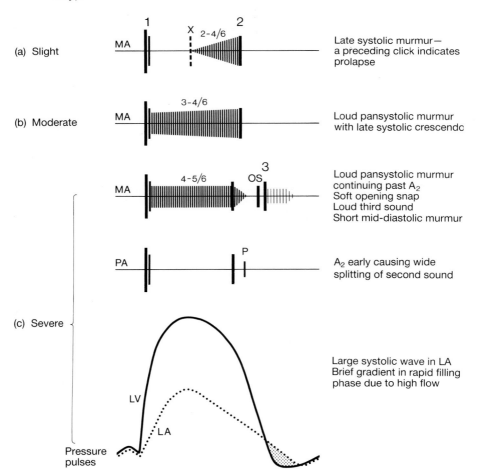

Fig. 4.17. Mitral regurgitation — auscultatory findings. MA = mitral area; PA = pulmonary area; X = click; OS = opening snap; 3 = third sound.

Chest radiography

Dilated LV (preloaded ventricle), atrial appendage and atrium (high LA pressure), upper lobe vein diversion (pulmonary arterial resistance greater in lower lobes).

Echocardiography and Doppler scanning

1 Rheumatic regurgitation causes thickened cusps (see Fig. 4.14): prolapsed cusps are large and thin and prolapse into the left atrium (Fig. 4.19a & b): the ischaemic valve appears normal.

2 Degree of regurgitation — deduced from the size of the LV, the stroke volume and LA size.

3 Left ventricular function — affects prognosis.

Cardiac catheterization and angiocardiography

Left ventriculography confirms the degree of regurgitation and of contractility of the LV. In the older age groups a coronary arteriogram is an essential prelude to surgery.

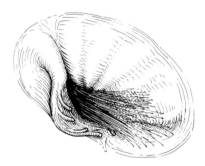

Fig. 4.18. Ruptured chordae of posterior leaflet of mitral valve with regurgitating jet passing anteriorly under 'hood' of leaflet.

Associated lesions

A regurgitant prolapsing valve is seldom associated with significant disease of another valve although the tricuspid valve may show minimal changes at postmortem. In Marfan's syndrome the collagen abnormality is more severe, mitral regurgitation is more rapidly progressive and the aorta and its ring are nearly always dilated and aortic dissection frequent. With rheumatic heart disease, the aortic and tricuspid valves are often affected. In ischaemic heart disease the coronary disease is usually more important than the mitral regurgitation.

Complications

Ventricular ectopics are frequent with prolapsing valves but ventricular tachycardia, fibrillation and sudden death are rare. With increasing age and LA enlargement *atrial fibrillation* is the rule. Important *thrombo-embolism* is rare,

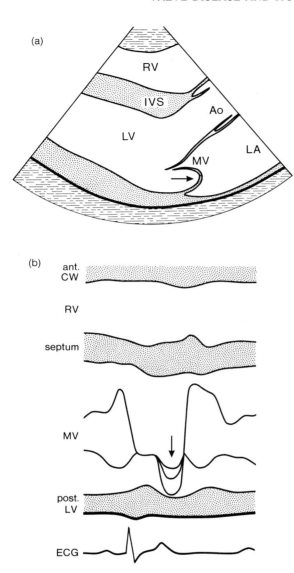

Fig. 4.19. Redundant mitral cusps (a) Parasternal long axis two-dimensional echo showing prolapse of the posterior mitral leaflet (arrow). (b) M-mode echo showing mid-systolic prolapse (arrow). Ao = aorta; IVS = interventricular septum; MV = mitral valve; CW = chest wall.

though minor platelet emboli secondary to platelet aggregation in the folds of large cusps occur. *Infective endocarditis* occurs more frequently with mild mitral regurgitation than with any other lesion (5%).

A small proportion of patients with prolapsing valves suffer chordal rupture (Fig. 4.18) causing a sudden increase in regurgitation and *LV failure* which is frequently transient. *Pulmonary hypertension* is less common than in mitral stenosis (lower mean LA pressure) but occurs exceptionally in patients with small left atria.

Assessment of severity

No *symptoms*, except palpitations from ectopics, until LV function becomes abnormal. The *intensity of the systolic murmur* is no indication of severity, but a late systolic murmur indicates that the regurgitation is slight. A third sound and mid-diastolic flow murmur confirm severity. LV size and stroke volume on echo are measures of severity, confirmed by an LV injection of *contrast medium*.

Differential diagnosis

Aortic stenosis. An aortic ejection murmur may be maximal at the apex, but finishes before A_2, though A_2 may disappear when the valve is calcified, and the shape of the murmur is only apparent on a phonocardiogram. The associated slow-rising carotid pulse, greater LV hypertrophy and calcium in the aortic valve differentiate it.

Ventricular septal defect. The pansystolic murmur is maximal at the tricuspid area, but differentiation may be difficult.

Tricuspid regurgitation. Inspiratory pansystolic murmur at the fourth left interspace.

Prognosis

Mild regurgitation

Good except for risk of infective endocarditis, and chordal rupture in redundant prolapsed cusps (relatively rare). Tendency to gradual increase in regurgitation in older subjects.

Severe regurgitation

Well tolerated initially as there is little resistance to LV outflow. Eventually LV failure though LV contractility may appear good on echo due to the diminished afterload. If surgical repair is left too late, abolition of regurgitation results in sudden increase in afterload which a poor LV may not tolerate.

Ischaemic regurgitation

The prognosis is of the underlying coronary disease unless acute (p. 119).

Treatment

Medical

Control of AF with digoxin, diuretics and vasodilation for LV failure. Prophylaxis against infective endocarditis (p. 107). Ventricular ectopics are ignored unless multiple or associated with ventricular tachycardia. Systolic hypertension is treated as it increases regurgitation.

Surgical

Indications for surgery

 Symptoms (dyspnoea) and severe regurgitation confirmed by echo and angio. Poor LV function may preclude surgery.

Technique

 1 Rigid or calcified valve — mitral valve replacement. Choice of valve (pp. 262–263). Advantage of valve replacement is that the valve is immediately competent. Disadvantage — mitral valve disease is replaced with prosthetic valve disease plus risk of anticoagulant related bleeding.

 2 Mobile valve — mitral valve repair.

  (a) *Rheumatic valve.* Full commissurotomy; mobilize posterior cusp by dividing shortened secondary chordae; refashion valve ring to fit cusp size, e.g. insert Carpentier–Edwards valvoplasty ring (Fig. 4.20b).

  (b) *Redundant mitral leaflet prolapse.* Excise redundant cusp section (Fig. 4.20a); adjust length of chordae to ensure cusp apposition: valvoplasty ring (Fig. 4.20b).

(a)

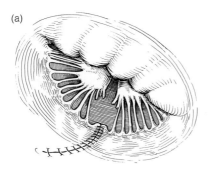

(b)

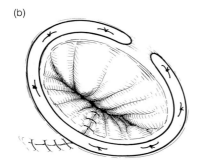

Fig. 4.20. (a) Redundant section excised and edges of cusp sutured. (b) Carpentier–Edwards valvoplasty ring inserted.

Results

   Mortality. Valve replacement 6%, valve repair 2%, greater with LV failure.
   Paraprosthetic leak 2% (higher in prolapsing valves).
   Residual mitral regurgitation (significant) in mitral valve repair 5%. Re-
   operation in mitral valve repair 2% per year.

PULMONARY STENOSIS

Aetiology

   The only cause, apart from rarities such as invasion by tumour, is congenital (see
   Chapter 9 for other types of stenosis).

Haemodynamics, clinical presentation and treatment
(see pp. 187–190)

PULMONARY REGURGITATION

Aetiology

   As pulmonary arterial diastolic pressures are normally so low, pulmonary
   regurgitation is confined to patients with pulmonary hypertension, congenital
   absence of the pulmonary valve or following surgical valvotomy.

Clinical presentation and management (see p. 190)

TRICUSPID STENOSIS

Aetiology and pathology

Rheumatic

   In the adult, aetiology is nearly always rheumatic with mitral and aortic valves
   also involved.

Carcinoid (rare)

   With carcinoid tumours of the small intestine and hepatic secondaries.

Congenital

Clinical presentation

Symptoms

   Fatigue (low cardiac output): hepatic pain, ascites, dependent oedema (raised
   RA pressure).

Clinical examination

Jugular venous pressure

   Giant 'a' wave (RA hypertrophy) if in sinus rhythm, and slow 'y' descent
   (delayed atrial emptying).

Auscultation

A presystolic murmur in the tricuspid area, increased on inspiration. With AF diagnosis is difficult, particularly as mitral valve disease is almost invariably present.

Electrocardiography

RA hypertrophy (P pulmonale; p. 293).

Echocardiography and Doppler ultrasound

Thickened tricuspid leaflets and stenotic jet.

Cardiac catheterization and angiography

End-diastolic gradient (small) across thickened valve.

Surgery

Indications

Almost always associated with mitral valve surgery.
- Symptoms
- Gradient at cardiac catheterization

Technique

1 *Mobile valve.* Make it bicuspid by dividing the two commissures between septal leaflet and others: refashion ring (e.g. insert Carpentier valvoplasty ring) to fit cusp size and shape.

2 *Rigid valve.* Carry out a valve replacement only as last resort because of its poor long-term results.

TRICUSPID REGURGITATION

Aetiology and pathology

Right ventricular failure from any cause is accompanied by dilatation of the tricuspid ring, causing tricuspid regurgitation. *Rheumatic disease*, usually with some stenosis also, causes distortion of the cusps and dilatation of the valve ring. Congenital tricuspid regurgitation occurs in *Ebstein's anomaly* and *endocardial cushion defects* (pp. 180, 191). Infective endocarditis is rare in the right heart except in mainline drug addiction.

Haemodynamics

The RV pressure pulse is transmitted to the RA, producing large systolic waves which can be seen in the neck and felt on palpating the liver. The cardiac output falls.

Clinical presentation

Almost always secondary with symptoms of the primary problem, e.g. mitral stenosis or pulmonary vascular disease.

Symptoms

Fatigue (reduced cardiac output): hepatic pain, ascites and dependent oedema (raised RA pressure).

Clinical examination

Pulse. AF almost invariable.

Jugular venous pressure. High with a large systolic wave seen in the neck. The 'y' descent is sharp.

Cardiac impulses. The hyperkinetic RV causes marked pulsation at the lower left sternal edge — almost a 'rocking' movement of the heart.

Auscultation. Pansystolic murmur heard maximally at the lower end of the sternum (but with RV dilatation the murmur may be heard at the apex when it is difficult to distinguish from mitral regurgitation). Louder on inspiration.

Liver. Enlarged. Hepatic pulsation occurs synchronously with the systolic wave on the JVP.

Ascites (raised mean RA pressure). If regurgitation is severe.

Dependent oedema (raised mean RA pressure).

Electrocardiography

Usually AF and RV hypertrophy or right bundle branch block.

Chest radiography

Large heart (RA, RV): absence of pulmonary venous congestion in severe cases owing to reduced forward flow.

Echocardiography

Enlargement of the right heart with abnormal tricuspid cusps. Doppler scanning shows regurgitant jet.

Cardiac catheterization and angiography

Thickened cusps and tricuspid regurgitation on RV injection of contrast.

Differential diagnosis

Ebstein's anomaly (p. 191). The RV is underdeveloped and no RV pulsation can be felt. Associated right bundle branch block causes wide splitting of the first sound; loud tricuspid closure with an opening snap and a ventricular filling (flow) murmur; echo and angiocardiography confirm the diagnosis.

Ventricular septal defect. Pansystolic murmur is louder — no systolic wave in JVP — left heart is overactive.

Prognosis

Tricuspid regurgitation itself is not usually disabling though forward output may be greatly reduced. The prognosis is that of the associated left heart problems or of the pulmonary hypertension.

Treatment

Medical
Control of the heart rate in the presence of AF; diuretics.

Surgical

Indications
Almost always associated with mitral valve surgery.
1   Longstanding tricuspid regurgitation — failing to respond to medical treatment.
2   Tricuspid regurgitation found at surgery for the mitral valve.

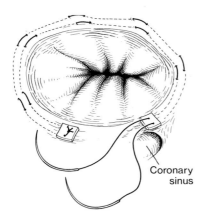

Coronary
sinus

Fig. 4.21. De Vega tricuspid valvoplasty.

Technique
1   Rheumatic regurgitation associated with mitral valve surgery.
(a) Dilated ring with mobile cusps. De Vega double circumferential suture in order to narrow ring (Fig. 4.21).
(b) Organically thickened valve. Make it bicuspid if also stenosed, mobilize cusps and refashion ring, e.g. by inserting Carpentier valvoplasty ring.
(c) As a last resort — valve replacement. Avoid if possible as valve thrombosis and leaflet restriction is common with artificial valves in the right heart.
2   Mainline drug-related endocarditis. Excise without valve replacement because of risk of further prosthetic endocarditis from continuing drug abuse.
3   Congenital in endocardial cushion defect and Ebstein's anomaly (pp. 180, 191).

COMPLICATIONS OF VALVE DISEASE

Arrhythmia
See specific valve and Chapter 8.

Heart failure

See specific valve and Chapter 6.

Systemic thrombo-embolism

Systemic embolism signals a search for an intracardiac cause.

Origin of systemic embolism

Mitral stenosis (even minimal). Thrombus formation, primarily in the LA appendage, often occurs with the first onset of AF and low cardiac output. Rare in sinus rhythm — except with paroxysmal AF.

Atrial fibrillation. Rare with lone AF but not uncommon in sino-atrial disease with alternating atrial arrhythmia and sinus bradycardia (bradytachy syndrome). Occurs with cardioversion of AF to sinus rhythm (anticoagulants should be given for 3 weeks beforehand).

Recent myocardial infarction. Rare with old infarcts, even with thrombus in LV aneurysm.

Left ventricle *dilated and hypocontractile,* even in sinus rhythm — e.g. dilated cardiomyopathy, end-stage coronary disease.

Calcific aortic stenosis. Fragments of calcium may become detached from a craggy, calcified aortic valve. Usually small and cause symptoms only when they obstruct an end-artery such as the retinal.

Mitral regurgitation. Thromboembolism rare because the regurgitant jet prevents left atrial stasis. With greatly enlarged cusps in floppy mitral valves, platelet aggregation may occur in valve 'backwaters', causing minor emboli.

Infective endocarditis. Friable vegetations embolize (p. 103)

Myxoma of the left atrium. Microscopy of the embolus identifies its origin. Tumour identified by echocardiography.

Prosthetic and bioprosthetic valves. Less with the latter.

Clinical presentation

Cerebral embolism

Abrupt onset of neurological deficit, often with rapid recovery.

Visceral embolism

1 Spleen — left hypochondriac pain and friction rub.
2 Kidneys — loin pain and haematuria.
3 Mesenteric arteries — acute abdomen, ileus and melaena.

Peripheral embolism

Sudden pain and loss of function of limb. Pallor, coldness, anaesthesia and absent pulses. Differentiated from thrombosis and atheromatous narrowing by the absence of a previous history of claudication, etc.

Differential diagnosis of site of origin of systemic embolism

In the absence of an intracardiac cause for embolism, the most likely site is an atheromatous plaque, particularly in the carotid system.

Prevention of systemic embolism

Anticoagulation therapy with warfarin or allied antiprothrombins in patients at risk. Prothrombin time is kept at two to three times the normal level and is measured by an experienced laboratory every 4–8 weeks (more frequently initially or after any gastro-intestinal upset or antibiotics, causing variation in absorption).

This is routine after prosthetic valve replacement; is ideally carried out before onset of AF in mitral stenosis (older age and large LA); and is carried out after mitral valvotomy if there is low cardiac output, AF, and large LA.

Treatment of systemic embolism

Cerebral embolism

1 Maintenance of cerebral blood flow by sustaining the blood pressure and treating heart failure (oxygen, digitalis, etc.).
2 Anticoagulation for prevention of further emboli may do more harm from intracerebral bleeding than good from prevention of propagated thrombus in the brain. It should be delayed for 2–3 weeks.
3 Reduction of surrounding oedema with steroids (e.g. dexamethazone).

Visceral embolism

1 Splenic and renal embolism — conservative (as cerebral).
2 Mesenteric embolism — embolectomy if early or, if late, resection of gangrenous bowel.

Peripheral embolism

1 *Conservative.* If limb is clearly viable, anticoagulation is begun with heparin, and continued with warfarin. Heart failure is treated if present. The limb is kept level (to prevent oedema), at room temperature (to lower oxygen demands), and the rest of the body is warmed with heat and alcohol (to cause reflex vasodilation of the limb).
2 *Embolectomy.*
   (a) Indications. Almost always required for a saddle (aortic bifurcation) embolus, almost never for brachial embolus. In lower limb embolism, if the limb does not appear viable (still pale, cold, paralysed and anaesthetic) 6 hours after the onset, embolectomy is indicated.
   (b) Technique. An incision is made at or below the point where the pulse disappears. Proximal and distal clot is removed with a Fogarty (balloon tipped) catheter until bleeding is free from both ends, when the artery is sutured.

Infective endocarditis

Definition

Microbiological invasion of a heart valve or an area of endocardium or arterial intima.

Classification

Infective endocarditis (IE) can be classified by:

1 Clinical presentation, e.g. acute or subacute.
2 Infecting organism.
3 Site — valve (normal, abnormal, prosthetic) or congenital abnormality.
4 Population, e.g. drug addiction.

Pathogenesis

Aetiology

1 Intimal damage from turbulent flow.
(a) Aortic valve abnormality (even minimal) — bicuspid, regurgitant, stenotic.
(b) Mitral valve abnormality — regurgitation (however slight); infection on pure mitral stenosis is rare (no high velocity jet).
(c) Left to right shunts with high velocity jets — ventricular septal defect (on the wall of the RV where the jet impinges), patent ductus arteriosus (on the pulmonary artery). Infective endocarditis does not occur when the jet is of low velocity as in atrial septal defect.

2 Foreign bodies in the circulation, e.g. prosthetic valves, biological valves (sutures), endocardial pacing wires (p. 165).
3 Intravenous drug addiction — right heart valves.
4 Virulent organisms, e.g. *Staph. aureus*.

Microbiology

Native valve endocarditis

The commonest infection overall is still that involving a previously abnormal heart valve with a *'viridans'* streptococcus derived from the mouth. In only about 15% of cases does it follow dental extraction but in most cases the existing *gums* or teeth are unhealthy. Enterococci, such as *Streptococcus faecalis*, are less common than *'viridans'* streptococci and usually come from the genito-urinary tract though seldom directly attributable to instrumentation. *Strep. bovis* seems to be associated with colonic pathology.

Endocarditis that involves a previously healthy valve is caused almost always by *Staph. aureus*, a virulent, aggressive pathogen, the organism gaining entry through a minor skin lesion and presenting with acute septicaemia often with meningism. When acquired in hospital, it results from intravenous lines, wounds or haemodialysis.

Prosthetic valve endocarditis

Prosthetic valve endocarditis (PVE) differs in its pathogenesis depending upon whether it occurs early (within three months of surgery) or late. Early PVE is usually caused by staphylococci, either *Staph. aureus* and *Staph. epidermidis*. The organism is acquired in the theatre. With *Staph. aureus* the wound is usually overtly infected. Late PVE involves organisms that are similar to those of native valve endocarditis, i.e. predominantly *'viridans'* streptococci, though a wide variety of organisms can be involved.

Drug addiction

In drug addiction, IE commonly affects the normal right heart causing tricuspid regurgitation, but where there is a pre-existing valve lesion, other valves may be involved. The predominant pathogen is *Staph. aureus*.

Pathology

Organisms invade the damaged valve, endocardium or arterial intima, and, together with platelets and fibrin, form large friable vegetations in which the organism is protected both from the normal defence mechanisms and to some extent from antibiotics in the blood-stream.

1 *Valve regurgitation* from destruction of cusp tissue and rupture of chordae tendineae. Discrete holes in cusps are particularly characteristic of IE.

2 *Perivalvular abscesses* follow extension of infection into valve ring and myocardium, causing sinuses, fistulae, septal defects and abnormalities of conduction.

3 *Embolism* occurs when a fragment of the vegetations becomes detached: systemic embolism from vegetations on the left side of the heart, and pulmonary infarcts from the tricuspid or pulmonary valve, ventricular septal defect or patent ductus arteriosus. The infarcts of IE do not suppurate, with rare exceptions in the lungs, spleen and brain.

4 *Mycotic aneurysms.* When the muscular wall of a medium-sized artery is infected from embolism to the vasa vasorum causing localized weakening and aneurysm formation. Occasionally mycotic aneurysms rupture.

5 *Glomerulonephritis* may be immunological.

6 *Myocardial failure.* Toxic myocarditis, micro-emboli.

Clinical presentation

In a patient with an abnormal valve or high velocity left to right shunt, any unexplained fever or period of ill-health suggests infective endocarditis. Rare in children probably because teeth and gums are usually healthy.

Symptoms

1 *Toxaemic symptoms.* Malaise, anorexia, weight loss, night sweats, arthralgia and general aches and pains.

2 *Embolic symptoms.* Attacks of abdominal pain (splenic, renal or mesenteric infarcts), hemiplegia, monoplegia, loss of vision in one eye (cerebral embolism) chest pain, haemoptysis (pulmonary infarcts).

3 *Cardiac failure.* Dyspnoea, orthopnoea, oedema (valve regurgitation and toxic myocarditis).

4 Unexplained CNS symptoms.

Clinical examination

Signs due to an infective process

1 Pyrexia, usually low grade and intermittent, but may be absent particularly in the elderly.

2   Pale complexion due to the development of anaemia from toxic depression of the bone marrow.
3   Splinter haemorrhages (fine purple streaks under the nails from multiple small emboli or immune complex aggregates). These are often absent and may occasionally be present in normal subjects.
4   Finger clubbing when therapy is delayed.
5   Splenomegaly (small and soft in early cases, large and firm later).

Embolic signs
1   *Osler's nodes (cutaneous emboli).* Tender, small, erythematous swellings on the pads of fingers and toes, sides of the fingers and on the thenar and hypothenar eminences. Janeway lesions are non-tender, flat, red swellings on palms of hands and soles of feet.
2   *Cerebral emboli.* Retinal haemorrhages with white centres in the optic fundi (Roth spots): other emboli, e.g. hemiplegia.
3   *Red cells in the urine.* Focal embolic or immunological glomerulonephritis. Often unnoticed unless the urine is centrifuged.
4   *Absent pulsation* in a smaller artery such as the posterior tibial or radial artery (embolism of that vessel).

Cardiac signs
Evidence of a lesion predisposing to IE is almost invariably present. Murmurs may vary from day to day, particularly in acute endocarditis. With a congenital bicuspid aortic valve, however, the only abnormal sign may be an aortic ejection sound.

Investigation
1   *Blood culture.* Isolation of the infecting organism is vital to effective treatment. Antibiotics should *never* be given until two or three blood cultures have been taken. In the absence of a positive blood culture there is always some doubt about the diagnosis and about the choice of antibiotic for therapy. Where previous antibiotics have been given, it may be difficult to grow the organism — several blood cultures should be done over a few days. Organisms such as *Coxiella burnetii* (Q fever) and *Chlamydia psittaci* can only be detected serologically.
2   *Blood.* The peripheral blood shows an elevated ESR, progressive normochromic normocytic anaemia and, rarely, a mild leucocytosis.
3   *Urine.* The urine may contain red cells on microscopy, particularly if centrifuged.
4   Echocardiography may show vegetations on the cusps; adjacent sinuses and fistulae may be demonstrated; myocardial function is assessed. Useful for serial assessment of progress, particularly in acute endocarditis.
5   Cardiac catheterization and angiography are seldom needed and may induce embolism.

Clinical presentation of acute infective endocarditis
In acute staphylococcal IE, the patient is septicaemic, very ill and may progress from normality to death in 48 hours. Pulmonary oedema from rapid valve

destruction and multisystem failure (renal, hepatic, CNS) are common. Tender muscles (multiple emboli) are a particular feature.

Prognosis

Despite appropriate antibiotics, IE still has a significant mortality rate. This is much higher for acute than subacute IE, but overall it approaches 25%. This mortality should be reduced by early referral for surgery for gross valve lesions.

Prophylaxis

Although antibiotic prophylaxis has never been of proven benefit, it is conventionally given to patients with cardiac lesions liable to become infected to cover dental procedures, tonsillectomy, instrumentation of the genito-urinary tract, childbirth and surgery of the large bowel.

Dental therapy

Recommended antibiotic cover for dental therapy such as extraction, scaling or periodontal surgery, against the *'viridans'* streptococci is 3 g amoxycillin by mouth 1 hour before the procedure: penicillin-allergic patients should receive 1.5 g erythromycin by mouth 1–2 hours before the procedure and a further 0.5 g 6 hours later. Gum hygiene is very important.

Genito-urinary instrumentation, gynaecological and large bowel surgery

Gentamicin 120 mg is given with amoxycillin (1 g) intramuscularly just before induction of anaesthesia to provide protection against enterococci.

Cardiac surgery

Prophylaxis is primarily antistaphylococcal, and varies widely in cardiac units both in type of antibiotic and duration of prophylaxis. An effective regimen is 500 mg of flucloxacillin 6 hourly for 48 hours, the initial dose being given with premedication and a further dose given before closing the chest.

Treatment of infective endocarditis

Infective endocarditis is almost always fatal unless the infecting organism is eradicated with appropriate antibiotics. The advice of a microbiologist should always be sought in determining the appropriate antibiotic regimen which should be bactericidal for the pathogen and given intravenously. It is useful to determine the bactericidal activity in the patient's serum against the infecting organisms once antibiotics have been started. Such tests ('back titrations') predict bacteriological but not clinical cure.

Choice of antibiotic

Infective endocarditis caused by sensitive streptococci can probably be satisfactorily treated with 2 weeks of penicillin plus low dose gentamicin though antibiotics are often given for longer. Less sensitive streptococci and staphylococci should be treated for 4 weeks. The following is a summary of the recommendations of the Working Party of the British Society for Antimicrobial Chemotherapy (*Lancet*, 1982; **2**:1323–1326, 1985; **2**:815–817).

Dosage of antibiotics

Streptococci

Sensitive strains. Intravenous benzylpenicillin 2 megaunits 4 hourly plus intravenous gentamicin — dose will depend on age, weight and renal function but should achieve 1 hour serum concentration of 3–5 mg/litre and trough serum concentration of < 1 mg/litre. Two weeks' treatment has been shown to be effective. If further treatment is required after 2 weeks, oral amoxycillin is given (1 g t.d.s.) for a further 2 weeks.

Less sensitive strains including Strep. faecalis. The regimen above is given for 4 weeks. Gentamicin assay *must* be performed at least twice weekly to monitor levels.

For patients allergic to penicillin the advice of a microbiologist must be sought. Vancomycin 1–2 g daily intravenously, and controlled by blood assay, will usually be needed, sometimes including gentamicin also.

Staphylococci

Flucloxacillin 2 g 4 hourly intravenously: plus fusidic acid 500 mg 8 hourly orally or gentamicin.

Dental treatment

Any patient with newly diagnosed 'viridans' streptococcal IE should have an early dental opinion sought so that any necessary procedure can be undertaken coincidentally with the start of antibiotic therapy.

Surgery

Early surgery with replacement of the infected valve is advised for uncontrolled infection (unresponsive pyrexia, persistently positive blood cultures despite appropriate antibiotic therapy), deteriorating valve regurgitation (particularly aortic regurgitation), and perhaps actual or incipient embolism (large vegetations on echo). Mortality is higher than for elective surgery and paraprosthetic leak more common because oedematous tissue holds sutures poorly and paravalvular abscesses may have destroyed the valve ring itself. Earlier surgical intervention is essential if the current unsatisfactory mortality of IE is to be reduced.

Surgery for residual lesions after cure of endocarditis has the same prognosis as elective surgery, so ideally one should wait 6 weeks if the patient's general condition allows, because the previously oedematous valve ring becomes fibrous and then holds sutures well.

Treatment in acute staphylococcal infective endocarditis

Early identification of the causative organism and institution of antibiotics is critical. If the presentation is primarily of acute septicaemia, multisystem failure may require intermittent positive pressure ventilation for pulmonary oedema; protection of the kidneys, e.g. dopamine; and circulatory support, e.g. adrenaline. Immediate valve replacement to remove the infective focus and correct acute valve regurgitation may be life-saving.

Chapter 5
Ischaemic Heart Disease

Obstructive coronary artery disease is the commonest cause of death in Europe and the USA, accounting for one-third of all male, one-quarter of all female deaths and over half of all sudden deaths.

PATHOGENESIS
Patches of intimal damage, most frequently in the proximal coronary arteries, lead to the formation of atheromatous plaques. Narrowing or obliteration of the lumen causes myocardial ischaemia. Sudden complete obstruction of a major artery is usually due to disintegration of a plaque following an intimal tear with secondary thrombosis. Its effect depends on the state of the other arteries and the patency of the collateral circulation and varies from:
- *Nil*, or minimal with unrecognized symptoms
- *Angina of effort*, if the flow at rest is sufficient to preserve the myocardium
- *Myocardial infarction*, if the flow at rest is insufficient to preserve the myocardium
- *Sudden death*, which is usually due to ventricular fibrillation

HAEMODYNAMICS
Significant reduction of blood flow does not occur until the lumen is narrowed to < 50%. With critical stenosis without good collateral flow, the increased systolic blood pressure and heart rate required by exertion or emotion causes ischaemia of the myocardium and diastolic stiffening which impairs ventricular filling. This is associated with a transient rise of left atrial (LA) and pulmonary venous pressure, S–T depression on the ECG, angina in the majority of cases and sometimes dyspnoea. Thrombosis of a major artery without a good collateral circulation causes infarction. Small infarcts make little difference to myocardial efficiency but are life-threatening if accompanied by arrhythmias such as ventricular tachycardia (VT) or fibrillation (VF). Large or multiple infarcts cause impairment of both left ventricular (LV) contraction and filling, progressing to LV failure. The scar resulting from an old infarct may be a cause of electrical instability and arrhythmia.

AETIOLOGY
The basic cause of obstructive arterial disease is unknown but the following are important factors:
1 *Male sex*. The disease is more frequent in males than females.
2 *Genetic disposition*. Family history of coronary disease.
3 *High serum cholesterol level* below the age of 50, especially when associated with low high-density lipoprotein (HDL) levels. Above the age of 50, elevated

cholesterol has little significance. Familial hyperlipidaemia (rare) is associated with high levels of cholesterol and a greatly increased risk of coronary disease.

4 *Heavy cigarette smoking* probably accounts for the greater incidence in manual workers who smoke more than the professional classes.

5 *Hypertension*, both diastolic and systolic.

6 *Other factors:* diabetes, myxoedema, obesity, lack of exercise, and possibly stress.

CLINICAL PRESENTATION

Ischaemic heart disease presents in different ways:

- Angina pectoris (ischaemic cardiac pain)
- myocardial infarction
- heart failure without angina — uncommon
- arrhythmia — uncommon
- asymptomatic — abnormal ECG at routine examination

ANGINA PECTORIS

Symptoms

Angina pectoris of effort (ischaemic cardiac pain)

Myocardial ischaemia is caused by gradual reduction of lumen, usually of more than one vessel, or acute obstruction with a good collateral circulation preventing infarction. It also occurs in aortic stenosis, hypertrophic cardiomyopathy, occasionally in dilated cardiomyopathy, and rarely and mysteriously in women with no evidence of heart disease except possibly T wave changes on the ECG. It is exacerbated by anaemia.

A careful history of the characteristics of the chest discomfort or pain is critical.

Site

Typically mid-sternal, radiating *across* the chest, down the arms and up to the angle of the lower jaw, but may radiate to left chest, left scapula, wrist or throat. It may be confined to any one of these areas.

Causation

Increased cardiac work from increased systolic blood pressure and heart rate. Typically this is from walking uphill, exacerbated by carrying a briefcase (isometric exercise increases systolic blood pressure), or after meals or in cold weather. It may wake the patient at night, perhaps because of dreaming or restless sleep. In severe cases it is brought on by lying down (increased venous return), or stooping.

Type of pain

Tightness, gripping, crushing — varies from severe to merely an unpleasant sensation.

Relief

Within 2 min after stopping exertion or taking nitroglycerine. Nocturnal episodes are relieved by sitting up or standing.

Second wind phenomenon

After exertional warming-up, angina is less easily provoked because of a reduction of cardiac work related to a fall in peripheral vascular resistance.

Angina at rest (unstable angina)

1   Brief episodes of angina at rest — resulting from spasm or transient thrombotic obstruction followed by natural lysis.
2   Prolonged and repeated episodes of angina at rest without infarction (unstable angina, acute coronary insufficiency). Usually associated with severe disease and impending infarction.

Coronary spasm (Prinzmetal's angina)

Repeated attacks of prolonged spasm without infarction, associated with widespread S–T elevation, described originally by *Prinzmetal*; in about half these patients there is associated coronary stenosis.

Clinical examination

In the absence of an LV aneurysm or cardiac failure, examination is usually negative. Evidence of abnormal lipid metabolism is occasionally present — arcus senilis before the age of 50; xanthelasma (cholesterol deposits in the regions of the eyes); cholesterol nodules on the tendons of the hands, sometimes causing thickening of the Achilles tendon. Anaemia, coincidental cerebrovascular and peripheral vascular disease and diabetes need to be looked for.

Electrocardiography (p. 293)

Resting

Usually normal if no previous infarct but S–T and T wave changes for the first few weeks or months after the onset of angina (Fig. 14.23) and then may return to normal, probably due to regression of areas of focal ischaemia. Depression of S–T during angina, and not infrequently without, in severe cases.

Exercise (p. 39).

Myocardial ischaemia caused by exercise on a treadmill or bicycle usually causes S–T depression linked to the angina (Fig. 2.1). Occasionally exertion causes S–T depression without pain (silent ischaemia). S–T depression in women, however, may have no significance.

Echocardiography (two-dimensional)

For assessing LV dimensions, contractility and ejection fraction; for localizing regional wall abnormalities; and for differentiating cardiomyopathy from multiple infarcts in patients with heart failure.

Serum lipids

Elevation of serum cholesterol and low density lipoprotein (LDL), useful in prediction of risk but only before the age of 50 (except with very high levels as in familial hyperlipidaemia).

Nuclear medicine (p. 55)

1 *Nuclear ventriculogram.* Ventricular contraction at rest is normal unless there has been previous infarction. Regional dyskinesia may be displayed after exertion.

2 *Thallium scanning* may show areas of ischaemia on exertion but is not particularly sensitive and false positives occur.

Invasive investigations

Coronary arteriography

Through a brachial or femoral catheter, contrast medium is injected into each coronary artery with multiple views recorded by cinephotography. This is the most important test of the severity and localization of coronary disease, and is essential whenever coronary artery surgery or angioplasty is being considered. Risk is now negligible. Unfortunately a precise estimate of flow through a narrow vessel is not possible.

Ventriculography

Contrast medium is injected via the catheter into the LV to give a precise picture of ventricular function at rest.

Intracardiac pressures

Elevated LV end-diastolic, LA, and pulmonary arterial (PA) pressures confirm LV failure. The anoxic myocardium becomes less compliant and the 'a' wave may·be elevated without failure. There is transient elevation of LV end-diastolic pressure, LA and PA pressures during episodes of myocardial ischaemia.

Differential diagnosis of angina

Chest and left arm pain from extracardiac causes are frequent in the general population and are exacerbated by anxious thoughts of a possible cardiac origin. Common causes are:

Root pain

Discomfort anywhere in the chest, even substernal, with or without radiation to the arm, or the arm alone may be affected. The commonest cause is cervical spondylosis or an acute disc lesion. The pain is unrelated to exertion, lasts too long and may be exacerbated by jolting, movement and coughing. With chronic cervical spondylosis there is often a long history of repeated episodes, the discomfort is usually worst in the left chest and arm and lasts for hours at a time.

Pericardial pain

Central, substernal and exacerbated by inspiration and coughing. It is often partially relieved by leaning forwards.

Pleural pain

Right- or left-sided and related to inspiration and coughing. With diaphragmatic pleurisy the pain may be in the shoulder.

Dyspepsia

Usually long-standing, mainly epigastric and related to food. With *oesophageal reflux* from hiatus hernia, however, the pain is substernal and is worse lying down. It tends to last for hours and to be associated with acid regurgitation. Oesophageal pain radiates vertically rather than horizontally. *Colonic spasm* may produce pain in the upper left or right chest and may cause brief stabs of pain. Occasionally the pain of myocardial infarction is epigastric in site.

Herpetic pain

May precede the rash.

Prognosis of angina

Variable. Uncertain when recent or crescendo. Good when mild and chronic (90% survive 8 years). Bad when severe (50% survive 5 years). Good in the rare cases (usually women) without coronary disease.

Treatment of angina pectoris

General aspects

Alteration of lifestyle to avoid effort pain:
1   No smoking.
2   Diet — correct obesity: reduce animal fats.
3   Regular daily rhythmic exercise (e.g. walking), short of provoking pain.
4   Hyperlipidaemia — low calorie and animal fat diet with substitution of unsaturated fat. If severe, lipid lowering agents, such as ion exchange resins (e.g., questran).
5   Diabetes and myxoedema. Careful control.
6   Avoid overtiredness and stress.
7   Correct anaemia.

Drugs

1   *Vasodilators.* Oral nitroglycerine or spray is best used prophylactically before exertion likely to cause pain, and is rapidly absorbed from the mouth. Long-acting vasodilators (absorbed through the gastro-intestinal tract or the skin) in severe cases, but may induce tolerance. Headache may be a problem.
2   *Beta-blocking drugs*, e.g. propranolol — effective in reducing oxygen consumption of the myocardium by slowing heart rate, reducing systolic blood pressure and myocardial contractility. Relatively contra-indicated in heart failure and asthma and peripheral vascular disease.

3 *Calcium antagonists*, e.g. verapamil, diltiazem or nifedipine reduce myocardial oxygen requirements and are useful as an adjunct to β-blockers or when these have side-effects. Nifedipine particularly useful for coronary spasm (Prinzmetal).

Anticoagulants

A daily small dose of aspirin (e.g. 70 mg) appears to reduce the incidence of coronary thrombosis because of its action as an antiplatelet stickiness agent, and is routinely used following coronary artery surgery to promote graft patency. Long-term anticoagulants (anti-thrombins such as warfarin) are not widely used in cor-onary artery disease except to prevent thrombo-embolism in patients with dilated ventricles or to prevent pulmonary embolism when prolonged bed rest is required.

Percutaneous transluminal coronary angioplasty (PTCA)

Balloon angioplasty

Insertion of a balloon under radiographic control into coronary stenoses to dilate or split them.

Indication

Localized proximal incomplete block in coronary arteries with angina not responding to medical treatment or positive exercise test.

Contra-indications

Total occlusion of arteries (balloon cannot be passed through obstructions unless recent): diffuse and distal disease: long stenoses: stenoses involving important side branches.

Results

1 Success in relieving chronic angina — 70%.
2 Complications such as infarction 5–8%.
3 Mortality — 0.1–1% (depending on experience of operator).
4 Recurrence — up to 30% at one year: second PTCA successful in 80%.

Laser angioplasty

Laser heated catheter tips to vaporize blocks in arteries are under trial.

Coronary artery surgery (Fig. 5.1)

Indications for surgery

Coronary artery stenosis of > 50% in the presence of:
- Severe angina not responding to medical treatment
- Marked S–T depression of exercise ECG
- Left main stem stenosis
- Severe triple vessel disease
- Angina with LV dysfunction (poor prognosis with medical treatment)

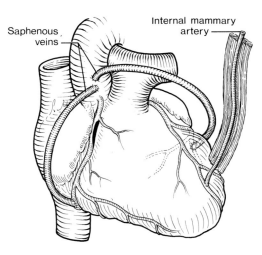

Fig. 5.1. Coronary artery bypass grafts.

Contra-indications

Mild angina with normal exercise test and normal ejection fraction (> 50%): recovered infarction free of symptoms or with only mild symptoms and normal ejection fraction.

Technique (Fig. 5.1)

Coronary artery bypass grafts (CABG). Either a reversed segment of saphenous vein is anastomosed between the aorta and each affected coronary artery distal to the obstruction, or whenever possible, the internal mammary artery is used (better long-term patency).

Results of coronary bypass grafts

Operative mortality

With normal ventricular function — < 1%: poor ventricular function — 5%.

Longevity

Same as medical management in single and double vessel disease: better in left main stem stenosis and severe triple vessel disease.

Myocardial infarction

Peri-operative — 6%: late — same as medical management, but fewer fatal infarcts.

Relief of angina

- *At one year*: complete relief — 90%, partial — 5%, none — 5%.
- *At 10 years*: complete relief — 50%, partial — 25%, none — 25%.

Recurrence of angina is due to progression of native coronary artery disease or to atheroma and thrombosis of saphenous vein grafts. The latter is significantly less with internal mammary artery grafts.

MYOCARDIAL INFARCTION

Sudden complete obstruction of a major coronary artery by thrombus results in infarction of the area supplied by the vessel unless the collateral circulation is adequate. Obstruction of the left anterior descending coronary artery causing anterior infarction is the most common and also the most serious. Rarely, infarction is secondary to embolism or to contusion from trauma.

Clinical presentation

Symptoms

There may be a previous history of past infarction or increasing angina of effort. Often there have been recent brief spells of ischaemic pain at rest.

1   Pain.

Similar to angina but usually starts at rest with its duration varying from a half to 12 hours. The pain varies from severe to minimal tightness and is sometimes absent.

2   Nausea, sweating and vomiting from a vagal reaction, particularly at the onset.

3   Dyspnoea from LV failure with large infarcts — occasionally at onset masking the pain.

Clinical examination

Findings vary from normal to shock from low cardiac output.

1   *Rhythm* varies from regular with tachycardia and a few extrasystoles to multiple ectopics, VT and VF. Atrial fibrillation (AF) is usually unimportant.

2   *Blood pressure* is often elevated at first (from emotion) and later falls.

3   *Jugular venous pressure* is normal, unless there is complicating heart failure.

4   *Heart sounds.* Tachycardia may cause summation of atrial and third sounds. At slower rates, atrial sound.

Electrocardiography (Chapter 14 p. 293, Figs 14.24–14.30)

Diagnostic if significant area of necrosis. Initially S–T elevation in the area affected, rapidly followed by loss of R (Q waves) with full thickness infarcts and T inversion later. With small infarcts, ECG changes may be confined to T inversion and delayed 1–3 days.

Confirmatory evidence of myocardial necrosis

1   Reaction of the body to necrotic muscle:

(a) Pyrexia — appearing on the second day and subsiding over the next few days.

(b) Leucocytosis — maximal during the first few days.

(c) Pericardial friction rub — fleetingly present early.

(d) Erythrocyte sedimentation rate — maximum in the second week.

2   Enzymes released by the necrotic muscle.

Serum glutamic oxaloacetic transaminase (SGOT, normal range 10–35 units)

Increased within 12 hours, peak levels between 18–36 hours, back to normal within 3–4 days. Other conditions causing a raised SGOT are hepatic congestion, primary liver disease, skeletal muscle disease, shock, myocarditis, pericarditis, pulmonary embolism, tachycardia, direct current shock, ingestion of oral contraceptives or clofibrate.

Serum lactic dehydrogenase (LDH)

Increased 24–48 hours from onset of pain, peak activity 3–6 days, normal range after 8–14 days. Also raised in congestive heart failure, haemolytic anaemia, megaloblastic anaemia, acute and chronic liver disease, renal disease, neoplastic disease, pulmonary embolism, shock. The iso-enzyme LDH is a more specific indicator of myocardial infarction.

Serum creatine phosphokinase (CPK)

Increased within 6–8 hours of myocardial infarction, reaches a peak of two to tenfold in 24 hours and declines to normal within 3–4 days. Also markedly raised in muscular dystrophy, inflammatory disease of muscle, alcohol intoxication, diabetes mellitus, convulsions, psychosis and after intramuscular injections. Its iso-enzyme, CKMB, is more specific.

Complications of acute myocardial infarction

Arrhythmias

Ventricular — multiple ectopics; VT; VF.

Accelerated idioventricular rhythm.

Supraventricular — AF and flutter. Usually benign.

Bradycardia

(a) Sinus — rarely extreme.

(b) Atrioventricular block: (i) Follows 10% of inferior infarcts. Transient due to AV nodal ischaemia. The idioventricular rhythm is usually high in origin with a narrow QRS and is seldom very slow; and (ii) Rarely follows a large anterior infarct which in itself has a poor prognosis. The anterior infarct interrupts first the right bundle and then the left, producing broad complex, slow, idioventricular rhythm.

Heart failure and shock

Dyspnoea and pulmonary venous congestion on X-ray — often transient.

Shock — after large infarcts, with low blood pressure, cardiac output and arterial oxygen tension.

Ruptured interventricular septum

Pansystolic murmur, differentiated from mitral regurgitation by Doppler ultrasound and cardiac catheterization.

Mitral regurgitation

Occurs especially after inferior infarcts involving papillary muscle. Loud, apical, pansystolic murmur — confirmed by Doppler scanning.

Ventricular aneurysm (especially following large anterior infarcts).

Myocardial rupture

Death from tamponade follows (unless immediate surgery takes place).

Embolism

1 *Systemic* from endocardial thrombus formation, particularly in the first few days.
2 *Pulmonary* from leg vein thrombosis related to low cardiac output and immobilization.

Differential diagnosis of myocardial infarction

Dissection of the aorta (p. 250)

Pain radiating to back; venous pressure may be elevated from leak into pericardial sac; ECG and enzymes relatively normal; early diastolic murmur from aortic regurgitation. Femoral or other pulses reduced.

Pulmonary embolism (p. 219)

Central substernal pain is uncommon. Pleuritic pain if complicated by pulmonary infarction. Raised jugular venous pressure (JVP).

Root pain (from disc displacement)

Immediate prognosis of myocardial infarction

Mortality 60%, half dying (usually of VF) before reaching hospital unless a special local organization for rapid transfer is available. Hospital mortality 25%, reduced to 12% by intensive therapy units.

Treatment of acute myocardial infarction

General

Bed rest with monitoring and DC cardioversion immediately available (p. 322), in an intensive care unit (ITU) for 1–3 days with ambulation after 5–7 days, later for large infarcts and LV failure. Sedation if necessary.

Reduction of infarct size

Thrombolysis

Since myocardial infarction is almost always a result of thrombotic obstruction of a major coronary artery, the early use of thrombolytic drugs is essential. Heparin and antiprothrombins have been unsuccessful in the past but the early use of streptokinase reduces mortality and infarct size. All patients who present within

6 hours of the onset of chest pain should receive aspirin 150–300 mg and 1.5 megaunits of streptokinase intravenously over 1 hour (preceded by chlorpheniramine 10 mg and hydrocortisone 100 mg in 100 cc of 5% dextrose to suppress allergic reactions.) Other lytic drugs, such as urokinase or tissue plasminogen activator (TPA) may prove superior, particularly when therapy is delayed, but are very expensive. Early therapy is essential as irreversible changes in the myocardium occur after 4 hours.

Re-occlusion has been a major problem but the early use of aspirin 75 mg daily and heparin are proving successful. Early angiography and balloon dilatation are less effective than the conservative policy outlined which has the advantage of being easy to practise without specialized equipment, and can be started without delay. Improvements in thrombolytic therapy are likely in the near future.

Vasodilators
Intravenous nitrates unless contra-indicated by hypotension.

Early use of β-blockers
Still under trial.

Arrhythmias

Multiple ventricular ectopics
Lignocaine 100 mg intravenously as a bolus followed by 100–200 mg per hour for 36 hours. Adverse reactions are drowsiness and convulsions.

Ventricular tachycardia (20% of patients)
As above or *practolol* intravenously up to a maximum of 25 mg. *Sodium phenytoin* (may cause phlebitis in the injected vein, and nausea, vomiting, dizziness and nystagmus), *bretylium tosylate*, *procainamide*, or the insertion of a *temporary cardiac pacemaker* to drive the heart at a fast rate. *DC countershock* (p. 322) for resistant VT.

Ventricular fibrillation (2%)
DC countershock followed by *lignocaine*, then *procainamide* 500 mg 4 hourly for up to 3 weeks.

Accelerated idioventricular rhythm (20%)
Characterized by a ventricular rate of between 50–100 beats per minute. Usually benign, requiring no specific treatment.

Atrial fibrillation and flutter (usually benign)
Digitalization or DC countershock.

Bradycardia
1   *Sinus bradycardia.* If extreme, intravenous *atropine* 0.6 mg.
2   *Atrioventricular block* (p. 160). Inferior infarcts — pacing seldom required except with slow rates unresponsive to atropine. Anterior infarcts require endocardial pacing — the wire should be inserted early, e.g. for right bundle

branch block with lengthening P–R or left axis deviation. Endocardial potentials are low and care is required to avoid inappropriate pacing (p. 164).

Heart failure

Digoxin is not very effective unless AF is present — beware digitalis arrhythmia. Diuretics. Vasodilators.

Shock

May require cautious infusion of dextrose to maintain high filling pressure. Vasodilators reduce afterload if blood pressure is not too low. Dopamine or dobutamine for low cardiac output: in severe cases intra-aortic balloon counter-pulsation.

Surgery

Indicated for complications of myocardial infarction.

Left ventricular aneurysm (Fig. 5.2a)

1 *Indications for surgery.* Left ventricular failure not responding to medical treatment (usually late when patient ambulant) — little risk of late rupture.
2 *Technique* (Fig. 5.2b). Excise aneurysm on cardiopulmonary bypass with cardioplegic arrest; CABG to other critically stenosed coronary arteries.
3 *Results.* Depend on amount and contractility of remaining myocardium: peri-operative mortality — 5–7%; relief of dyspnoea is better than postoperative echo- and angiographic ventricular function would predict.

Mitral regurgitation

1 *Indication for surgery.* Left ventricular failure not responding to medical treatment.
2 *Technique.* Replace or repair valve with concomitant CABG (Figs 4.16 and 5.1).
3 *Results.* Peri-operative mortality (15%) is higher than for other causes of mitral valve replacement (associated acute myocardial infarct). Relief of symptoms depends on extent of infarcted myocardium.

Ruptured interventricular septum

1 *Indications for surgery.* Ideally wait 3 months until edges of defect are fibrous but only if haemodynamics are adequate: operate early for 3 : 1 shunt or LV failure.
2 *Technique.* Open LV through infarct: patch defect with Teflon felt-supported sutures and Dacron patch on high pressure (LV) slide.
3 *Results.* Peri-operative mortality of acute anterior defect — 10–20%: posterior defect — 20–40%. Dehiscence of patch is common (friable myocardium).

Management of recovered infarct

The risk of further infarction gradually recedes and becomes small after 6 months. Beta-blockers reduce the risk and are recommended for 2 years. A small dose of aspirin (about 75 mg) preventing platelet aggregation also reduces the further attack rate and probably should be taken indefinitely.

Long term prognosis is excellent if symptoms are absent or mild with good ventricular function (ejection fraction of more than 50%). Poor with impaired LV function, severe angina and marked S–T depression on an exercise test performed 7–10 days after attack. Anxiety states are common and require strong reassurance.

(a)

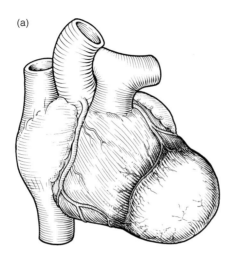

(b)

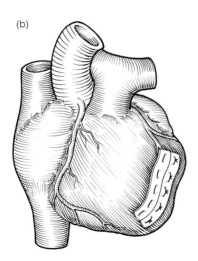

Fig. 5.2 (a) Left ventricular aneurysm. (b) Excised left ventricular aneurysm.

OTHER CLINICAL PRESENTATIONS OF MYOCARDIAL ISCHAEMIA

Heart failure without angina

A late stage of coronary disease in which the myocardium has been severely scarred by multiple infarcts or by a large infarct with an aneurysm.

Arrhythmia

Repeated ventricular tachycardia following recovery from infarction: paroxysmal or established AF: and sino-atrial disease and atrio-ventricular block may all be due to chronic coronary disease.

Asymptomatic coronary artery disease

Electrocardiography as part of a routine examination for business executives, airline pilots or for insurance may show abnormalities which are due to symptomless coronary artery disease. About 25% of patients over the age of 50 who have coronary arteriograms preceding valve replacement have coronary stenoses without symptoms to suggest the disease. Symptomless myocardial infarction is not uncommon, particularly in diabetics.

Chapter 6
The Myocardium and Heart Failure

THE MYOCARDIUM

Histology

The myocardium consists of columns of striated muscle fibres arranged as a syncytium. Each fibre has an outer membrane, the sarcolemma, surrounding the bundles of myofibrils between which are mitochondria. Each myofibril (Fig. 6.1) contains the contractile proteins, actin and myosin, interrupted at intervals by Z lines. Between the Z lines is the functional myocardial unit, the sarcomere.

The sarcolemma is invaginated by transverse tubules in the Z line continuous with the extracellular space. Longitudinal tubules close to the myofibrils dilate into cisternae which approximate to, but do not join, the transverse tubules.

Biochemistry and physiology

Biochemistry

Actomyosin complex

Myosin and actin can combine reversibly to form actomyosin, which is the fundamental mechanism of myocardial contraction. Cross bridges between the

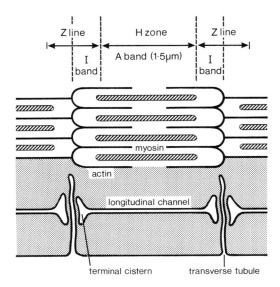

Fig. **6.1.** Diagrammatic representation of the myofibril.

actin and myosin develop in the overlap region between them, causing one filament to slide over the other.

Contraction

Depolarization of the sarcolemma causes an electric potential which is conducted through the transverse tubules to the cisternae and the longitudinal channels which release calcium ions. Troponin in the resting state has an inhibitory effect on actin via tropomyosin but this effect is inactivated by troponin's binding of calcium. Calcium catalyses the breakdown of adenosine triphosphate (ATP) by the ATPase of myosin which releases energy for contraction of the actomyosin complex. High-energy phosphate is generated from aerobic respiratory processes in the mitochondria.

Relaxation

Calcium ions are then again actively taken up by the sarcoplasmic reticulum and relaxation of the myofibril occurs as the myofibrillar calcium concentration falls.

Electrical activity (see Electrocardiography p. 267).

The myocardium, unlike skeletal muscle, has the property of spontaneous rhythmicity, fastest at the sino-atrial node at the upper part of the right atrium, from which the impulse spreads through the atrium to the AV node in the atrial septum in front of the coronary sinus and to the AV bundle (of His) which runs on the left side of the top of the muscular septum and splits into left and right bundles.

Cardiac output

The cardiac output is a product of heart rate and stroke volume and is normally 3 litres per minute per square metre of body surface area. Stroke volume depends on the filling pressure (preload, volume load), peripheral resistance (impedance, afterload) and myocardial contractility.

Preload

Frank-Starling's law of the heart states that the mechanical energy set free on passage from the resting to the contracted state is a function of the resting length of the muscle fibre, itself a function of the volume of blood in the ventricle prior to contraction (preload). Atrial contraction, when properly timed, augments ventricular filling and contraction. Increase in preload (e.g. aortic and mitral regurgitation) causes dilatation and, secondarily, hypertrophy. Ischaemia of the myocardium from coronary artery stenosis decreases compliance of the left ventricle (LV) without dilatation. Infarction produces secondary fibrosis and eventually dilatation and failure.

Afterload

The resistance against which the ventricle contracts is termed 'afterload'. Increase in afterload (e.g. hypertension, aortic stenosis) causes hypertrophy, and only following failure does the heart dilate.

Contractility

> Defined as the force of contraction independent of the effect of filling pressure. Increased contractility is produced by inotropic agents such as sympathetic tone, adrenaline, isoprenaline, dopamine, and, minimally, by increase in heart rate and afterload; reduced contractility follows damage to the myocardium from ischaemia, hypoxia or such drugs as β-blockers and calcium antagonists.

PRIMARY ABNORMALITIES OF THE MYOCARDIUM

> Not as common as myocardial abnormalities secondary to scars and infarcts from coronary disease (Chapter 15) and severe valve disease (Chapter 4).
>
> Primary myocardial diseases include dilated (congestive) cardiomyopathy; hypertrophic (including obstructive) cardiomyopathy; and acute disorders from immunological reactions, infections and toxins and postpartum.

Dilated (congestive) cardiomyopathy

Aetiology

> Alcohol — prolonged heavy drinking; amyloid disease; familial; previous myocarditis (e.g. Chagas' disease, Coxsackie virus); diabetes; unknown (the majority).

Histopathology

> Diffuse, non-specific, interstitial fibrosis (except amyloid which is rare). Left ventricle (LV) usually more affected than RV.

Clinical presentation

Symptoms

> Dyspnoea on exertion appears gradually and progresses. Rarely symptoms are sudden in onset due to tachyarrhythmia. Occasionally exertional chest tightness, but typical angina favours coronary disease.

Clinical examination

Arterial pulse

> Usually normal. Atrial fibrillation (AF) particularly in the alcoholic group; ventricular ectopics, single or in short runs, not abolished by exercise; ventricular tachycardia.

Jugular venous pressure

> Elevated except in mild cases or following diuretic therapy.

Apex beat

> Displaced with associated LV hypertrophy.

Auscultation

Loud third sounds (LV and RV failure). Dilated ventricles may cause secondary mitral and tricuspid regurgitation. P_2 is loud from pulmonary hypertension secondary to LV failure.

Electrocardiography

Almost invariably abnormal with T inversion, bundle branch and occasionally AV block.

Chest radiography

Cardiac enlargement, easily detectable if previous films are available for comparison. Exceptions are amyloid disease and endocardial disease. Pulmonary venous congestion in *severe* cases.

Echocardiography

Large, poorly contracting LV with reduced aortic and mitral valve motion indicating low stroke output (Fig. 6.2). Functional mitral regurgitation detected by Doppler ultrasound.

Cardiac catheterization and angiocardiography

Seldom required except to exclude coronary disease. Dilated, uniformly poorly-contracting ventricle with normal coronary arteries. Raised LV diastolic pressure and secondary pulmonary hypertension.

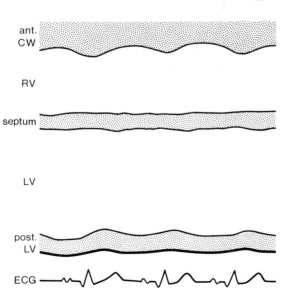

Fig. 6.2. M-mode echo in dilated cardiomyopathy showing greatly dilated hypocontractile LV.

Endomyocardial biopsy
Rarely diagnostic except in amyloid disease.

Complications
Left ventricular and eventually RV failure: thrombo-embolism, particularly with AF: ventricular tachycardia and fibrillation.

Differential diagnosis

Aortic stenosis
In aortic stenosis with a low cardiac output, the ejection murmur may become soft or disappear, but calcium may be seen in the aortic valve and the ejection murmur reappears as the patient improves.

Coronary artery disease
Multiple infarcts or ischaemic fibrosis — identified by a history of exertional angina or infarction, abnormal Q waves on the ECG, asymmetrical contraction of the LV on echocardiography and coronary angiography.

Prognosis
Based on the course of the disease and the state of the LV as visualized by serial echoes.

The downhill course may be slow and occasionally may be arrested, particularly if sinus rhythm can be preserved or if alcohol is the cause and is stopped. Heart failure resistant to diuretic therapy carries a bad prognosis.

Treatment
- Limitation of physical activity — some recommend bed rest for months
- Digitalis and control of arrhythmias
- Diuretics
- Afterload reduction — vasodilators to lower peripheral vascular resistance, e.g. hydralazine, nitrates, prazosin, captopril, enalapril
- Cardiac transplantation — for intractable cardiac failure

Hypertrophic (obstructive) cardiomyopathy (idiopathic hypertrophic subaortic stenosis) Figs 6.3 and 6.4

The area most affected is the septum in the LV outflow tract, which led to its first description as 'asymmetric hypertrophy', and later as idiopathic hypertrophic subaortic stenosis but any portion of the ventricles, even the right, may be affected, or the hypertrophy may be diffuse. Electron microscopy reveals disarray of giant myocardial cells with whorls to a degree that is not found with other causes of hypertrophy.

The disease is familial with dominant inheritance. Frequently there is a history of sudden death in relatives in middle age.

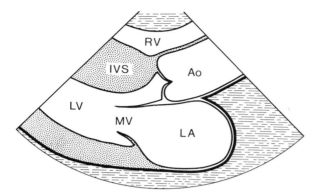

Fig. 6.3. Parasternal long axis echocardiogram of hypertrophic cardiomyopathy. The grossly thickened interventricular septum protrudes into the LV outflow tract below the aortic valve.

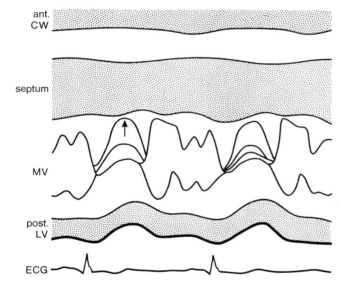

Fig. 6.4. M-mode echo of hypertrophic cardiomyopathy. The interventricular septum is grossly thickened (> 3 cm). The mitral valve impinges on the septum in diastole and there is systolic anterior motion (SAM — arrow).

Haemodynamics

In many patients normal at rest. The combination of gross septal hypertrophy and systolic anterior movement of the mitral valve towards the septum may lead to mid-systolic LV outflow obstruction and mitral regurgitation.

Clinical presentation

Symptoms

Sudden death may be the first presentation. More often there is exertional *dyspnoea*, eventually progressing to LV failure. *Angina* occurs in brief episodes, not always related to exertion, (hypertrophy of heart muscle beyond its blood supply). *Arrhythmia* and *syncope* are common.

Clinical examination

Arterial pulse

Sharp upstroke from the grossly hypertrophied LV before mid-systolic obstruction occurs. AF late in the course of the disease has a profoundly deleterious effect on haemodynamics.

Jugular venous pulse

Large 'a' wave indicating obstruction to RV inflow in a patient with LV disease suggests hypertrophic cardiomyopathy.

Apex

LV hypertrophy.

Auscultation

Loud, often palpable, atrial (fourth) sound (LV hypertrophy). Aortic ejection murmur (often displaced to right). Phonocardiography shows that the murmur stops before A_2, excluding primary mitral regurgitation (Fig. 1.15e).

Electrocardiography

LV hypertrophy — the pattern is often bizarre with steep T inversion which may affect inferior as well as lateral leads. Deep Q waves in any lead (Fig. 6.5). Rarely in mild cases the ECG is normal.

Chest radiography

Normal until the LV dilates from failure.

Echocardiography

Diagnostic method of choice. Septum greatly and often asymmetrically thickened (Fig. 6.3); LV cavity diminished; systolic anterior motion of the anterior cusp of the mitral valve towards the septum; (Fig. 6.4); inward movement of the aortic valve cusps soon after initial ejection (Venturi effect from subvalvar obstruction).

Cardiac catheterization and angiocardiography

Seldom required. In cases with obstruction, gradient at subvalvar level, increased by vasodilators, e.g. isoprenaline, and decreased by vasoconstricting drugs, e.g. phenylephrine (LV outflow held open longer). Angiography demonstrates the hypertrophied septum, but not as clearly as the echo.

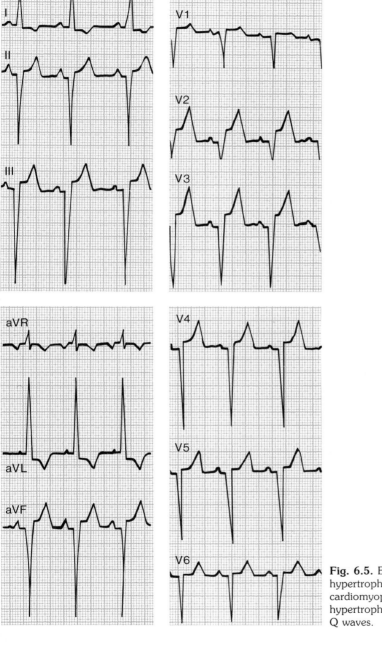

Fig. 6.5. ECG in hypertrophic obstructive cardiomyopathy. Gross LV hypertrophy. Large bizarre Q waves.

Differential diagnosis

1 From *aortic valve stenosis*, by the sharp upstroke on the arterial pulse, by echo and by cardiac catheterization. Family history helpful.

2 From *dilated cardiomyopathy*; by absence of cavity dilatation.

Prognosis

Risk of sudden death is considerable, particularly in those with symptoms and a family history. Small in mild cases such as those discovered by routine echocardiography in members of an affected family.

Treatment

Medical

Left ventricular failure is treated with diuretics and digoxin. Beta-blockers reduce outflow obstruction (reduced contractility of outflow tract), but may cause failure if the myocardium is badly affected. Arrhythmia is probably best treated with amiodarone.

Surgical

With modern medical management, surgery is rarely indicated except for severe symptoms with persistent large gradients across the subaortic stenosis in spite of therapy. On cardiopulmonary bypass a gutter is cut through the stenosis (Fig. 6.6).

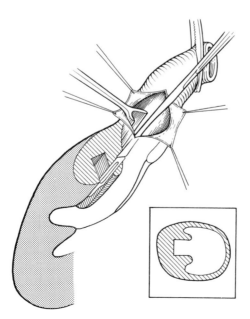

Fig. 6.6. Surgical relief of outflow obstruction in hypertrophic obstructive cardiomyopathy by 'guttering' the septum.

Acute disorders of the myocardium (myocarditis)

Aetiology and pathology

May be an immunological reaction to infection elsewhere (e.g. acute rheumatic fever), due to a virus infection, or secondary to a toxin. The acute attack may not be recognized clinically and the end result, perhaps years later, is a dilated cardiomyopathy with a rapid downhill course.

Immunological reaction

Acute rheumatic fever, which is a reaction of endothelial surfaces to a throat infection from the β-haemolytic streptococcus. While flitting arthritis is the main feature, the myocardium, heart valves and pericardium are involved in half the cases. The myocardium is never involved unless the heart valves are also affected (p. 65).

Infective

Mild myocarditis, recognized only by ECG abnormalities, occurs in a small proportion of patients with influenza or any of the acute exanthemas. The Coxsackie virus is the commonest cause of more severe attacks. Rickettsial infections occur in the Rocky Mountains of the USA and Chagas' disease in tropical South America.

Toxins

Acute myocardial damage is seen after the excessive intake of many toxins including alcohol, and with the administration of many drugs. ECG changes are often seen with tricyclic depressants. More serious damage may occur with cytotoxic chemotherapy, e.g. adriamycin.

Clinical presentation

Symptoms

No specific symptoms. Viraemia causes fever, tachycardia and generalized muscle aches, pericardial pain and in severe cases heart failure (usually biventricular so that pulmonary oedema is rare).

Auscultation

Abnormal ventricular filling sounds. Pericardial friction rub. Evidence of valve disease always in acute rheumatic carditis.

Electrocardiography

Frequently shows widespread T inversion arrhythmia and occasionally conduction defects (especially in Chagas' disease).

Echocardiography

Left ventricle dilated and contracts poorly with or without pericardial effusion.

Chest radiography

Cardiac enlargement in severe cases. Pleural involvement with some infections.

Specific tests

Rising antibody titres are the usual method of diagnosis of an infective agent. A high erythrocyte sedimentation rate (heart failure lowers it) and a rising antistreptolysin titre are invariable in acute rheumatic fever. Endocardial biopsy seldom gives specific information or differentiates acute myocarditis from a dilated cardiomyopathy. The cause of acute myocardial damage is often in doubt.

Treatment

- Immediate withdrawal of toxic agents
- Control of arrhythmia
- Aspirin and steroids for the immunological group; effective symptomatically but may not shorten the natural course of the disease
- Prolonged reduction in physical activity (even up to 1 year)
- Vasodilators to reduce cardiac work

HEART FAILURE

Inability of the myocardium to maintain normal haemodynamics, at first on exertion and later at rest. Failure to achieve a normal ejection fraction of > 50% leads to increased residual volume, raised ventricular end-diastolic pressure and raised atrial and venous pressures. Most commonly the LV is first affected and failure causes raised pulmonary venous pressure, secondary pulmonary hypertension and eventually RV failure, with raised jugular venous pressure (JVP), hepatic congestion and oedema. Simultaneously the low cardiac output causes diminished renal blood flow, sodium retention and oedema.

Aetiology of heart failure

Heart failure may be due to primary myocardial disease, but is more commonly due to myocardial damage from coronary artery disease or is the end result of increased ventricular work from valve disease or hypertension. (For congenital heart disease see Chapter 9).

Factors which precipitate failure include arrhythmias (fast or slow), respiratory infection, sodium retaining drugs, pulmonary embolism, pregnancy and too rapid administration of parenteral fluids, particularly in the elderly.

Heart failure is divisible into LV failure, RV failure and biventricular failure.

Left ventricular failure

Raised diastolic pressure in the LV, left atrium (LA) and pulmonary veins. Acute symptoms occur when the LV fails in the presence of a relatively intact RV.

Clinical presentation of left ventricular failure

Symptoms

Except with acute myocardial infarction or an acute tachyarrhythmia superimposed on ventricular disease, exertional dyspnoea appears gradually and progressively increases in severity with orthopnoea, paroxysmal nocturnal dyspnoea (PND) and eventually pulmonary oedema (p. 2).

Clinical examination
Often less helpful than the history.

Pulse
Rhythm may be normal but any arrhythmia may occur. Blood pressure — usually normal unless the cause is hypertension, but low output and tachycardia may cause reflex increase in systemic vascular resistance and mild elevation of diastolic pressure.

Jugular venous pressure
Normal with pure LV failure.

Cardiac impulses
Apex usually displaced (LV dilatation) and sustained (LV hypertrophy) except when failure is secondary to acute myocardial infarction when they are normal.

Auscultation
Loud third sound at the apex (elevated LA pressure increasing the rate of rapid filling). An atrial (fourth) sound does not indicate failure. There may be summation of atrial and third sounds from tachycardia or a long P–R interval making interpretation difficult. In the pulmonary area P_2 is abnormally loud from pulmonary hypertension. Left ventricular dilatation may cause mitral regurgitation.

Electrocardiography
Abnormal (with rare exceptions in cardiomyopathy).

Chest radiography
Cardiac enlargement except in endocardial fibrosis and *acute* myocardial infarction. In severe cases, upper lobe vein diversion, Kerley's lines and pulmonary oedema (p. 53).

Echocardiography
Increased dimensions of the LV (except with endocardial fibrosis). Poor contraction. Large LA.

Cardiac catheterization and angiocardiography
Seldom necessary. Elevated LV end-diastolic, LA and pulmonary artery pressures. Left ventriculogram confirms echo findings.

Complications
Systemic thrombo-embolism from the dilated and poorly contracting LV or LA, particularly in the presence of AF. Peripheral venous thrombosis and *pulmonary*

embolism are frequent because of the low cardiac output. *Ventricular arrhythmias* are common. Low renal blood flow may cause *renal failure*.

Differential diagnosis

Respiratory dyspnoea, particularly bronchial asthma, may be difficult to differentiate unless history available since left ventricular failure may cause bronchospasm. Chest X-ray and lung function tests may implicate respiratory disease. The cause of LV failure may be masked by a low cardiac output, e.g. the murmur of aortic stenosis may temporarily disappear.

Prognosis

Worst when due to aortic stenosis or diffuse myocardial fibrosis from coronary disease. Comparatively good when failure is precipitated by change of rhythm or acute mitral regurgitation from chordal rupture.

Right ventricular failure

Raised diastolic pressures in the RV, right atrium (RA) and systemic venous system.

Aetiology

Usually pulmonary hypertension except for rare cases of RV outflow obstruction and isolated tricuspid valve abnormalities. The pulmonary hypertension is usually secondary to LV failure or mitral obstruction: other causes are primary or embolic pulmonary hypertension and Eisenmenger's syndrome (Chapter 10).

Clinical presentation

Symptoms

Often minimal apart from oedema which may have been reduced or abolished by diuretics. The symptoms of LV failure may diminish when the RV fails with tricuspid regurgitation, because of reduction of RV output to the LV.

Clinical examination

Pulse

Often sinus rhythm if LA not enlarged. Atrial fibrillation usual when left-heart disease with LA enlargement is the primary cause, but may also occur with pulmonary embolism.

Jugular venous pressure

Elevated JVP: later large systolic waves from tricuspid regurgitation.

Cardiac impulses

Right ventricular hypertrophy — hyperkinetic with tricuspid regurgitation.

Auscultation

Right ventricular third sound (atrial fourth sound indicates hypertrophy only). Later a tricuspid pansystolic murmur (dilatation of tricuspid ring). P_2 loud and delayed particularly when venous pressure is high.

Hepatic enlargement, ascites, and dependent oedema

Electrocardiography

Right axis deviation and RV hypertrophy (p. 289), which may be masked by LV hypertrophy. Large P waves (P pulmonale) in leads 2, 3, aVF and V1 (RA hypertrophy — p. 293).

Chest radiography

Large heart: pleural effusions.

Echocardiography

Right ventricular dilatation but diagnosis more difficult than for LV.

Chest X-ray

Large heart: pleural effusions.

Cardiac catheterization and angiocardiography

Useful for diagnosis of pulmonary hypertension and embolism. Injection of contrast medium may be dangerous by causing systemic vasodilatation in the presence of low cardiac output.

Complications

Tricuspid regurgitation; cardiac cirrhosis (prolonged venous hypertension).

Biventricular failure

May be due to end-stage of LV disease when LV failure has been followed by pulmonary hypertension and RV failure; or due to cardiomyopathy or acute myocarditis affecting both ventricles equally. Severe attacks of pulmonary oedema are rare as RV output is reduced at the same time as LV output.

Differentiation from constrictive pericarditis may be difficult.

Treatment of heart failure

The principles are: removal of cause; reduction of cardiac work (e.g. vasodilators); diuretics; control of arrhythmia; improvement of myocardial contractility; administration of oxygen; positive pressure ventilation; aortic counterpulsation; transplantation.

Removal of cause

For example: control of thyrotoxicosis and systemic hypertension; correction of anaemia; treatment of alcoholism and nutritional deficiencies; and cardiac surgery for valve lesions or congenital defects.

Reduction of cardiac work

Rest in bed and chair — leg muscles should be used regularly to avoid phlebothrombosis and pulmonary embolism. Prolonged rest for several months may improve cardiomyopathy. Afterload reduction (p. 260) or intermediate positive pressure ventilation (IPPV) (p. 260) if treatment fails.

Diuretics

Diuretics act by reducing sodium by selective tubular activity. Thiazide diuretics are the first choice. Frusemide (40 mg) and bumetanide (1 mg) are more potent and may be given in larger doses. Overdiuresis is avoided and sodium levels watched to avoid excessive dehydration (sodium in the diet is reduced).

Simultaneous potassium loss is counteracted by concurrent administration of amiloride (5 mg), aldosterone antagonists (spironolactone, 25–50 mg q.d.s.), or potassium tablets.

Gout may be precipitated and diabetes exacerbated.

Control of arrhythmia

Tachyarrhythmia often precipitates heart failure in mitral stenosis, or with LV hypertrophy or fibrosis — shortening of diastole from tachycardia reduces ventricular filling and elevates LA pressure. Associated loss of atrial contraction (e.g. AF) is particularly harmful in aortic stenosis and hypertrophic cardio-myopathy.

Digoxin

Load with 2–3 mg orally over 2 days and then 0.25 mg daily, depending on lean body weight and renal function. May be given intravenously in emergency.

Digitalis toxicity — cumulation due to impairment of renal excretion is common in the elderly and with coincidental quinidine administration — serum levels are useful (range 0.5–2.5 ng/ml). Signs of toxicity — nausea, ventricular ectopics, nodal rhythm, regular atrial tachycardia with variable block and complete AV block.

Avoid coincidental low potassium which may precipitate VF.

Calcium antagonists

These, e.g. Verapamil 40–120 mg t.d.s. are safer than digoxin except for its hypocontractile effect on the myocardium. Often used in combination with digoxin to slow ventricular rate in AF.

Beta-blockers

Slow ventricular rate but depress myocardial contractility and are relatively contra-indicated in heart failure.

Improvement of myocardial contractility

Digoxin is the first choice but improvement may only be temporary. In emergencies intravenous dopamine, dobutamine and adrenalin may be used.

Vasodilators

Hydralazine, nitrates, intravenous sodium nitroprusside (for emergencies). The angiotensin converting enzyme inhibitors (captopril and enalapril) are the most useful. Care is required to avoid hypotension.

Oxygen administration

To improve hypoxia in pulmonary oedema.

Intermittent positive pressure ventilation

Temporarily effective for LV failure by reducing cardiac work and pulmonary oedema.

Intra-aortic balloon counterpulsation

To tide over a period of acute low output.

Cardiac or heart and lung transplantation

The last resort but now a practical possibility (p. 265).

Management of specific types of heart failure

Acute left ventricular failure

1 Nurse in upright position with legs dependent to reduce venous return, oxygen by face mask for hypoxia.
2 Drugs.
　　(a) *Intravenous morphine* reduces pulmonary oedema by venodilation and sedation.
　　(b) *Intravenous nitroglycerine* or other rapidly acting vasodilators to reduce afterload.
　　(c) *Intravenous diuretics* (e.g. frusemide) to reduce pulmonary oedema.
　　(d) *Intravenous aminophylline* (0.25–0.5 g) for secondary bronchospasm.
3 Intermittent positive pressure ventilation to reduce cardiac work and pulmonary oedema.

Heart failure in infancy

Symptoms

In an infant any degree of respiratory distress will be most evident during feeding while cyanosis is most prominent on crying.

Growth

A child whose heart is coping with a volume overload from a large intracardiac shunt, or whose left ventricle is pressure overloaded grows poorly. This failure to thrive can be monitored on a growth centile chart.

Clinical signs

1 A low cardiac output is reflected both by its direct consequences (hypoten-

sion, floppiness, low urine output) and by evidence of compensatory sympathetic overactivity (pallor, restlessness, sweating, cool peripheries).

2   Because their venous system is so compliant, infants do not develop marked elevation in their venous pressure. Hepatomegaly is a feature of heart failure in babies but peripheral oedema is rare. Equally, fine crackles (crepitations) are seldom heard when babies with left-sided lesions go into heart failure.

3   Since a growing thoracic cage moulds itself over an enlarged heart, a precordial bulge indicates underlying cardiomegaly. If the lungs have been stiff for a long time, the diaphragmatic insertion to the ribs can be visible as a groove — Harrison's sulci.

Treatment

The treatment rationale is the same as for adults. Drug doses are calculated by body weight and may need frequent adjustment during periods of rapid growth — e.g. infancy.

Chapter 7
Systemic Hypertension

Diastolic blood pressure persistently > 100 mmHg (*see* p. 15 for method of measurement), lower in childhood and pregnancy. In many normal subjects, transient rises above this level are common, particularly when visiting the doctor.

Elevation of *systolic pressure* without a rise in diastolic pressure is common in the elderly because of loss of elasticity of the aorta and arteries, with a figure of 100 + age in years the upper limit of normal. Recently, however, systolic pressure has been found to be a better predictor of mortality than diastolic pressure; it is possible that there is an association with atheroma, and certainly with increased left ventricular (LV) work.

AETIOLOGY AND PATHOLOGY

Diastolic hypertension is due to increased resistance (impedance) to blood flow in the small arteries and arterioles, probably at first due to spasm and later to thickening of the muscle layers. The LV hypertrophies.

Renin, an enzyme produced in the kidney, produces angiotensins which are potent vasoconstrictors, and are a primary stimulus for the adrenocortical production of aldosterone, which at distal tubular level causes retention of sodium and water. Disorders of this system play a part in the mechanism of production of renal hypertension, but not of primary hypertension. The main practical importance of the renin angiotensin cascade is the value of inhibitors (e.g. captopril and enalapril) of the enzyme which converts angiotensin I to angiotensin II, a potent constrictor of resistance vessels.

Essential hypertension

Primary (essential) hypertension is common, often with a family history, and appears to be due to an interaction between genetic and environmental factors. It may run a *benign* course for decades, particularly in women, but in general its progress depends on the average diastolic pressure. A very high pressure associated with retinopathy, papilloedema, raised intracranial pressure and renal failure is termed *malignant* or accelerated hypertension: this syndrome is now rare, probably because of successful therapy early in its course.

Secondary hypertension

Other less common causes of hypertension are:

Renal hypertension

Hypertension of renal origin is relatively rare and occurs with:
1   Acute nephritis.
2   Chronic glomerulonephritis (late, usually in association with renal failure).

3 Chronic pyelonephritis and other types of parenchymal disease.
4 Renal artery stenosis (fibromuscular hyperplasia in the young; atheroma in older patients).
5 Congenital polycystic kidneys.
6 Diabetic nephropathy.

Endocrine disorders

1 *Phaeochromocytoma.* A rare, usually benign, tumour of the chromaffin system and usually sited on one of the suprarenal glands. Secrete adrenaline and noradrenaline and cause attacks of sweating, palpitation and headache. Hypertension may be paroxysmal or sustained.
2 *Cushing's syndrome.* Hypercortisolism from a tumour of the anterior pituitary or adrenal causing moon facies, central truncal obesity, muscular weakness, purple striae, acne, hirsutism and hypertension.
3 Acromegaly.
4 *Primary aldosteronism* (Conn's syndrome). Usually caused by an adrenal adenoma and associated with low serum potassium and muscular weakness.
5 Hyperparathyroidism.

Pregnancy

Toxaemias and eclampsia. Also in susceptible subjects from contraceptive pills with a high oestrogen content.

Collagen diseases

Polyarteritis nodosa may produce renal hypertension.

Coarctation of the aorta (see p. 239)

The congenital narrowing is usually at the site of the ductus arteriosus. Only upper limb blood pressure is elevated and the femoral pulses are small or absent.

Drug interactions

For example, between monamine-oxidase inhibitors and food containing tyramine (some cheeses); sympathomimetic drugs interaction; excessive alcohol.

CLINICAL PRESENTATION

Symptoms

Usually *asymptomatic* and picked up at a routine examination. Sometimes morning *headache* (cervical spondylosis can do the same). Anxiety symptoms secondarily elevate the blood pressure and moderate hypertension can aggravate pre-existing migraine. Malignant hypertension causing retinopathy and papill-oedema may present with visual defects, headache and hypertensive encephal-opathy (confusion, agitation, lethargy, nausea and vomiting).

Clinical examination

Blood pressure

A single elevated reading in a symptom-less patient cannot be evaluated. Repeated diastolic pressures of 100 mmHg or more, particularly in a young male, require further investigation. Continuous monitoring of blood pressure while the patient continues his normal life is ideal, but technically is difficult to achieve, and in practice, a minimum of three blood pressure readings are taken at different times of the day by someone to whom the patient is accustomed, e.g. the family doctor on a home visit.

Fundi (Fig 1.4; and pp. 15 and 16)

Retinal haemorrhages and exudates (retinopathy) indicate that the hypertension is severe; papilloedema that it is malignant. The degree of irregularity of the lumen of the arterioles correlates with the average diastolic pressure and is absent in transient hypertensives. Arteriovenous crossing changes ('nipping') are found in hypertension, but mild degrees are also seen in normal elderly subjects.

General examination

The femoral pulses are checked to exclude coarctation. The abdomen is examined to exclude renal tumours, polycystic kidneys and bruits indicative of renal artery stenosis.

Cardiac impulses

Left ventricular hypertrophy only in sustained hypertension.

Auscultation

The aortic component of the second heart sound is abnormally loud. An atrial (fourth) sound is evidence of LV hypertrophy. Aortic regurgitation, usually slight, may occur if the hypertension has stretched the aortic root. If the LV fails and dilates, a pansystolic murmur of secondary mitral regurgitation may appear. There may be a soft ejection murmur from aortic cusp thickening.

Urine examination

Albuminuria suggests renal involvement and is rare in essential hypertension. In acute nephritis there will be red cells and casts.

Electrocardiography

LV hypertrophy (see Fig. 14.18) indicates sustained hypertension. Increased voltage in the chest leads is the first sign, but is only *sensitive as a change* since voltage is also influenced by chest wall thickness. S–T depression with T flattening and inversion is more specific to sustained hypertension if hypertrophy from other causes (e.g. hypertrophic cardiomyopathy and aortic stenosis) can be excluded.

Echocardiography

Thick (> 1 cm) posterior wall and septum. Dilated aortic root. With failure, the LA and LV dilate.

Special investigations

Serum creatinine, urea and electrolytes are checked at the initial screening. Other tests are not normally performed unless there are pointers to secondary hypertension or if the patient fails to respond to hypotensive therapy. These include estimation of plasma and 24 hour urine *catechol amine metabolites* for phaeochromocytoma, with localization by ultrasound and CT scan.

COMPLICATIONS

1   Cerebrovascular accident — thrombotic or haemorrhagic and including sub-arachnoid haemorrhage from a berry aneurysm.
2   Coronary atheroma and thrombosis.
3   Dissection of the aorta.
4   Left ventricular failure.
5   Renal failure — rare except with renal hypertension or the malignant phase of essential hypertension.
6   Hypertensive encephalopathy — transient exacerbation of hypertension, usually already severe, causing diffuse and reversible cerebral symptoms, particularly headache, confusion, agitation or lethargy, nausea, vomiting and visual disturbance.

ASSESSMENT OF SEVERITY

Retinopathy and papilloedema indicate severe or malignant hypertension requiring admission to hospital and intensive therapy. In general, the severity is assessed by repeated blood pressure readings and by the degree of LV hypertrophy assessed clinically and from the ECG and echocardiogram. Radiological enlargement of the LV and uncoiling of the aorta are ancillary signs, but in old age the aorta becomes uncoiled without hypertension.

DIFFERENTIAL DIAGNOSIS

Sustained hypertension

The most important problem is to separate transient hypertension or 'hypertonia' in anxious subjects from sustained hypertension. Many blood pressure readings are required. Irregularity of lumen of retinal arterioles and evidence of ventricular hypertrophy including an atrial sound, are evidence of sustained hypertension.

Causes of hypertension (pp. 141, 142)

PROGNOSIS

Expectation of life is reduced both with diastolic and systolic hypertension even of mild or moderate degree if sustained.

The prognosis of severe hypertension and particularly of malignant hypertension has been dramatically improved by modern therapy. The incidence of cerebrovascular accident has been greatly lowered. The increased incidence of coronary disease in mild hypertensives remains the major problem, but is probably being reduced by careful therapy.

TREATMENT OF HYPERTENSION

Lifestyle and diet

Mental tranquillity is achieved by a more placid way of life and even psychotherapy. Weight reduction in the obese, avoidance of heavily salted foods and excessive alcohol. These measures may be sufficient in mild cases.

Diuretics

The thiazides (e.g. bendrofluazide 5–10 mg *mane*) are the most effective, and after 6 months the serum potassium should be checked and if necessary increased, e.g. by adding amiloride 5 mg.

Beta-blocking drugs

Beta-blockers (e.g. atenolol 50 or 100 mg o.d.) usually form the basis of therapy in the more severe hypertensives, but may produce troublesome side-effects such as bronchospasm, drowsiness, depression, a cold periphery or aggravation of claudication. Ventricular failure is a relative contra-indication.

Calcium antagonists

Calcium antagonists, e.g. nifedipine slow release 20 mg b.d. or verapamil 160 mg b.d., often in combination with other drugs.

Angiotensin-converting enzyme inhibitors

Angiotension-converting enzyme (ACE) inhibitors (e.g. captopril 25 mg t.d.s. and enalapril 10–20 mg daily), often in association with diuretics but without additional potassium. There may be a dangerous fall in blood pressure if the patient has been depleted of sodium by diuretics or has acute renal failure in the presence of renal artery stenosis.

Peripheral vasodilators (e.g. hydralazine)

Programme

In practice a start is made by modification of lifestyle, avoidance of highly salted foods and reduction of obesity. A thiazide diuretic or a small dose of β-blocker is then added, the choice depending on the psychology of the patient. The aim is to reach a diastolic pressure below 95.

Failure to respond requires larger doses of β-blocker (unless contra-indicated by side-effects) and the addition or substitution of other drugs such as the calcium antagonists or ACE inhibitors. Alpha methyl dopa (250 mg t.d.s.) still has a place in heart failure and pregnancy with hydralazine (25 mg t.d.s.) as a peripheral dilator.

Malignant hypertension requires admission to hospital and immediate treatment.

ACUTE HYPOTENSIVE THERAPY FOR MALIGNANT HYPERTENSION

Hypertensive emergencies are rare. For extreme hypertension or development of complications such as hypertensive encephalopathy, the aim is to reduce the pressure smoothly to a safe level while avoiding a rapid or excessive fall which can lead to cerebral or myocardial infarction.

Oral therapy

Alpha methyl dopa 500 mg every 3 hours to a maximum of 2 g is effective. Or, nifedipine 10 mg given sublingually (patient bites into capsule and holds contents beneath tongue); it is effective in 20 min and can be repeated as necessary.

Intravenous therapy

If more urgent (e.g. hypertensive encephalopathy, dissecting aneurysm) intravenous labetalol is given in 50 mg aliquots injected over 1–2 min and repeated as necessary every 5 min to a maximum of 200 mg. Sodium nitroprusside is preferred if LV failure is present or suspected; the dose is 0.5 μg/kg/min initially, increasing as necessary to a maximum of 8 μg/kg/min. Long continued infusions may give rise to cyanide toxicity. Phentolamine is the specific antidote for a hypertensive crisis due to phaeochromocytoma.

Chapter 8
Disorders of Rhythm

CONDUCTING SYSTEM AND CLASSIFICATION

Physiology of conducting system (see also p. 267)

Atrial conduction (Fig. 14.5)

Cardiac depolarization originates in the *sino-atrial (SA)* node at the junction of the right atrial (RA) appendage and the superior vena cava (SVC). The node is under rate control from the sympathetic and parasympathetic systems. Depolarization of the RA produces the first part of the P wave on the ECG and of the left atrium (LA) the second part. The impulse passes inferiorly through the RA musculature to reach the *atrioventricular (AV)* node in the interatrial septum in front of the coronary sinus orifice. At the junction a small His deflection can be displayed on an endocardial (cavity) ECG but is too small to be identified on the surface ECG.

P–R interval

Between onset of P and onset of QRS (120–200 msec). Made up of P to His (55–145 msec) and His to QRS deflections (30–55 msec). The P–R interval allows time for ventricular filling following atrial contraction. The AV node acts as a filter rejecting high-rate atrial impulses.

One in a thousand of the population has a bypass with the possibility of an accelerated pathway between atrium and ventricle: it is possible for a circus movement to cause tachycardia (p. 307).

Ventricular conduction (Fig. 14.5)

After the AV node the activation potential passes rapidly down the specialized His conducting tissue, splitting into a small right bundle with no branches until nearing its periphery, and a large left bundle with numerous divisions arising early in its course. The left bundle divides into anterior and posterior hemibundles. The width of the QRS complex seldom exceeds 80 msec in normal subjects.

Classification of arrhythmia

Disorders of rhythm can be classified clinically into three groups; irregular rhythm; tachycardias; and bradycardias.

Haemodynamic effects of arrhythmia

The *effect* of irregular rhythm at normal rates is small. Tachycardia > 150, particularly in older subjects with impairment of ventricular filling, causes shortening of diastole and cardiac output falls. Bradycardia < 40 also limits output unless the heart can accommodate the increased stroke volume, e.g. athletic training.

IRREGULAR RHYTHM

Sinus arrhythmia

Normal respiratory reflexes often induce sinus slowing during inspiration in children and young adults.

Ectopic beats

Half the normal population have premature beats from an ectopic focus which may be supraventricular (Fig. 8.1) or ventricular (Fig. 8.2). Momentary refractoriness after this ectopic may cause omission of the next beat and a prolonged diastole with increased stroke volume of the following beat. The sequence may be repeated causing coupling (bigeminy — Fig. 8.3). Awareness of irregularity (palpitation) often causes anxiety but ectopic beats *as an isolated abnormality* are rarely of significance. Atrial ectopics may however precede atrial fibrillation (AF) and ventricular ectopics, particularly from multiple foci, may be evidence of ischaemic ventricular disease, electrolyte disturbance or drug intoxication and may precipitate ventricular tachycardia (VT) and even fibrillation (VF).

Clinical recognition

Atrial ectopics

Atrial premature beats are often interpolated without causing omissions and differentiation from AF may be difficult (p. 10).

Ventricular ectopics (premature ventricular contractions, PVCs) (Fig. 8.2)

Retrograde transmission of the impulse often causes delayed atrial contraction against a closed tricuspid valve and therefore irregular cannon waves in the jugular venous pulse (JVP). Exertion and tachycardia tend to abolish ectopics in normal subjects, but to increase them in patients with myocardial disease.

Coupling (bigeminy)

This is due to a premature ventricular contraction following each sinus beat.

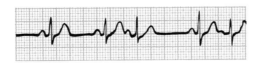

Fig. 8.1. Premature atrial ectopic beats (third complex) causing omission of next sinus beat. Difference in P wave and P–R interval, but identical QRS indicating normal transmission from AV node.

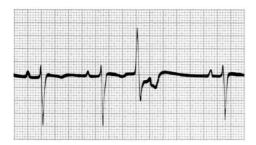

Fig. 8.2. Ventricular ectopic beat (third beat) — premature, causing failure of conduction of next sinus beat. Absent preceding P and broad bizarre QRS indicates non-His conduction. (P occurs at expected time here.)

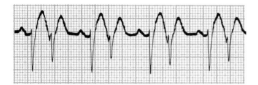

Fig. 8.3. Coupling (bigeminy) due to a premature ventricular ectopic following each sinus beat. Greater prematurity results in diminished LV filling and the ectopic beat may be impalpable.

Diminished LV filling may make the ectopic beat impalpable and extreme bradycardia may be misdiagnosed unless auscultation is used to detect the premature beat (Fig. 8.3).

Treatment

None with no underlying cardiac abnormality. When secondary to acute ischaemia, ventricular disease, electrolyte abnormality, toxic drugs or recent cardiac surgery, particularly if the ectopics are multifocal in runs of three or more, myocardial depressants are required (p. 156).

Atrial fibrillation (see under Tachycardia p. 152)

Second-degree atrioventricular dissociation

The P wave is sporadically not conducted (see Figs 8.12, 8.13). May be the first sign of progressive disease of the conducting tissue (p. 159).

TACHYCARDIAS

Tachycardias may be sinus, supraventricular (including AF and flutter), or ventricular.

Sinus tachycardia (> 90 beats per minute)

Seldom of primary cardiac origin — usually emotional, variable in rate and slowing during sleep. May be a manifestation of thyrotoxicosis or secondary to fever or low cardiac output.

Supraventricular tachycardias (SVT)

Atrial tachycardia (Fig. 8.4)

Regular brief attacks are common in the general population. They may be secondary to an AV nodal bypass causing a re-entry circus movement precipitated by an ectopic beat — the short-circuit may be revealed by a short P–R interval as evidence of pre-excitation. Typically this is associated with a slurred upstroke to the QRS, the Wolff–Parkinson–White (WPW) syndrome (p. 307, Fig. 8.5 and Figs 14.31–14.34).

Clinical presentation

Episodes of rapid, regular palpitation at rates of 130–250, usually in an otherwise normal subject. May cause hypotension if the ventricular rate is fast causing too short a diastole for adequate ventricular filling, particularly in older subjects.

Onset. Sudden and unexpected and usually at rest with no immediate emotional stimulus.

Duration. Seconds to hours and even days.

Cessation. Sudden but may not appear so to the patient if followed by a sinus tachycardia.

Accompanying symptoms. In older subjects, hypotension and ischaemic pain.

Precipitating factors. Often none but more likely to occur during periods of emotional stress causing ectopic beats.

Diagnosis

Usually clear-cut from the history. Ideally from ECG taken during an attack or on a patient-activated recording system. A 24 hour tape is usually too short to catch an attack.

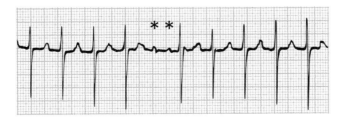

Fig. 8.4. A paroxysm of supraventricular tachycardia (rate 135). P waves may be difficult to see on a surface lead but are revealed in a break in rhythm here (*).

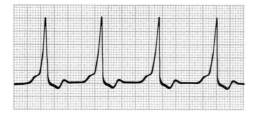

Fig. 8.5. Wolff–Parkinson–White syndrome. Pre-excitation of His system shown by a short P–R interval and slurred upstroke of QRS. In this example the P wave passes straight into the upstroke, and apparent duration of QRS is 0.14 s.

The ECG usually shows a normal QRS complex. If atrial rate is too fast to be conducted down the right bundle branch, there is aberration and a right bundle branch block (RBBB) pattern causing confusion with VT. P waves can usually be seen in some leads (V1–V2) and multiple simultaneous leads may identify them; they usually have a regular 1 : 1 relationship to the QRS. An oesophageal or cavity ECG shows the exact relationship. With 2 : 1 or greater block, digitalis toxicity is a likely cause.

Differential diagnosis
• *Sinus tachycardia.* Seldom so fast nor sustained at the same speed for long periods.
• *Ventricular tachycardia.* Irregular cannon waves in the neck and wide splitting of sounds, usually occurring in a patient with myocardial disease. Differentiation of VT from SVT with aberration may be difficult.

Prognosis
Normal in the absence of underlying heart disease. Attacks stop eventually and never cause permanent sequelae (temporary T inversion).

Treatment
Valsalva and carotid massage. Often the patient can stop an attack, particularly near its onset, with deep breathing or the Valsalva manoeuvre of forced expiration against a closed glottis in the supine position. Carotid sinus massage with firm posterior pressure is also often effective.

Drugs. Sedatives and sleep often stop the attacks spontaneously. Intravenous verapamil (5 mg) is the drug of choice. Beta-blocking drugs are also effective (e.g. i.v. practolol). DC cardioversion is occasionally needed.

Patients with frequent and severe attacks of SVT often have the WPW syndrome (p. 307). Attacks may be stimulated and an appropriate preventive drug identified by electrophysiological studies. In severe cases ablation of the pre-excitation pathway may be achieved by selective shock therapy through an endocardial electrode or by mapping and surgical incision of the pathway.

Prevention of attacks

Strong reassurance that the attacks are harmless is the single most important therapy. Avoid stimulants (black coffee, tea, emotional upsets). Continuous medication should be reserved for patients with prolonged and frequent attacks; verapamil, β-blockers, digoxin, quinidine and other depressant drugs may be tried. A patient away from home may travel with an ampoule of verapamil and a syringe.

Nodal tachycardia

Diagnosis

Regular but seldom as fast as atrial tachycardia. The P wave is usually inverted and delayed because of retrograde conduction, occurring just before or during the QRS and difficult to recognize on a surface trace. The diagnosis is then made by seeing regular cannon waves in the JVP, or on a cavity or oesophageal ECG.

Treatment

Verapamil or quinidine-like drugs such as disopyramide.

Atrial fibrillation (Fig. 8.6)

Completely irregular. Rapid, unco-ordinated and functionless atrial contraction. The usually increased ventricular rate causes shortening of diastole, reduction in ventricular filling and fall in output and blood pressure. This is accentuated by loss of atrial contraction, particularly when ejecting into a hypertrophied LV, e.g. aortic stenosis or hypertrophic cardiomyopathy.

Aetiology

1 Primary dysfunction of the SA node.

(a) Lone atrial fibrillation. Ventricular rate sometimes not fast with little reduction in output and discovered by chance. No evidence of underlying cardiovascular disease (echocardiogram needed to exclude early myocardial disease), may be paroxysmal at first, later permanent. Prognosis good. No treatment required except a nodal slowing drug, e.g. digoxin, if ventricular rate is fast.

(b) Bradytachy (sick sinus) syndrome (p. 157).

2 Secondary to increased atrial pressure and size.

(a) Mitral stenosis. AF almost invariable after age 40, earlier in populations

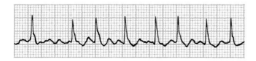

Fig. 8.6. Atrial fibrillation (lead I). Complete irregularity of QRS complexes and therefore of pulse. P waves are replaced by rapidly occurring and irregular waves often most clearly seen in leads V1 and V2.

with low standards of living. Ventricular rate usually fast, with low cardiac output and risk of thrombo-embolism.

(b) Reduced compliance of LV; e.g. cardiomyopathy (including mild dilated), aortic stenosis, acute infarction, ischaemic fibrosis.

3 Secondary to alcohol (and occasionally other toxins). May be paroxysmal and eventually chronic.

4 Secondary to thyrotoxicosis, which may be mild and difficult to diagnose.

5 Secondary to congenital defects — e.g. atrial septal defect (ASD) causing atrial dilatation.

Clinical presentation

Symptoms

May be symptom-less if ventricular rate is not fast. With mitral stenosis or myocardial disease, there are symptoms of a low cardiac output and rise of LA pressure (fatigue and dyspnoea).

Clinical examination

• *Pulse* completely irregular and usually fast with irregularity increased by exertion

• *Jugular venous pulse*. Loss of 'a' wave ('c' and 'v' remain). May be elevated if AF is not lone

• *Auscultation*. Essential for establishing that irregularity is complete since beats following a short diastole do not produce a pulse but produce sounds

• *Differentiated from ectopics* by absence of cannon waves and regular pattern to the irregularity on auscultation.

Electrocardiography

The P waves are replaced by up to 400 irregular 'f' waves per min, varying in amplitude and timing (Fig. 8.6). Transmission to the ventricles is only partially blocked at the AV node causing usually an irregular tachycardia.

Echocardiography

To exclude mitral stenosis and LA and LV enlargement.

Treatment

1 None — if ventricular rate not fast. Drugs contra-indicated in bradytachy syndrome (p. 157).

2 Drugs.

• *Digoxin* to control ventricular rate, particularly on exertion — digitalization with 0.25 mg q.d.s. for 2 days followed by 0.25 mg daily. (Less in elderly or with renal impairment.)

• Other AV node suppressants. *Verapamil* 40–80 mg t.d.s., or β-*blocking drugs*, unless ventricular function is poor

• *Anticoagulants* in mitral stenosis, cardiomyopathy and the bradytachy syndromes. Not indicated for lone AF

3 DC cardioversion (*see also* p. 322)

The heart is depolarized momentarily, abolishing all electrical activity and sinus rhythm is re-established in well-selected cases, at least temporarily.

• Indications. In cardiomyopathy, mitral regurgitation or lone AF if attacks not recurrent, LA is not large and patient is young. Also if the cause has been removed, e.g. thyrotoxicosis, chest infection, mitral stenosis

• Contra-indications. Mitral stenosis unless minimal, severe LV disease, AF for > 1 year as further attacks of AF will occur

• Technique of DC cardioversion:

(a) *Anticoagulants* given for 3 weeks beforehand to avoid thrombo-embolism. An anti-arrhythmic drug, e.g. quinidine may be given just before and continued afterwards (e.g. kinidurules 1 t.d.s.) to reduce recurrence. Digitalis is discontinued for 36 hours before cardioversion.

(b) *Sedation* with short duration anaesthetic or intravenous sedative.

(c) *Large electrodes* placed to the right of the sternum and over the apex.

(d) *DC shock*. 100–400 joules according to body size given at the peak of the R wave of the ECG, timed automatically to avoid the upstroke of the T wave which may precipitate VF (p. 322).

Prevention

Long-acting quinidine (e.g. kinidurules 1 t.d.s.) or other quinidine-like drugs, amiodarone (when justifiable), β-blockers, lowering LA pressure (e.g. mitral valvotomy).

Atrial flutter (Fig. 8.7)

Regular rhythm. Regular 'f' waves around 300, with regular transmission to ventricles with block (e.g. 2 : 1 causing a rate of 150, 4 : 1 a rate of 75). Variations in block may occur suddenly and fast ventricular rates cause acute hypotension. Paroxysmal atrial tachycardia with varying block has to be differentiated (p. 155) because it is usually a sign of digitalis toxicity.

Clinical diagnosis

May be mistaken for sinus rhythm as pulse is regular.

Electrocardiographic pattern

Large 'f' waves best seen as a saw tooth pattern in inferior leads and V1; may

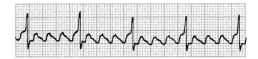

Fig. 8.7. Atrial flutter with 4 : 1 block and ventricular rate of 102. Regular tachycardia with usually a constant rate and regular pulse, but sometimes changing block so that rate suddenly doubles or halves, or varies, but is not *completely* irregular.

be invisible in lead 1 or in a monitoring lead placed transversely. Unlike paroxysmal atrial tachycardia, atrial flutter is seldom lone. Paroxysmal atrial tachycardia with block has more normal P waves.

Treatment
Control of ventricular rate by digitalis, plus verapamil or β-blockers. Can be converted to sinus rhythm by DC cardioversion (p. 233) — or rarely with quinidine with greater difficulty.

Prevention
As for AF.

Ventricular tachycardia
Regular fast rhythm (Fig. 8.8) Fast rates may produce syncope or degenerate into VF. Usually slower than SVT, associated with myocardial disease and more dangerous because of the absence of rate control from the AV node.

Diagnosis

Clinical examination
Irregular cannon waves (no relation between atrial and ventricular contraction). Splitting of first and second sounds.

Electrocardiography

Surface ECG
Broad, bizarre complexes resembling a ventricular ectopic, but in runs of more than five complexes. Differentiation from SVT may be difficult if there is RBBB pattern but VT is usually more disorganized, often slightly irregular, and no P waves can be seen preceding QRS.

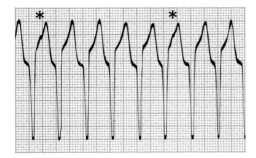

Fig. 8.8. Ventricular tachycardia. Broad complex tachycardia (rate 170) arising from the ventricular portion of the conducting tissue. In this example dissociated P waves are visible (*).

Endocardial ECG

Shows no His deflection preceding QRS. An attack with similar morphology of QRS may be precipitated by appropriate endocardial stimulation.

Prognosis

That of the underlying cause and, in the rare cases without ventricular disease, whether or not VT progresses to VF.

Treatment

For the acute attack: intravenous lignocaine, amiodarone, disopyramide and, best, DC countershock (Chapter 15).

Prevention

Drugs

Myocardial depressants, e.g. procainamide, amiodarone, quinidine, flecainide and tocainide. Amiodarone (600 mg daily for 2 weeks, and then 100–200 mg) is the most effective and the least depressant, but side-effects include light sensitivity, thyroid dysfunction and pulmonary fibrosis. No effect is expected for 2 weeks and its effect is thereafter prolonged. It activates warfarin and retards digoxin excretion.

When random drug regimes fail, electrophysiological studies are undertaken, tachycardia provoked and the most effective protective drug identified.

Ablation of the trigger area (endocardial shock or surgical)

When drug therapy fails.

Ventricular fibrillation

Fast irregular unco-ordinated contraction (Fig. 8.9) with no cardiac output. Usually a terminal rhythm unless immediately reversed. Irreversible brain damage after 4 min (or less if low output beforehand). (See also under cardiac arrest, pp. 319–322).

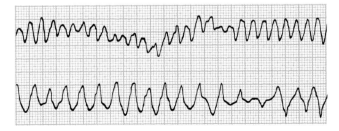

Fig. 8.9. Ventricular fibrillation (2 examples). Fast irregular broad waves without co-ordinated contraction and thus no cardiac output.

BRADYCARDIAS

Sinus bradycardia

Physiological variant due to strong vagal tone or athletic training. Rate as low as 50 at rest and 40 during sleep with sinus or Wenckebach omissions (p. 158), and parasinus, nodal or ventricular escape beats.

Lazy sinus

Bradycardias and sinus omissions at rest in the absence of athletic training. Rate increases normally with exertion or excitement. Benign.

Sino-atrial disease (bradytachy, sick-sinus syndrome)

Diagnosis

Abnormalities in the SA node usually produce AF (see Fig. 8.6), but atrial tachyarrhythmias may alternate with profound sinus bradycardias and sinus omissions causing dizziness and syncope (Fig. 8.10). Thrombo-embolism occurs in 1/5 of cases.

A chronic low-grade syndrome usually of unknown aetiology with possibly years between spells. Monitoring by a patient-activated machine for prolonged periods may be required for diagnosis. May also be a transient complication of acute myocardial infarction.

Treatment

No drugs should be given in the bradytachy syndrome because depressants and nodal blockers (digitalis, verapamil, β-blockers) worsen the bradycardia and stimulants (ephedrine, isoprenaline) increase the tachycardia. As prognosis is good, pacing is only required when symptoms are severe or for safety at work (e.g. up ladders) or driving. If simple ventricular pacing is used (p. 164) the rate should be set at a slow pace (e.g. 50) so that the unit only comes into action for severe bradycardia — otherwise competition with sinus rhythm will result in fluctuation of blood pressure depending on the timing of atrial contraction. Physiological pacing with an atrial-triggered system overcomes this problem but not that of atrial dysrhythmias. Depressant drugs for tachycardias should only be used after installation of a pacemaker. Anticoagulants are considered.

Carotid sinus syncope

Pressure over the normal carotid sinus induces vagal stimulation and sinus

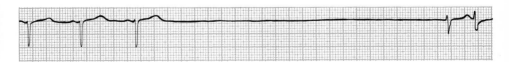

Fig. 8.10. Sino-atrial disease. Sinus bradycardia with sinus omissions and escape beats.

slowing. A hypersensitive reflex may occasionally be evidence of an abnormal tendency to bradycardia and syncope without pressure on the neck. Rarely a tumour of the carotid body may cause syncope, particularly on neck pressure.

Atrioventricular conduction delay (Heart block)
May be first, second or third degree.

First degree atrioventricular block (Fig. 8.11)
Prolonged P–R interval (> 0.20 s).

Aetiology
Seldom of clinical significance, and unlikely to progress, when an isolated abnormality, unless delay of 0.40 s or more. May be associated with an acute illness (e.g. acute rheumatic fever, diphtheria), myocardial infarct, or drugs such as digoxin. Prolonged His — QRS section of P–R is more likely to be abnormal (delay distal to AV node).

Clinical examination
Loud mid-diastolic ventricular filling sound due to summation of the atrial sound on preceding third sound (p. 32).

Treatment
None required but avoid nodal suppressants (e.g. digitalis).

Second degree atrioventricular block

Types

Mobitz type 1 (Wenckebach omission, Fig. 8.12)
Gradually increasing P–R intervals culminating in an omission. When isolated, usually physiological and due to increased vagal tone and abolished by exercise and atropine.

Mobitz type 2 (Fig. 8.13)
1 Sporadic sudden omissions without preceding increase in P–R interval indicate AV conduction disease (Fig. 8.13a).
2 Continuous 2 : 1, 3 : 1, 4 : 1 AV block (Fig. 8.13b). Liable to cause symptoms and to increase in severity.

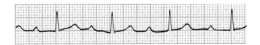

Fig. 8.11. Atrioventricular block of first degree — P–R interval prolonged (0.36 s., normally up to 0.2 s). No effect on rhythm. Atrial sound audible.

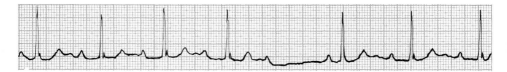

Fig. 8.12. Atrioventricular block of second degree (Wenckebach or Mobitz type 1 variety). Increasing P–R intervals and finally a complete omission. Usually due to increased vagal tone and, if the only abnormality, usually benign. In this case a transient change following inferior infarction (ischaemia of AV node).

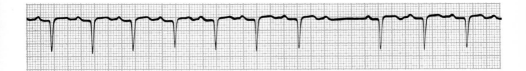

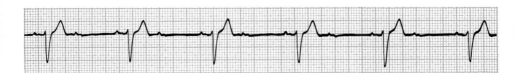

Fig. 8.13. Atrioventricular block of second degree — Mobitz type 2 variety. QRS omissions not preceded by lengthening P–R in previous cycles. There may be random omission of QRS complexes (beat 8) despite normally recurring P (A), or there may be regular omissions such as 2 : 1 (B) which caused a regular bradycardia of 43; the non-conducted P wave in mid-diastole caused a loud ventricular filling sound (summation of atrial and third sounds).

Clinical presentation

1 *Symptoms.* As third degree but less severe.

2 *Clinical examination* Pulse omissions with no premature beat (even on auscultation) to explain them. With 2 : 1 block there is regular bradycardia and a loud summation ventricular filling sound in diastole because of summation of the premature atrial and third sounds.

Treatment

Episodes of dimming or loss of consciousness associated with bradycardia require pacing. Even tachycardias provoked by preceding bradycardias will be abolished by pacing. Wenckebach omissions, provided that they are isolated, seldom require attention.

Third degree (complete) atrioventricular block (Fig. 8.14)

Usually causes bradycardic symptoms, particularly syncope. P waves continue, unrelated to regular slow idioventricular rhythm. Rates are 30–50/min depending the position of the pacemaker in the His system — a narrow QRS and higher rate indicates a site near the AV node and a more stable rhythm which may accelerate on exertion. A wide QRS indicates a peripheral site, is slower, unaffected by exertion and tends to be unstable.

Clinical types

Acute atrioventricular block

Complicates myocardial infarction (occasionally caused by digitalis poisoning, diphtheria and virus infections). Occurs 1–3 days after 15% of *inferior myocardial infarcts* because of transient AV node ischaemia, sinus rhythm returning a few days later. QRS is usually narrow and rate is 50–60 — syncope and permanent AV block are rare. Occasionally complicates *anterior infarction* because of interruption of both bundles causing a distal (broad QRS) and unstable idioventricular rhythm. Prognosis is bad because of the size of the infarct and liability to standstill and VF.

Chronic atrioventricular block

Common in elderly age groups due to idiopathic bilateral bundle branch fibrosis (50%). Other causes include chronic coronary disease (especially ages 55–65); calcium from aortic valve or mitral annulus spreading into the conducting tissue; sarcoid disease; Chagas' disease; gumma; congenital (with relatively good prognosis).

Clinical presentation

Symptoms

1 *Attacks of alteration of consciousness.* Recurrent syncopal (Stokes–Adams) attacks, or dimming of consciousness due to extreme bradycardia and asystole (80%), or VT and VF (20%). Occur without warning in two-thirds. Sudden pallor may be accompanied by epileptiform convulsions (cerebral anoxia), followed by flushing with return of the heart beat due to accumulation of vasodilating metabolites. Disorientation and other cerebral symptoms (particularly in the elderly) result from the low cardiac output of the extreme bradycardia.

2 *Dyspnoea.* The demand for an increased stroke volume may produce biventricular failure, particularly when the heart muscle is also damaged (but no paroxysmal nocturnal dyspnoea as both ventricles are affected).

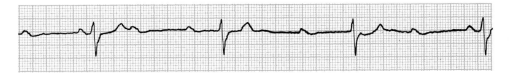

Fig. 8.14. Atrioventricular block of third degree with complete dissociation between atria and ventricles, each contracting independently. Bradycardia (32 here) with no, or little, acceleration with exertion.

Clinical examination

Regular fixed bradycardia rate 30–50. With high idioventricular rhythms (narrow QRS, usually congenital), the rate may increase with exercise. Variable cannon waves in neck and varying intensity of first heart sound (varying AV relationship p. 27). Variable ventricular filling sounds in diastole occur when atrial contraction coincides with rapid filling phase (p. 32).

Twenty–five per cent of patients with Stokes–Adams attacks are in sinus rhythm at the time of clinical examination, making diagnosis difficult, but almost invariably there is BBB and its association with syncope suggests paroxysmal complete block, though ventricular disease causing high rate VT must also be considered.

Treatment of atrioventricular block (see Tables 8.2, 8.3)

Acute inferior infarction block

Give intravenous atropine. Temporary pacing occasionally required for very slow rates.

Acute anterior infarction block

Early temporary pacing is required and may have to be permanent if block remains. Endocardial potentials may be low and care is required to avoid inappropriate pacing (p. 164).

Chronic block

Pacing is almost always required except for symptomless congenital block with a narrow QRS. Drug therapy with long-acting isoprenaline seldom has a place.

Differential diagnosis of causes of recurrent attacks of loss or dimming of consciousness (Table 8.1)

Simple faints

These are differentiated by the history (heat, food, alcohol, pregnancy, low blood pressure, emotion and familial tendency). Onset is gradual and associated with nausea and sweating. Pallor and bradycardia are long lasting and an ECG may show momentary complete cessation of all electrical activity. Symptoms are made worse if the patient is held vertical or sitting.

Sino-atrial disease

Attacks of bradycardia usually result in dimming of consciousness or momentary unsteadiness rather than loss of consciousness accompanied by a fall. A 24 or 48 hour tape is seldom diagnostic as the attacks may be separated by weeks. A patient activated monitoring system which runs continuously for 2–3 weeks is more valuable. Normal patients, however, with strong vagal tone may have sleeping rates below 40 with blocked atrial beats and parasinus rhythm. Paroxysmal atrial arrhythmias, in addition, point to the sick sinus syndrome.

Atrioventricular disease (p. 158)

ECG almost invariably shows BBB.

Paroxysmal tachycardia

High rate, occasionally atrial (with WPW pre-excitation), usually ventricular with evidence of myocardial disease.

Postural hypotension

Not uncommon in the elderly and diagnosed by the history and fall in blood pressure on standing.

Table 8.1. Causes of repetitive syncope or near syncope

1	**Epilepsy**	EEG may be normal
2	**Circulatory**	
	(a) *Obstructive carotid disease* (with emboli)	Seldom syncope — transient focal signs in CNS
	Vertebrobasilar	Seldom syncope
	Aortic stenosis	
	HOCM	
	Fallot	} Usually exertional
	Primary pulmonary hypertension	
	Pulmonary embolism	
	Intracardiac tumour	
	(b) *Autonomic*	Simple faint
		Postural hypotension
		Cough syncope
	(c) *Arrhythmia*	
	Bradycardia	
	SA disease	ECG often normal
	Carotid sinus	Rare
	AV disease	Usually BBB
	Tachycardia	
	VT — high rate (180 +)	Secondary to bradycardia
		Coronary disease
	VF	Cardiomyopathy
		Idiopathic (rare)
		Drugs — potassium
		WPW (rare)

HOCM = hypertrophic obstructive cardiomyopathy

Labyrinthine disorders

These are characterized by spinning or rotation rather than dimming of consciousness.

Epilepsy

May have an aura, is sudden, and the patient is flushed with no pallor or bradycardia. Convulsions do not distinguish epilepsy unless they are focal.

ARTIFICIAL CARDIAC PACEMAKERS

Repeated brief electrical stimuli depolarize the ventricles (or the atria). Pacing through an intact chest wall requires large voltages and, even through an electrode impacted in the RV, the voltage of an effective artificial impulse is about 5 V instead of the physiological few mV (Fig. 8.15). A summary of management is given in Tables 8.2 and 8.3.

External pacemakers

Always temporary.

With external electrodes

Large voltages (100–200 V) cause painful contraction of chest wall muscles and are only used in an emergency or for prophylaxis against ventricular standstill during anaesthesia for surgical procedures on unpaced patients with disease of the conducting tissues. The electrode should be as large as is practical.

With internal electrodes

Transvenous or placed directly on the ventricle at surgery. Useful for low voltage temporary pacing or standby following myocardial infarction or cardiac surgery. May be used for days or weeks but there is then risk of septicaemia (usually Staphylococcal) and even endocarditis as the endocardial electrode abrades the tricuspid leaflets.

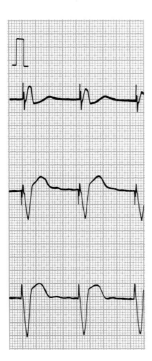

Fig. 8.15. Pacing the ventricles. Each artificial stimulus is followed by a broad QRS indicating depolarization of the ventricle by a non-His pathway.

Internal pacemakers

Permanent.

Types of pacemaker

The mode of operation of a pacemaker is described by a three-letter code:

1   Chamber paced (A = atrium, V = ventricle, D = double chamber).

2   Chamber sensed.

3   Mode of response (I = inhibited, T = triggered, D = atrial sensing triggers ventricular stimulation, ventricular sensing inhibits stimulation of atria, ventricles or both) — to avoid competition with spontaneous QRS complexes.

Usually the RV is paced with the same electrode used for sensing, so that the impulse is inhibited by a spontaneous QRS (VVI pacemaker). The rate may be set — usually 70–72 (haemodynamic disadvantage during exertion), or may be made to speed up on exercise. Sequential pacing with atrial followed by ventricular contraction is achieved by a second electrode sensing atrial depolarization (VDD). This has the advantage of achieving variation of rate according to need; atrial dysrhythmia may cause problems, but complicated means have been devised to avoid this.

Technique of pacing

Temporary pacing

Endocardial pacing with external unit (Table 8.2)

Endocardial wire inserted percutaneously below the clavicle into the subclavian vein and impacted in the RV under x-ray control and connected to an external pacemaker. For complete AV block with slow rates following infarction, particularly large anterior, it is essential to measure threshold daily and never to pace at more than twice the threshold. Endocardial potentials with a large infarct may be low and the pacemaker may not be inhibited by a spontaneous QRS; inappropriate pacing on the vulnerable part of the T wave may cause VF; continuous fast pacing is then advisable, a technique which can also be used to suppress ectopics.

After pacing there is transient T wave inversion (as with paroxysmal tachycardia).

Table 8.2. Temporary pacing — indications

Acute anterior infarct with:
1   Sinus rhythm with bifascicular block or P–R ↑
2   AV block
Acute inferior infarct + AV block
Only if symptoms or severe bradycardia despite atropine
Stable AV block
For anaesthesia, etc.

Epicardial pacing after cardiac surgery

Pacing wires inserted onto RA and RV and passed through the skin to cover postoperative bradycardia.

Permanent pacing

Endocardial pacing (Table 8.3, Fig. 8.15)
    The method of choice. The electrode is impacted into the RV under local anaesthesia via the jugular venous system with the pacing unit placed in a subclavicular pocket.

Epicardial pacing
    An electrode is sewn on to a ventricle. Seldom used except at cardiac surgery.

Complications of pacing

Failure to capture the ventricle (Fig. 8.16) or a rising threshold.
    Caused by poor electrode contact (e.g. displacement), a broken wire or loss of unit power, e.g. battery failure.

Table 8.3. Permanent pacing — indications

Complete AV block — unless asymptomatic and:
   1 Congenital and unchanging
   2 Narrow QRS with acceleration on effort
   3 Elderly and stable
Second-degree AV block if syncope or near syncope
BBB (right or left) if syncope or near syncope with no other explanation
SA disease if:
   1 Severe symptoms
   2 Associated AV disease

Local infection
    Of pacemaker pocket or subcutaneous part of the wire. Rare except at second procedure (e.g. for displacement of electrode) — ideally requires complete removal of old system and a new system on the other side.

Septicaemia
    Usually with tricuspid valve endocarditis. Rare except with mainlining drug addicts or prolonged external endocardial pacing. All intravascular foreign material has then to be removed and replaced with an epicardial system, followed by a 4 week course of bactericidal drugs.

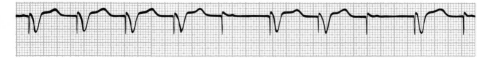

Fig. 8.16. Failure to capture. The fifth and eighth pacing stimuli are not followed by a depolarization QRS.

Pacemaker follow-up

Although pacemakers are now remarkably reliable, meticulous follow-up in an experienced unit is essential for long-term success. The pacemaker is validated at the time of insertion and checked by external measurement with an oscilloscope annually. Batteries last 5–10 years. Impending battery failure detected by change in power, wave form or rate of the stimulus.

Prognosis of paced patients

Depends on the cause of the initial bradycardia. With isolated disease of the conducting system (not uncommon), a normal lifespan is expected.

Chapter 9
Congenital Heart Disease

Congenital heart disease affects 8/1000 live births.

AETIOLOGY AND PREVENTION
The heart is formed by the ninth week of gestation, making environmental influences on the foetal heart less important after the first 2 months.

Maternal influences
1   *Maternal systemic disease.* Diabetes (increased incidence of structural heart disease and/or a characteristic hypertrophic cardiomyopathy); lupus erythematosus (associated with congenital complete heart block).
2   *Maternal infection.* Rubella, other viral infections.
3   *Drugs.* Thalidomide, warfarin, phenytoin.
4   *Maternal radiation.*

Genetic predisposition
1   Associated with some chromosomal defects, e.g. Turner's syndrome, Trisomy 21.
   Heart disease in Down's syndrome. 30% have congenital heart disease. Commonest lesion is atrioventricular (AV) septal defect, then isolated ventricular septal defect (VSD), Tetralogy of Fallot, primum atrial septal defect (ASD) and AV septal defect with Tetralogy of Fallot. Constitute about 5% of critical heart disease in infants.
2   In siblings and offspring of patients with congenital heart disease (risk about 5%).
3   Associated with multiple non-cardiovascular congenital abnormalities.

Prevention
1   *Avoidance of drugs/radiation.*
2   *Rubella immunization.*
3   *Antenatal ultrasound.* Foetal cardiac abnormality can be recognized on antenatal ultrasound examination from about 18 week's gestation, in time for termination of the pregnancy to be considered if the malformation is serious. This diagnostic facility is offered mainly to mothers with previous children affected by congenital heart disease.

FREQUENCY OF SPECIFIC MALFORMATIONS
The following lesions are the most commonly encountered in clinical practice:
• VSD (commonest defect)
• ASD

- Persistent ductus arteriosus (PDA)
- Tetralogy of Fallot (commonest cyanotic defect)
- Pulmonary valve stenosis
- Aortic coarctation
- Transposition of the great arteries (commonest cyanotic defect in the neonatal period)
- Hypoplastic left heart (commonest cause of cardiac death in the first week of life)

LEFT TO RIGHT SHUNTS

Sites
Communications occur at:
- *Atrial level* (e.g. ASD)
- *Ventricular level* (e.g. VSD)
- *Great artery level* (e.g. PDA, aortopulmonary window)
- *From great artery to atrium or ventricle* (ruptured sinus of Valsalva aneurysm, coronary-cameral fistula)
- *From ventricle to atrium* (Gerbode type of VSD, left ventricle (LV) to right atrium (RA))
- *Multiple levels* (e.g. AV septal defect)

Haemodynamics of left to right shunts
Oxygenated blood flowing across the defect into the lower pressure right heart arrives in the pulmonary bed and is returned to the left atrium (LA). All chambers and vessels overloaded by the shunt dilate and hypertrophy to cope with the volume load. An ASD overloads RA and right ventricle (RV), a persistent ductus overloads the LA and LV while a VSD overloads both ventricles.

The magnitude of the shunt depends on: the size of the defect; the pressure difference across the defect; and the relative resistances in the systemic and pulmonary beds.

Complications of left to right shunts
1   *Cardiac failure.* From volume overload of the involved ventricle or ventricles.

2   *Infective endocarditis.* Related to high-velocity jets roughening the endocardium. High risk with small VSD, very low risk with large ASD.

3   *Increasing pulmonary vascular resistance (PVR).* The pulmonary vascular bed is progressively damaged by excessive pulmonary artery (PA) pressure and pulmonary blood flow. Medial thickening and later intimal changes serve to raise the PVR and limit the blood flow through the lungs. Pulmonary vascular disease eventually becomes irreversible even if the cause of the vascular stress is relieved by closing the left to right shunt (Eisenmenger syndrome).

Atrial septal defects

Types of atrial septal defect (Fig. 9.1)

1   *Patent foramen ovale.* Present in all neonates and remains a potential atrial communication in 20% of adults. *In utero* much of the most oxygenated blood returning from the placenta via the inferior vena cava is diverted through the foramen ovale to be ejected from the LV.

2   *Secundum ASD.* Commonest, situated in the middle of the atrial septum.

3   *Sinus venosus defect.* High ASD often associated with anomalous drainage of the right upper and middle lobe pulmonary veins into the superior vena cava or high RA.

4   *Primum ASD.* The inferior margin of the atrial septum, normally anchoring the atrioventricular valves, is missing. This is part of the 'family' of defects called 'atrioventricular septal defects'.

5   *Partial anomalous pulmonary venous drainage.* Right or left pulmonary veins can drain to the RA, with or without an associated ASD.

Haemodynamics (Fig. 9.2)

Typically, ASDs are large so that no pressure gradient develops across them. The direction of shunting thus depends on the relative compliances (resistance to filling) of the RA and RV compared with the LA and LV. At birth, the two

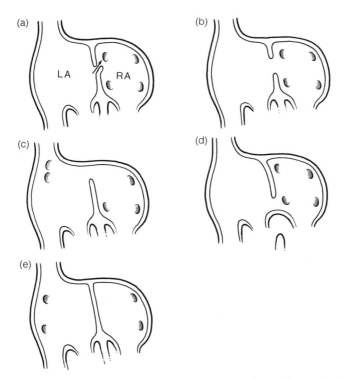

Fig. 9.1. Types of ASD. (a) Patent foramen ovale. (b) Secundum ASD. (c) Sinus venosus ASD. (d) Primum ASD. (e) Partial anomalous pulmonary venous drainage.

(a)

(b)

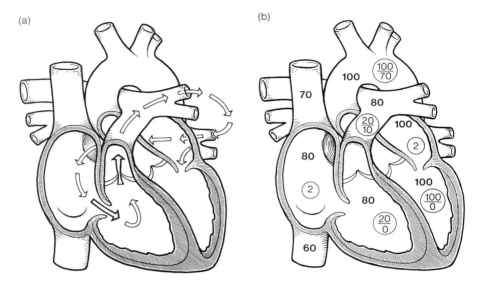

Fig. 9.2. (a) Left to right shunt at atrial level. Murmurs correspond to high tricuspid and pulmonary flows. (b) Oxygen saturations and pressures (circled) in ASD.

ventricles are equally thick and no shunting occurs. Normally the pulmonary vascular resistance falls after birth allowing the RV to thin. As it does so, it becomes more compliant and able to accept more blood in diastole.

Much of the blood returning to the LA recirculates through the atrial defect while some crosses the mitral valve normally to fill the LV. Normal left ventricular output is maintained because the pulmonary venous return is excessive. The systemic blood flow is within normal limits but the pulmonary flow may be more than three times normal.

Clinical presentation of secundum atrial septal defect

Symptoms

Typically the patient is asymptomatic until atrial arrhythmias related to the longstanding RA distension supervene. This is rare in childhood but more common in middle age. Occasional children suffer recurrent chest infections, related to the excessive pulmonary blood flow.

Clinical examination

General

Normal

Pulse and blood pressure

Normal unless complicated by atrial fibrillation (AF).

Jugular venous pressure
Normal

Precordial impulse
Left parasternal heave (hyperkinetic RV).

Auscultation (Fig. 9.3)

Second sound. Widely split (delay of P_2) because of prolongation of RV systole due to the volume load. The split remains fixed during respiration, both A_2 and P_2 being equally delayed so that the interval between them remains fixed (pp. 29, 30).

Murmurs of the defect. None. The defect is large, with no pressure gradient across it.

Flow murmurs. Increased flow across the tricuspid and pulmonary valves accounts for a short mid-diastolic ventricular filling ('flow') murmur in the tricuspid area and an ejection murmur in the pulmonary area. Murmurs are soft but louder on inspiration as the venous return increases.

Electrocardiography
1   Right axis deviation.
2   rSR′ in lead V1 (partial right bundle branch block, mild RV +)

Chest radiography
1   *Pulmonary plethora* (excessive pulmonary blood flow).
2   *Enlarged right heart.* RA, ventricular mass and PA prominent (increased flow through these chambers).

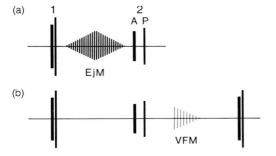

Fig. 9.3. ASD heart sounds and murmurs. (a) Pulmonary area. (b) Tricuspid area. EjM = ejection murmur. VFM = ventricular filling murmur.

Echocardiography

The ASD can be visualized. The interventricular septum 'moves' with the RV because of the right ventricular volume overload (reversed 'paradoxical' septal motion).

Cardiac catheterization

Not usually performed unless there is concern about a high pulmonary vascular resistance or more complex heart disease. An increase in oxygen saturation in the atria compared with the cavae shows the level of the shunt. The right-sided pressures are normal, unless the pulmonary vascular resistance has risen.

Angiography

The ASD can be demonstrated by injection of contrast into a pulmonary vein, the plane of projection being chosen to profile the atrial septum.

Differentiating other types of atrial septal defect

This may require ultrasound examination, but other pointers are:
- *Sinus venosus defect*. Chest x-ray may show a bulge at the lower end of the superior vena cava (at the site of entry of anomalous entry of right upper lobe pulmonary veins)
- *Primum ASD*. Typically associated with a cleft and often incompetent mitral valve. Patients often more symptomatic with dyspnoea, recurrent chest infections and arrhythmias. Also differentiated by the presence of:
1 *Auscultation*. Apical pansystolic murmur of mitral regurgitation, if present.
2 *Electrocardiogram*.
  (a) *Left axis deviation*.
  (b) *Long P–R interval*. Both electrocardiographic abnormalities relate to associated abnormalities of the conducting system.
3 *Angiography*. A LV injection may show mitral regurgitation. The LV outflow tract looks narrow — a 'goose-neck deformity' due to the abnormal mitral valve attachment.

Partial anomalous pulmonary venous drainage

Same physical signs as secundum ASD.

Catheterization

The anomalously draining veins may be entered directly from the RA. Following the contrast through from a PA angiogram will demonstrate the anomalous pulmonary venous return. Occasionally the right pulmonary veins drain below the diaphragm to the inferior vena cava (Scimitar syndrome).

Treatment

Indications for surgery

Pulmonary to systemic flow ratio > 2 : 1. The aim of surgery is to prevent later progressive pulmonary vascular disease, arrhythmias and RV failure. Ideally elective operation is undertaken before a child goes to school.

Contra-indications and risk factors

Pulmonary vascular disease and severe mitral regurgitation.

Technique of operation (Fig. 9.4)

1   *Secundum defects.* Direct suture or closure of the defect with a patch.
2   *Sinus venosus defects* and anomalous pulmonary venous return. A patch is used to close the defect and redirect the anomalous pulmonary veins to the LA.
3   *Primum ASD.* Besides closing the defect with a patch, the mitral valve may require repair, or occasionally replacement.

Results

Uncomplicated secundum and sinus venosus defects

Morbidity or mortality levels below 2%, considerably higher in the presence of pulmonary vascular disease. Occasional complications relate to air embolism or damage to the sino-atrial node.

(a)

(c)

(b)

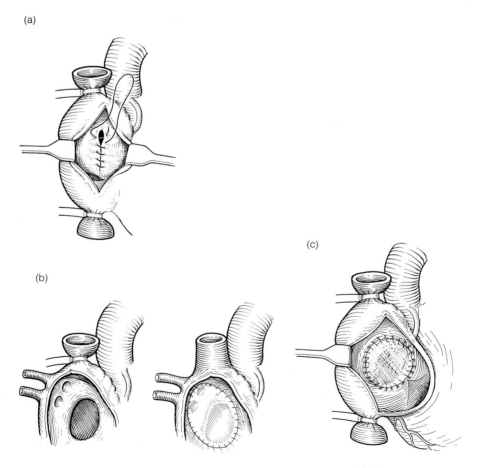

Fig. 9.4. Surgery of ASD. (a) Secundum. (b) Sinus venosus (c) Primum.

Primum atrial septal defect

Morbidity and mortality higher. Complications include complete heart block and residual mitral regurgitation which is poorly tolerated because the LA is small, owing to its previous decompression by the ASD.

Ventricular septal defects

Types of ventricular septal defects (Fig. 9.5)

Perimembranous

The commonest defect. The membranous septum is deficient. The defect can extend into the outlet, muscular or inlet septum. The bundle of His runs along the posterior margin of this defect.

Inlet

The septum between the tricuspid annulus and the insertion of the papillary muscles is deficient. The conduction tissue runs along the superior margin of this defect.

Subarterial

The septum immediately below and supporting the semilunar valves is deficient. These defects can be complicated by progressive aortic regurgitation.

Muscular

Holes in the muscular septum may be multiple. Unlike the other defects, they can be acquired after trauma or myocardial infarction.

Ventricular septal defect with overriding arterial valve

This is seen in the context of more complex congenital heart disease, e.g. Tetralogy of Fallot or truncus arteriosus.

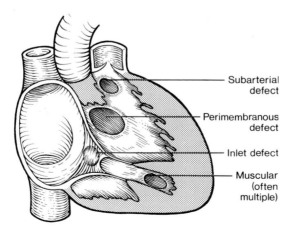

Fig. 9.5. Types of VSD.

Haemodynamics (Fig. 9.6)

The shunt

In ventricular systole, blood flows across the defect into the RV, through the pulmonary valve and into the low-resistance pulmonary bed. It returns to the LA and LV and some recirculates through the lungs. Thus both ventricles carry a volume overload and the LA is also dilated.

Magnitude of the shunt

Depends on:

1 *Size of the defect.* A small defect restricts the shunt.

2 *Pulmonary vascular resistance.* The level of pulmonary vascular resistance depends on how long the pulmonary bed has had a high PA pressure and blood flow. In infancy the PVR is low relative to systemic and the pulmonary flow high. In time, the pulmonary arterioles develop medial hypertrophy and intimal thickening which increases the resistance to flow (pulmonary vascular obstructive disease). Advanced vascular changes are irreversible, even if the VSD is surgically closed.

Clinical presentation of ventricular septal defect

Symptoms

Depend mainly on the pulmonary blood flow. A small shunt causes no symptoms; a larger shunt causes dyspnoea, recurrent chest infections and failure to thrive. An infant with a large VSD feeds poorly.

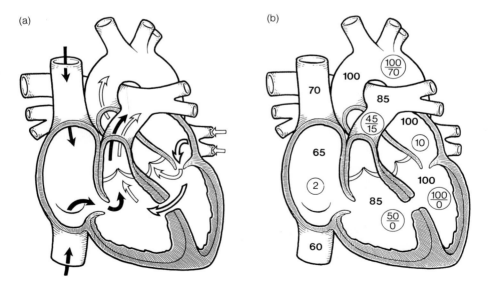

Fig. 9.6. (a) Haemodynamics of moderate-sized VSD. Murmurs correspond to flow through VSD and high mitral flow. (b) Oxygen saturations and pressures (circled).

Clinical examination

General

Normal or underweight, depending on the size of the defect. The sternum bulges if the underlying RV is enlarged in a growing child. There may be a groove in the ribs corresponding to the insertion of the diaphragm if the lungs have been chronically stiff because of pulmonary plethora — Harrisons's sulci. The patient is pink; if cyanosis is observed or mentioned in the history there must be concern that pulmonary vascular disease is restricting pulmonary blood flow and intermittently reversing the direction of the intracardiac shunt (Eisenmenger syndrome p. 215).

Pulse

Normal.

Jugular venous pressure

Normal but large liver in young child.

Precordial impulse

Left parasternal heave and forceful apical impulse (biventricular hypertrophy) if a significant shunt is present.

Auscultation (Fig. 9.7)

1   *Heart sounds.* The loudness of the second heart sound is an important key to the level of the resistance in the pulmonary circulation. If the VSD is large, systolic pressures in the LV, RV and PA are bound to be similar. Provided the resistance to pulmonary flow is still low, the pulmonary diastolic pressure remains low and P_2 is normal (the pulmonary valve closes in diastole!). As pulmonary vascular disease progresses, the pulmonary diastolic pressure rises and P_2 becomes louder.

2   *Murmur of the defect.*

(a) A tiny defect in the muscular septum may functionally close in late systole with the murmur confined to early systole.

(b) Moderate or large defect. Loud pansystolic murmur and thrill, maximal at the lower left sternal edge.

(c) If a large defect is not closed surgically and pulmonary vascular disease progresses, the flow across the defect decreases as the PVR rises and the murmur eventually disappears as the resistances in the systemic and pulmonary beds become balanced (Eisemenger syndrome).

3   *Flow murmurs.* If pulmonary flow is more than twice systemic flow, the excessive return through the mitral valve is audible as a mid-diastolic flow murmur. The pulmonary flow murmur is usually drowned in the pansystolic murmur.

Electrocardiography

May be normal in a small defect. In larger defects the findings depend on the stage of the natural history of the disease. While the PVR is low, the pulmonary

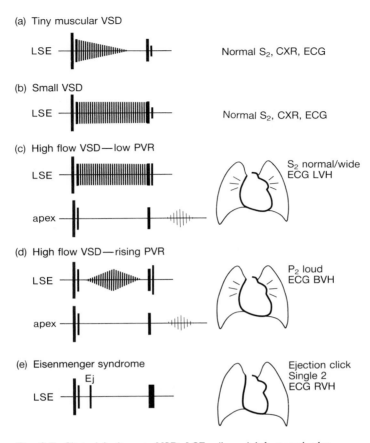

Fig. 9.7. Clinical findings in VSD. LSE = (lower) left sternal edge.

blood flow is high and the LV volume overloaded, the ECG showing LV hypertrophy. With the onset of pulmonary vascular disease the diastolic and mean PA pressures rise and the ECG will show RV hypertrophy as well. Once the PVR is high enough to prevent significant left to right shunt through the defect, the LV volume overload falls and the LV hypertrophy is lost, leaving pure RV hypertrophy.

Chest radiography

Heart size

Depends on the size of the left to right shunt. If this is large LA, LV, RV and PA are all enlarged. If the shunt is small, either because the VSD is small or because the patient has pulmonary vascular disease restricting the shunt, the heart size may be normal.

Lung fields

Pulmonary vascularity depends on the pulmonary blood flow and hence on the size of the shunt. The lung fields may be normal (small VSD), plethoric (larger VSD) or oligaemic with loss of perfusion of peripheral small vessels (pulmonary vascular disease, Eisenmenger syndrome).

Pulmonary artery

In the presence of pulmonary vascular disease the mean PA pressure is high, though the pulmonary flow may be normal or low. The dilated PA is usually prominent on the chest radiograph.

Echocardiogram

The site of the defect is visualized. If the shunt is large, LA, LV, RV and PA are dilated.

Cardiac catheterization

Small defects

Normal right heart and PA pressures. Oxygen saturation samples show a small 'step up' in oxygen saturation in the RV.

Large defects

Right ventricular and PA pressures are elevated. The proportion of 'left to right shunt' can be calculated from the appropriate oxygen saturations and the pulmonary vascular resistance is estimated from the pulmonary flow and the appropriate pressures (p. 60).

Angiography

Injection of contrast into the LV demonstrates the defect.

Natural history

Seventy-five per cent of small and 10% of large VSDs close spontaneously. Others become relatively smaller. Ten per cent of large VSDs develop RV outflow tract obstruction and come to behave like Tetralogy of Fallot, the patient eventually becoming cyanosed. Ten per cent of patients with large VSDs develop progressive pulmonary vascular disease during childhood and some develop circulatory failure and may die in infancy if the defect is not closed. About 0.5% of VSDs — often small — are complicated by infective endocarditis. About 2% of VSDs develop aortic regurgitation.

Treatment

Medical

The symptoms of excessive pulmor.ary flow may be controlled temporarily with diuretics. Sucking and breathing simultaneously is difficult for a dyspnoec baby, so solids are introduced early.

Surgical

Indications for surgery

1   Large defects causing heart failure uncontrolled by diuretics are closed at any age, including early infancy.

2   Even if well tolerated, defects associated with the features of progressive pulmonary hypertension are closed to prevent end-stage pulmonary vascular disease.

3   Development of infundibular obstruction (like Tetralogy of Fallot) warrants operation.

4   Small defects are closed after an attack of infective endocarditis to prevent recurrence.

5   Subarterial defects do not close spontaneously and are closed electively to prevent aortic regurgitation.

Otherwise the patient is followed in the hope that the defect will close spontaneously.

Technique

Closure of the defect (Fig. 9.8a). The defect is closed with a patch using cardiopulmonary bypass. It is approached via the RA (through the tricuspid valve), through a right ventriculotomy or occasionally through the PA. Sutures are placed away from the nearby bundle of His to avoid producing heart block.

Pulmonary artery banding (Fig. 9.8b). In small, frail infants and sometimes in complex congenital heart disease, the pulmonary flow is restricted by constricting the PA with a strong ligature. The band is tightened sufficiently to drop the PA pressure distal to the band to about 30 mmHg. Eventually the defect must be closed and the PA debanded on cardiopulmonary bypass.

(a)   (b)

VSD   Pulmonary artery

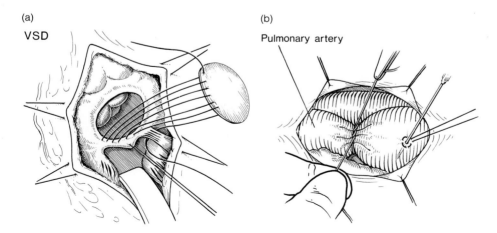

Fig. 9.8. Surgery for VSD. (a) VSD closure. (b) PA banding.

Results

Morbidity and mortality depend on the pulmonary vascular resistance, the pre-operative state of the patient and, to some extent, on the age at operation. An isolated VSD without elevation of the pulmonary vascular resistance above about 5 units is closed with a mortality below 5%.

Atrioventricular septal defect

Previously called the AV canal defect or endocardial cushion defect.

Anatomy

This consists of various combinations of: primum ASD; abnormalities of the atrioventricular valve from a 'cleft' mitral valve to a common AV valve; and inlet VSD. The 'complete' AV septal defect has an atrial component, a ventricular component and a common atrioventricular valve. It is common in patients with Down's syndrome (Trisomy 21).

Haemodynamics

The atrial and ventricular components of the defect allow a large shunt to develop when the pulmonary vascular resistance falls in early infancy. The common AV valve may become incompetent. The patients present with dyspnoea and failure to thrive in infancy. If unoperated in this phase, survivors develop pulmonary vascular disease which limits their intracardiac shunt and renders them less symptomatic for several years. The patient dies later with the Eisenmenger syndrome (p. 215).

Management (Fig. 9.9)

Surgical correction requires closure of the ASD and VSD with a patch, and reconstruction of the common AV valve to create competent 'mitral' and

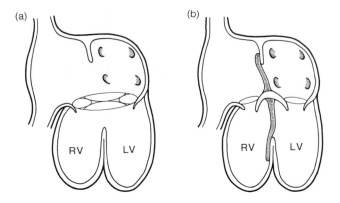

Fig. 9.9. Atrioventricular septal defect. (a) Complete. (b) Repair.

'tricuspid' valves. Surgical mortality is high, particularly if the pulmonary vascular resistance is elevated, and the risk of a residual haemodynamic defect after repair is significant.

Persistent ductus arteriosus

Foetal circulation (Fig. 9.10)

The ductus is derived from the sixth branchial arch and connects the left PA to the descending aorta.

In the foetus, oxygenated blood reaches the heart from the umbilical vein through the inferior vena cava. A flap of endocardium (the Eustachian valve of the inferior vena cava) deflects the blood across the foramen ovale into the LA. Crossing the mitral valve, it is ejected into the aorta and is distributed mainly to the head and neck.

The venous return from the head streams through the RA, across the tricuspid valve and is ejected into the main PA. The resistance of the pulmonary vasculature in the unexpanded lungs is high and most of this relatively desaturated blood arriving in the PA passes across the ductus to supply the lower body.

After birth

At birth the pulmonary vascular resistance is abruptly lowered as the lungs inflate and the ductus becomes obliterated over the next few hours or days. The duct closes by a prostaglandin dependent mechanism, the signal for closure being a

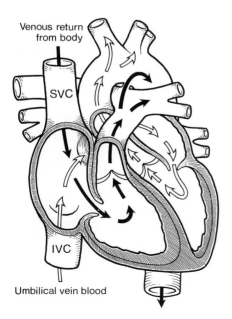

Fig. 9.10. Foetal circulation. SVC = superior vena cava. IVC = inferior vena cava.

rise in circulating oxygen levels. This 'programmed closure' is less likely to occur in very premature babies or those with perinatal asphyxia.

Haemodynamics of persistent ductus arteriosus (Fig. 9.11)

If the pulmonary vascular resistance is low, the aortic pressure exceeds the PA pressure throughout the cardiac cycle. Thus blood continually flows into the PA, returns to the LA and is ejected by the LV, a proportion then recirculating. The left heart is thus volume overloaded.

Clinical presentation

Symptoms

1   A premature baby is readily thrown into heart failure with tachypnoea and failure to thrive. If the ductus complicates the respiratory distress syndrome, it can substantially increase the work of breathing or the ventilatory requirements of the child.

2   A term baby rarely develops severe heart failure with a ductus but may be breathless with recurrent 'bronchitis' and failure to thrive.

3   Most commonly the child presents with no symptoms but with a continuous murmur.

Clinical examination

General

Normal unless the ductus is part of the rubella syndrome (cataracts, deafness, microcephaly, mental retardation).

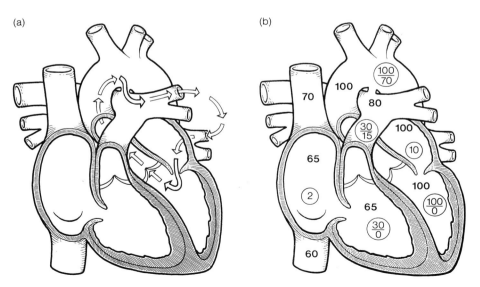

Fig. 9.11. (a) Haemodynamics of PDA. (b) Oxygen saturations and pressures (circled).

Pulse and blood pressure

Large amplitude pulse. The aortic diastolic pressure is low ('steal' from aorta into the PA) and the upstroke of the pulse sharp (large volume of blood ejected into an empty aorta).

Jugular venous pressure

Normal. There is no strain on the right heart.

Precordial impulse

Prominent apical impulse (dilated and hypertrophied LV).

Auscultation (Fig. 9.12)

Murmur of the defect. Continuous murmur, maximal under the left clavicle. With elevation of the PVR, the velocity of the left to right shunt lessens and the murmur may be confined to systole. With high PVR (Eisenmenger's syndrome) there is no shunt and no murmur.

Flow murmurs. Apical mid diastolic flow murmur (of excessive return across the mitral valve) is audible if the pulmonary blood flow is more than twice systemic.

Second sound. If the ductus is small, the diastolic pressure in the PA is low and P_2 normal and soft. The volume load of a larger ductus prolongs LV systole so that A_2 falls on P_2 and the second sound is single. Further delay of A_2 due to a large ductus causes a reversed split second heart sound (P_2 followed by A_2)

Electrocardiography

Normal or left ventricular hypertrophy, depending on duct size.

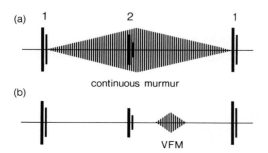

Fig. 9.12. Patent ductus arteriosus. Heart sounds and murmurs. (a) Second left intercostal space. (b) Apex. VFM = ventricular filling murmur.

Chest radiography
Dilatation of the PA, lung vessels, LA, ventricular mass and ascending aorta — due to increased flow through these structures.

Echocardiography
The ductus may be visualized. LA and LV are dilated.

Cardiac catheterization
Cardiac *catheterization* is usually not necessary to confirm the diagnosis. If performed from the femoral vein, a catheter manipulated into the PA often crosses the ductus. A 'step up' in oxygen saturations is found at PA level. The level of the PA pressure depends on the size of the shunt and the pulmonary vascular resistance.

Angiography
Blood flowing through a ductus is best visualized from an aortogram and may be the only way of demonstrating a duct when there is also a VSD partly accounting for increased oxygen saturation in the PA.

Prognosis

Small ductus
The main risk is infective endocarditis.

Large ductus
1   Can cause LV failure in infancy or occasionally later in adult life from prolonged LV overload.
2   Progressive pulmonary vascular disease.
3   Infective endocarditis.

Treatment

Medical
In the premature baby, a prostaglandin synthetase inhibitor, e.g. indomethacin, may promote duct closure.
NB In congenital lesions (e.g. pulmonary atresia) in which the circulation fails when the ductus closes, patency can be maintained by administering an infusion of prostaglandin.

Surgery
All persistent ducts are closed to prevent infective endocarditis.

Technique (Fig. 9.13)
Through a left thoracotomy the ductus is doubly ligated. Large ducts and those operated on in adult life are often divided.

(a)   (b)

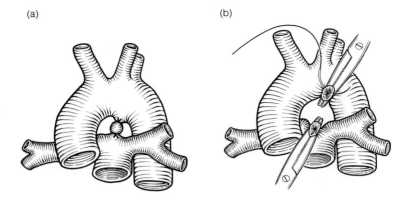

Fig. 9.13. Surgery for PDA. (a) Ligation. (b) Division.

Results
1 Mortality very low (< 0.5%)
2 Morbidity:
   (a) recanalization.
   (b) left recurrent laryngeal nerve palsy.

Other causes of a continuous murmur

Venous hum
Murmur often maximal under right clavicle, varies with position and disappears in the supine position.

Coronary-cameral fistula
A coronary artery branch empties into an adjacent cardiac cavity, commonly RA or RV. Such fistulae may close spontaneously or require surgical closure on cardiopulmonary bypass.

Aortopulmonary window (Fig. 9.14a)
Clinically similar to large ductus. The aortopulmonary communication can be big enough to equalize aortic and PA pressures and abolish the murmur. The window is visible on careful echocardiography or aortography. Patch closure requires cardiopulmonary bypass.

Sinus of Valsalva fistula (Fig. 9.14b)
Aneurysms of the aortic sinuses of Valsalva develop due to congenital deficiency of the media between the fibrous annulus of the aortic valve and the aorta itself. Occasionally they are mycotic or syphilitic in origin. The aneurysm projects into the adjacent cavity (right coronary sinus aneurysms bulge into the RV, non-coronary sinus aneurysms into the RA and the rarer left coronary sinus aneurysms into the LA). Unruptured aneurysms produce no haemodynamic disturbance.

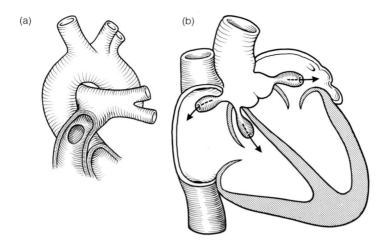

Fig. 9.14. (a) Aortopulmonary window. (b) Sinus of Valsalva fistula.

When these aneurysms rupture they produce a shunt from the aorta to the appropriate cavity with sudden cardiac failure associated with a new, typically continuous, murmur. The shunt is delineated by echocardiography and angiography and the aneurysm is excised and the aortic defect repaired surgically.

Vein of Galen fistula (and other cerebral arteriovenous malformations)
These produce a continuous murmur maximal in the head. Because of the low resistance of the fistula, the pulses are bounding and both LV and RV output high. Cause of profound heart failure in the neonate.

Systemic–pulmonary shunts
These are performed for cyanotic heart disease associated with a low pulmonary blood flow. Note the scar on the chest.

Major aortopulmonary collateral arteries
Originating in the descending aorta, these supply the pulmonary bed in some patients with pulmonary atresia and ventricular septal defect. The murmurs are widespread but maximal in the back and the child is cyanosed.

VALVE DISEASE IN CHILDREN

Congenital aortic valve disease
Aortic valve disease is most commonly congenital in origin so that patients can present in infancy (first year) or childhood. Presenting features vary with the degree of obstruction. The most severely deformed valves cause critical obstruction in the neonatal period (first month) while the least abnormal valves present with an ejection click with or without a murmur in asymptomatic children. The principles of management are discussed in Chapter 4.

Critical aortic stenosis in the neonate

A barely formed, 'mucoid' or dysplastic valve provides severe obstruction to LV ejection. At worst, perfusion of the body depends on blood reaching the aorta from the RV through the ductus. As the duct begins to close, systemic perfusion falls, the child becoming pulseless and acidotic. There may be virtually no murmur of blood crossing the stenosed aortic valve because the orifice is so small and the failing LV cannot generate sufficient power. The condition is amenable to treatment by balloon dilatation or surgery, though the mortality is high.

Hypoplastic left heart syndrome (Fig. 9.15)

The intra-uterine development of the whole left heart is disturbed, perhaps by premature closure of the foramen ovale. Though formed, the LA, mitral valve, LV and aortic root are small with survival being due to the systemic circulation *in utero* being provided mainly by the RV via the ductus. As the ductus closes after birth, the hypoplastic left heart proves too small to support the systemic circulation and systemic perfusion is lost. The condition is not usually amenable to corrective or palliative treatment.

Pulmonary valve stenosis

Aetiology

1   Almost always congenital in origin with thick deformed bicuspid or tricuspid valves. Sometimes associated with Noonan's syndrome (phenotype of Turner's syndrome, normal chromosomes).
2   Rheumatic involvement of the pulmonary valve is rare.
3   Carcinoid tumours of the small bowel with hepatic metastases are associated with acquired thickening of valves on the right side of the heart.

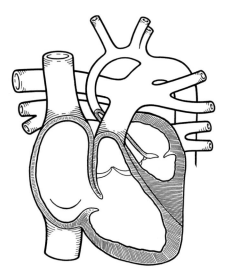

Fig. 9.15. Hypoplastic left heart syndrome.

Haemodynamics
The RV hypertrophies to overcome the obstruction to outflow. The post-stenotic dilatation of the PA distal to the valve is related to turbulence.

Clinical presentation

Symptoms
Usually asymptomatic, presenting with a murmur.

If obstruction is very severe, the cardiac output may be reduced and exertional syncope occasionally occurs.

If the obstruction is longstanding, the RV fails, requiring a high filling pressure (RA pressure).

Clinical examination

General
Normal unless Noonan's syndrome. Peripheral cyanosis in severe cases (low cardiac output).

Pulse and blood pressure
Normal.

Jugular venous pressure
Large 'a' wave (RA hypertrophy).

Cardiac impulse
Parasternal heave (RV hypertrophy), thrill in the pulmonary area.

Auscultation (Fig. 9.16 and p. 28)
- Pulmonary ejection click: the click disappears on inspiration in severe stenosis
- Loud pulmonary ejection murmur
- Second heart sound — as the obstruction progresses, RV ejection is prolonged and P_2 delayed and soft

Electrocardiogram
- P pulmonale (RA hypertrophy)
- RV hypertrophy

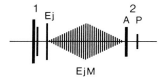

Fig. 9.16. Pulmonary valve stenosis. Heart sounds and murmurs in the pulmonary area. P_2 is delayed as stenosis becomes more severe. EjM = ejection murmur; Ej = ejection sound.

Chest radiography
- Prominent PA (post-stenotic dilatation)
- Ventricular mass is normal (unless a failing RV has dilated)
- RA dilatation

Echo/Doppler scan
The abnormal valve can be visualized and the severity of the stenosis estimated.

Treatment
Elevation of RV pressure above 60 mmHg requires treatment, even if the patient is asymptomatic.

Balloon dilatation of the pulmonary valve (Fig. 9.17)
Performed during cardiac catheterization. A wire is passed across the pulmonary valve and a balloon catheter positioned over it. The balloon is inflated, disrupting the fused commissures of the pulmonary valve and relieving the obstruction. This technique has replaced surgical pulmonary valvotomy, except in a few cases with very dysplastic valves.

Variants of pulmonary valve disease (Fig. 9.18)

Pulmonary valve stenosis with atrial septal defect
If the valve stenosis is severe and the RV very hypertrophied and stiff, desaturated blood shunts from right to left at atrial level, producing central cyanosis. On chest X-ray the lung fields are oligaemic. Repair requires cardiopulmonary bypass.

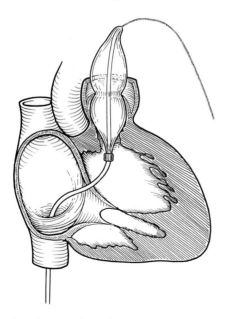

Fig. 9.17. Balloon dilatation of stenotic pulmonary valve.

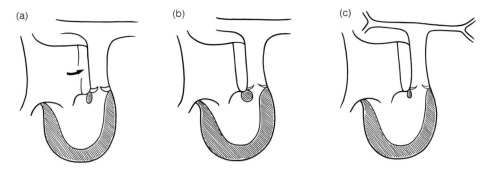

Fig. 9.18. Variants of pulmonary valve disease. (a) Pulmonary valve stenosis with ASD. (b) Pulmonary infundibular stenosis. (c) Pulmonary artery stenosis.

Pulmonary infundibular stenosis

A proportion of patients with VSD acquire pulmonary infundibular stenosis; the VSDs may then close, leaving significant infundibular obstruction alone. The presentation is similar to pulmonary valve stenosis but with no ejection click as the valve itself is normal and no post-stenotic dilatation of the PA. Surgical infundibular resection is needed if the obstruction is severe.

Pulmonary artery stenosis

Stenoses can occur in any part of the pulmonary arterial tree, most commonly at the bifurcation of the main PA or within the lung. Obstruction causes a corresponding degree of RV hypertension and, if severe or longstanding, RV failure. Intrapulmonary obstructions cannot be relieved surgically.

Associations
- *Rubella syndrome.* Cataracts; deafness; and microcephaly
- *Williams syndrome.* Supravalvar aortic stenosis; coarctation; renal artery stenosis; 'elfin facies'; hypercalcaemia; and mild mental retardation

Pulmonary regurgitation

Aetiology
- Rare congenital abnormality
- May complicate surgery to RV outflow tract (e.g. Fallot repair)
- Often present in severe pulmonary hypertension as a result of a dilated pulmonary valve ring

Natural history
When the lesion is isolated, the RV volume overload is well tolerated long term. Otherwise, the natural history is overshadowed by the associated cardiac or pulmonary vascular disease.

Differentiation from aortic regurgitation
- Absence of collapsing peripheral pulse

- RV hypertrophy and loud P_2
- In the absence of peripheral signs of aortic regurgitation or of pulmonary hypertension, the murmur is practically always due to mild aortic regurgitation

Treatment
- Congenital absence of pulmonary valve or post-valvotomy causing RV failure — homograft or xenograft valve replacement
- With irreversible pulmonary hypertension — heart and lung transplantation

Congenital mitral valve disease

Apart from AV septal defect, congenital malformations of the mitral valve are rare, though both congenital mitral valve stenosis and regurgitation can occur. Obstruction to LV inflow may also occur at supravalve level (supravalvar mitral membrane) or subvalve level (parachute mitral valve).

If one congenital malformation of the left heart is recognized, others are suspected — e.g. 'Shone syndrome', comprising supravalvar mitral stenosis, valvar or subvalvar aortic stenosis and aortic coarctation.

Congenital tricuspid valve disease

Ebstein's anomaly

Anatomy (Fig. 9.19)

The tricuspid valve is downwardly displaced into the RV, the posterior and septal leaflets being plastered down onto the RV wall. The part of the ventricle above the attachment of the valve becomes dilated and thin walled — the 'atrialized portion' of the ventricle. There is usually an ASD.

About 20% of patients have paroxysmal atrial tachycardia.

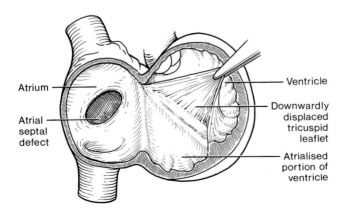

Fig. 9.19. Ebstein's anomaly.

Haemodynamics

The tricuspid valve is incompetent. In the presence of an ASD, much of the systemic venous return crosses to the LA, rather than through the inefficient right heart, causing central cyanosis.

Clinical presentation

Symptoms

Variable. Spectrum from profound cyanosis and cardiomegaly to pink with normal heart size. Some present mainly with supraventricular tachycardias.

Clinical examination

1   *General*. Cyanosis and clubbing. Usually progressive with age.
2   *Jugular venous pressure*. In the absence of an ASD, the tricuspid regurgitation causes mild elevation of the venous pressure and a systolic wave. An atrial defect, if present, decompresses the atrium.
3   *Cardiac impulse*. The LV may be hypertrophied (volume overload).
4   *Auscultation*. Split first heart sound (loud delayed tricuspid closure), split second heart sound (delayed P_2 due to right bundle branch block). There is often a tricuspid opening snap, a short ventricular filling murmur and an atrial (fourth) sound. Significant tricuspid regurgitation is accompanied by a prominent pansystolic murmur at the left sternal edge.

Electrocardiogram

Right atrial hypertrophy, right bundle branch block.

Chest radiography

Variable heart size from normal to huge.

Cardiac catheterization and angiography

Arrhythmias can make this procedure hazardous.

Prognosis

Variable; paradoxical embolism and arrhythmias are hazards.

Surgery

If symptoms are disabling, repair or prosthetic replacement of the tricuspid valve with closure of the ASD is sometimes appropriate.

COMPLEX CONGENITAL HEART DISEASE

Nomenclature of complex congenital heart disease

Even the most complex abnormalities can be described simply if a systematic approach is adopted.

The individual cardiac chambers are characterized according to their intrinsic morphology, not by their connections (e.g. a superior vena cava may be connected to a LA or an aorta to a RV). Because of their haemodynamic consequences, more attention is paid to abnormal connections (e.g. ventriculoarterial discordance) than to abnormal relations (e.g. aorta anterior to the PA).

Abnormalities of atrial arrangement are associated with structural heart disease as well as with cardiac malpositions, e.g. dextrocardia (apex of the heart in the right chest). First the atrial arrangement is described, then the atrioventricular connection, then the ventriculo-arterial connection.

Atrial arrangement (Fig. 9.20)

The right and left atria are morphologically distinct, the RA appendage having a broad base while the LA appendage is narrow and finger-like. The atrial arrangement almost always corresponds to the bronchial arrangement. The atrial arrangement may be:

1   *Situs solitus.* Usual atrial arrangement. RA on the right, LA on the left.
2   *Situs inversus.* Morphological RA on the left, LA on the right. Some patients with situs inversus have dextrocardia.
3   *Right isomerism.* Bilateral right atria (and right lungs, distinguishable on chest X-ray by the bronchial anatomy). The intra-abdominal consequences of this bilateral right sidedness is a mid-line liver and asplenia. Hearts with this atrial arrangement typically have complex congenital heart disease including anomalous *pulmonary* venous return.
4   *Left isomerism.* Bilateral left atria (and lungs). Intra-abdominally there is a mid-line liver and polysplenia. Typically these hearts have complex defects with anomalous *systemic* venous return.

Atrioventricular connection (Fig. 9.21)

The AV valve 'belongs' to its own ventricle so that a mitral valve empties into a LV and tricuspid to a RV. On angiography, the RV is trabeculated, the LV is smooth walled. Sometimes when there is only one ventricle, its morphology is indeterminate.

- *Atrioventricular concordance.* RA connects to RV, LA to LV
- *Atrioventricular discordance.* RA to LV, LA to RV
- *Absent AV connection.* Absent right (tricuspid atresia) or absent left connection (mitral atresia). When there is only one AV valve, there is only one normal-sized chamber in the ventricular mass
- *Double inlet ventricle.* If there is only one main ventricle, both AV valves may empty into it

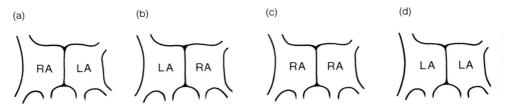

Fig. 9.20. Possible atrial arrangements. (a) Situs solitus. (b) Situs inversus. (c) Right isomerism. (d) Left isomerism.

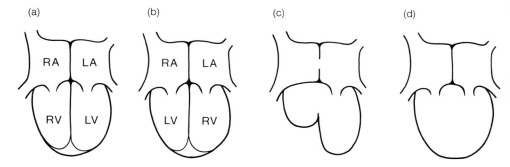

Fig. 9.21. Atrioventricular connection. (a) Concordance. (b) Discordance. (c) Absent. (d) Double inlet ventricle.

Ventriculo-arterial connection (Fig. 9.22)
- *Ventriculo-arterial concordance.* RV connects to PA, LV to aorta
- *Ventriculo-arterial discordance.* RV connects to aorta, LV to PA. Often called 'transposition'
- *Single outlet heart.* Pulmonary atresia, aortic atresia or truncus arteriosus
- *Double outlet ventricle.* Double outlet left, right or indeterminate ventricle

Once the connections are clarified, abnormal systemic or pulmonary venous return is specified, defects in the atrial and ventricular septa described and anomalies of the valves and of the great arteries listed. The position of the apex beat may also be noted (laevocardia or dextrocardia).

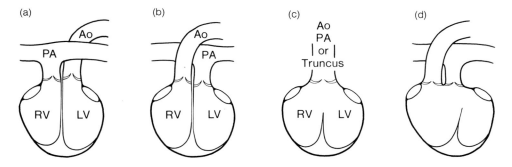

Fig. 9.22. Ventriculo-arterial (VA) connection. (a) Concordance. (b) Discordance. (c) Single outlet. (d) Double outlet. Ao = aorta.

CYANOTIC HEART DISEASE

Causes of cyanosis

A child with heart disease may be centrally cyanosed because of a shunt associated with:

Low pulmonary blood flow

There is little oxygenated blood circulating. Because they are oligaemic, the lungs are compliant and the child is not breathless at rest (e.g. any communication with associated pulmonary stenosis or atresia).

Transposition streaming

The systemic and pulmonary circulations operate in parallel, the cyanosis being mainly related to the unfavourable streaming of desaturated caval return into the aorta (e.g. transposition of the great arteries).

Intracardiac mixing of desaturated and saturated blood (so that some
desaturated blood reaches the aorta)

The level of cyanosis depends on the relative amounts of saturated and desaturated blood and hence on the pulmonary blood flow. If the pulmonary flow is high, cyanosis is mild but the child may be breathless at rest. Complete mixing can occur at atrial level (e.g. total anomalous pulmonary venous drainage), at ventricular level (all univentricular hearts) or at great artery level (e.g. truncus arteriosus).

Complications of cyanotic heart disease

- *Polycythaemia*. Mediated by hypoxic stimulus to erythropoetin production
- *Thrombosis* (e.g. cerebral). Related to polycythaemia, exacerbated by dehydration
- *Paradoxical embolism*. Intracardiac mixing gives potential for paradoxical embolism from systemic venous to systemic arterial bed
- *Cerebral abscess*. The intracardiac shunt allows bacteria from the systemic venous system to bypass the 'filter' normally offered by the lungs
- *Infective endocarditis*

Cyanotic conditions with a low pulmonary blood flow

Tetralogy of Fallot

The 'Tetralogy' consists of: VSD; overriding aorta; pulmonary stenosis; and RV hypertrophy.

Haemodynamics (Fig. 9.23)

The VSD is always large and unrestrictive so that the ventricular pressures are equal. The right ventricular outflow tract obstruction is at subvalvar (infundibular), valvar or supravalvar level and is of variable severity. The degree of right to left intracardiac shunting will increase when the systemic vascular resistance falls or the infundibular obstruction increases, e.g:

1   *Exercise*. Systemic vascular resistance falls with exercise. After exercise, the child may squat; this kinks the femoral arteries and acutely increases the systemic vascular resistance and so relieves the cyanosis.

2   *'Cyanotic spells'* correspond to an increase in infundibular obstruction. The

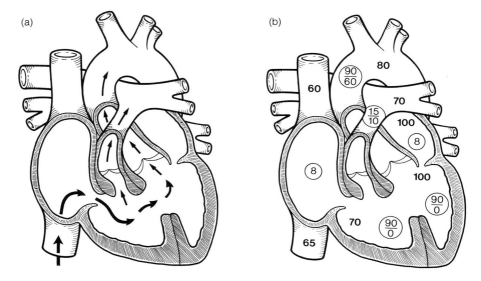

Fig. 9.23. Tetralogy of Fallot. (a) Right to left ventricular shunt. (b) Oxygen saturations and pressures (circled).

child becomes very blue, sometimes 'air hungry' and may collapse. Spells are sometimes precipitated by emotional upset and the anoxia can be severe enough to cause syncope or fits.

Clinical presentation

Symptoms

1   *Cyanosis and breathlessness.* The infundibular obstruction is usually mild at birth so it is unusual for a baby with Fallot's Tetralogy to present with cyanosis in the neonatal period. Many have overall left to right shunts at this age. Most come to notice later in the first year of life.

2   *Cyanotic attacks.* May be the presenting symptom, the child appearing pink between spells.

3   *Squatting on exercise.*

Clinical examination

General

Variable cyanosis, polycythaemia and clubbing.

Pulse and blood pressure

Normal.

Cardiac impulse

Palpable parasternal impulse (RV hypertrophy).

Auscultation (Fig. 9.24)

1 Ejection murmur of blood crossing the narrow RV outflow tract. A short murmur suggests that little blood is crossing and, in the unoperated patient, is associated with severe cyanosis.

2 Single second heart sound (aortic closure). P_2 is too late and too soft to hear.

3 There is no murmur from the VSD (too large).

Electrocardiogram

Right axis deviation and RV hypertrophy.

Chest radiography

- Normal heart size
- Pulmonary 'bay' (the normal bulge of the PA is absent because the PA, which carries little flow, is small)
- Pulmonary oligaemia (abnormally clear lung fields)
- Twenty-five per cent have a right aortic arch

Echocardiography

Shows the malformation.

Cardiac catheterization and angiography

This investigation is usually required before surgery to show the size of the PAs and to demonstrate the anatomy of the RV outflow tract. No attempt is made to enter the PA as this manoeuvre can precipitate a cyanotic spell.

Natural history

Besides being symptomatic from exercise intolerance, patients are at risk from the cerebral sequelae of cyanosis and paradoxical embolism.

Treatment

Medical

A severe spell requires treatment with agents to relax the infundibulum (e.g. propranolol or morphine) and/or to increase the systemic vascular resistance (e.g. noradrenalin). Oxygen does not help as the cyanosis is due to inadequate pulmonary flow. Cyanotic spells are prevented and treated using propranolol chronically. Persistent cyanotic spells are an indication for operation.

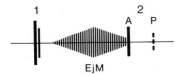

Fig. 9.24. Tetralogy of Fallot. Heart sounds and murmurs in the pulmonary area. EjM = ejection murmur.

Surgical

All patients require operation sooner or later. If they are symptomatic very early in life, a systemic to pulmonary shunt is performed.

1 *Systemic to pulmonary shunts.* All are performed through a thoracotomy incision and the shunt produces a continuous murmur.

(a) *Blalock Taussig shunt* (Fig. 9.25a). The subclavian artery is transected in the axilla, turned down and anastomosed end-to-side to the PA on that side. The arm pulse becomes absent on the side of the shunt.

(b) *Waterston shunt*. A small 'window' is made between the ascending aorta and right PA as they cross.

(c) *Pott's shunt*. Descending aorta to left PA 'window'.

2 *Total correction* (Fig. 9.25b)

(a) *Technique.* The VSD is closed with a patch so that the LV ejects only into the aorta. The RV outflow tract obstruction is relieved with another patch which may be carried across the pulmonary valve annulus if this is narrow. Such patients have pulmonary regurgitation postoperatively.

(b) *Mortality and morbidity.* Shunts are performed at low risk. In typical Fallot, mortality for total correction is about 8%.

Late morbidity relates to heart block, ventricular arrhythmias and late RV dysfunction, especially if there is residual RV outflow tract obstruction.

(a)   (b)

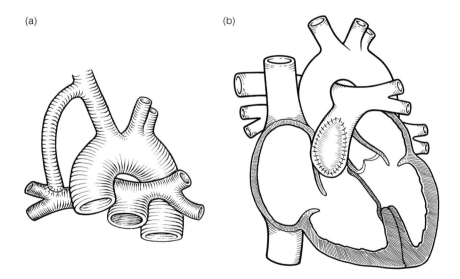

Fig. 9.25. Surgery for Tetralogy of Fallot. (a) Blalock Taussig shunt. (b) Complete repair.

Fallot variants

Pulmonary atresia with VSD

The intracardiac anatomy is similar to Fallot but there is no continuity at all between RV and main PA. Pulmonary blood supply is from a persistent duct (continuous murmur under the left clavicle) or from collaterals arising from the descending aorta (continuous murmurs maximal in the back). Correction requires a RV to PA conduit.

Absent pulmonary valve syndrome

The pulmonary valve mechanism is rudimentary, obstructive and incompetent and the pulmonary arteries hugely dilated. There is an ejection murmur and long early diastolic murmur of pulmonary regurgitation. There is typically a VSD with overriding aorta.

Pulmonary atresia with intact ventricular septum

Anatomy and haemodynamics (Fig. 9.26)

The tricuspid valve is patent but the pulmonary valve is atretic and the interventricular septum intact. Thus there is a 'way in' but no 'way out' of the RV. High RV pressures develop (e.g. 200 mmHg) and the RV muscle becomes extremely hypertrophied, encroaching on the RV cavity which becomes small. Most of the desaturated systemic venous return 'shunts' right to left at atrial level. The pulmonary blood supply depends on patency of the ductus.

Clinical presentation

The child presents in the first few days of life with cyanosis which becomes

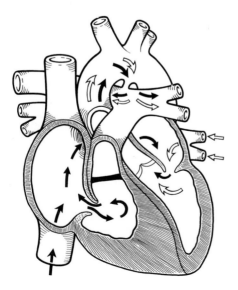

Fig. 9.26. Pulmonary atresia with intact ventricular septum. Anatomy and haemodynamics.

profound as the ductus begins to close. On auscultation a soft continuous murmur of ductal flow may be heard but, unlike pulmonary stenosis or tetralogy of Fallot, there is no ejection murmur corresponding to blood crossing a narrow RV outflow tract. The diagnosis is confirmed on two-dimensional echocardiography.

Management

- *Immediate*. A prostaglandin infusion is commenced to maintain patency of the ductus
- *Surgical*. A systemic–pulmonary shunt is performed. In some cases the atretic pulmonary valve can be excised, establishing continuity between RV and PA

Ebstein's anomaly (see p. 191.)

Pulmonary stenosis with atrial septal defect (see p. 189.)

Conditions with transposition streaming ('Transposition of the great arteries', TGA)

Situs solitus, AV concordance, ventriculo-arterial discordance. The term transposition is used because the aorta and pulmonary arteries have changed places, the aorta receiving mainly desaturated blood from the RV and the PA the mainly oxygenated blood from the LV. The systemic and pulmonary circulations function in parallel rather than in series and survival depends on there being some potential for mixing. Mixing is better at atrial than at ventricular level, better at ventricular than at great artery level.

'Simple' transposition ('Simple' implies no VSD)

Haemodynamics (Fig. 9.27)

The RV supplies the systemic circulation and thus operates at high pressure. The LV supplies the pulmonary circulation, so its pressure falls as the pulmonary vascular resistance falls postnatally. The 'unfavourable' streaming makes the infant profoundly cyanosed.

Presentation

This is the commonest cyanotic congenital heart defect presenting in the first week of life.
- *Symptoms*. The neonate is strikingly blue and management is urgent
- *Auscultation*. No murmurs, loud, single second heart sound (the aortic valve is anterior and near the stethoscope)

Electrocardiogram

Typically this is normal at presentation though the RV hypertrophy persists beyond the neonatal period.

(a)   (b)

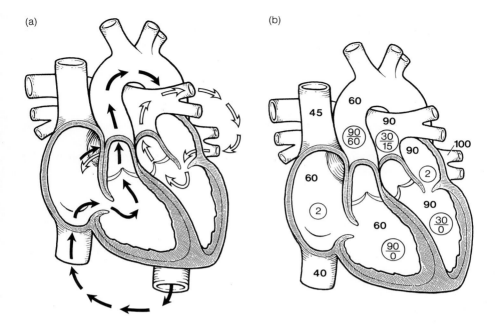

Fig. 9.27. Simple transposition. (a) Haemodynamics. (b) Oxygen saturations and pressures (circled).

Chest radiography

Cardiomegaly and plethora. This contrasts with the other large group of cyanotic neonates who have pulmonary atresia and therefore pulmonary oligaemia.

Echocardiogram

Demonstrates the aorta arising from the RV, PA from the left.

Management

Immediate

Cardiac catheterization and balloon atrial septostomy (Fig. 9.28). The first

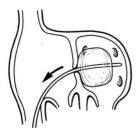

Fig. 9.28. Balloon atrial septostomy.

priority is to establish adequate intracardiac mixing by enlarging the natural patent foramen ovale into an ASD in the cardiac catheterization laboratory using a Fogarty catheter which is inflated in the LA and pulled back sharply to tear the atrial septum (balloon atrial septostomy). This improves the child sufficiently to allow him to thrive, if necessary, through the first 6 months of life.

Surgical options (Fig. 9.29)

1 *Arterial switch.* Aorta and PA are transected and reanastomosed, aorta to LV, PA to RV.

(a) *Advantages.* 'Corrective.' The LV supports the systemic circulation in the long term.

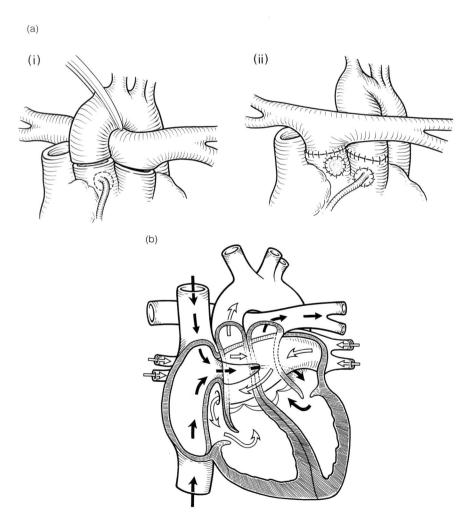

Fig. 9.29. Surgery for transposition. (a) Switch operation. (b) Interatrial repair.

(b) *Disadvantages*. Must be done in the first 2 weeks of life, before the LV regresses with the falling pulmonary vascular resistance. The coronary arteries must be transferred to the new aorta, a technically difficult manoeuvre in small babies. High early mortality, 10–30%.

2   *Interatrial repair (Mustard, Senning* operations). A 'baffle' made of pericardium or of the child's own atrial wall is created inside the atrium to divert the returning caval blood *behind* the baffle to the mitral valve and LV and PA with pulmonary venous return channelled *in front* of the baffle to the tricuspid valve, RV and aorta. The cyanosis disappears and the systemic and pulmonary circulations operate in series as normal.

(a) *Advantages*. Operation can be delayed as the LV will continue to serve the pulmonary circulation. The operation is usually undertaken at about 6 months of age. Technically easier, mortality < 2%.

(b) *Disadvantages*. The RV continues to supply the systemic circulation and there is concern that it may fail in middle age. The extensive atrial surgery is associated with chronic atrial arrhythmias.

Transposition with ventricular septal defect

The baby is not critically cyanosed at birth because of mixing at ventricular level. Surgery is needed in the first 6 months of life and involves arterial switch or interatrial repair and closure of the VSD.

Transposition with ventricular septal defect and pulmonary stenosis (Fig. 9.30a)

Cyanosis is the main problem and the child is palliated with a systemic to pulmonary shunt.

(a)   (b)

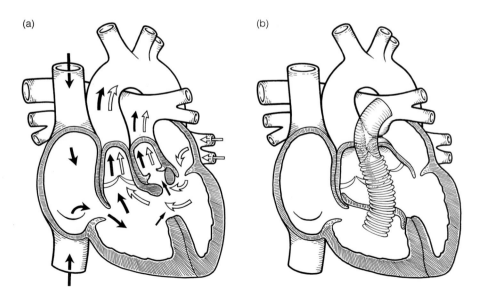

Fig. 9.30. Transposition with VSD and pulmonary stenosis. (a) Haemodynamics. (b) Rastelli operation.

Later a *Rastelli* operation (Fig. 9.30b) is performed: The VSD is closed in such a way that the LV ejects into the aorta. The proximal PA is closed and the RV is joined to the distal PA with a valved tube. In order to be able to insert an almost adult size conduit, the operation is delayed till the child is about 5 years of age.

Double outlet right ventricle (Fig. 9.31)

With subpulmonary ventricular septal defect ('Taussig Bing' anomaly)
Both great arteries arise from the RV, the posterior PA being nearer the VSD than the anterior aorta. Streaming is similar to that in transposition with VSD and management follows the same principles (closing the VSD to connect LV to PA and then performing a switch procedure).

With 'doubly committed' ventricular septal defect
Both great arteries arise from the RV, the VSD being adjacent to both arterial valves.

With subaortic VSD
Both great arteries arise from the RV, the aorta being nearer the VSD and LV. If there is subpulmonary stenosis in addition, this presents as Fallot's Tetralogy.

With 'uncommitted' ventricular septal defect
The VSD is remote from both great arteries and repair may involve an intraventricular tunnel or extracardiac conduit.

Cyanotic conditions with complete intracardiac mixing

Tricuspid atresia
Typically situs solitus, absent right AV connection, concordant ventriculo-arterial connection (about 20% have discordant ventriculo-arterial connection). The RV is rudimentary and an interatrial communication is always present.

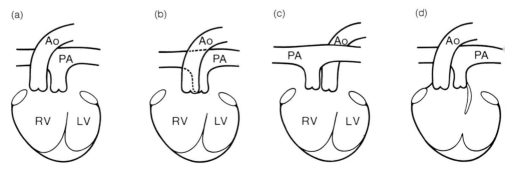

Fig. 9.31. Double outlet RV. (a) Subpulmonary VSD. (b) Doubly committed VSD. (c) Subaortic VSD. (d) Uncommitted VSD. Ao = aorta.

Haemodynamics (Fig. 9.32)

The only exit from the RA is via a patent foramen ovale or secundum ASD — an 'obligatory' right to left shunt. In ventriculo-arterial concordance (aorta from LV, PA from RV), blood reaches the RV and PA through a VSD, which is often small and limits pulmonary flow.

Clinical presentation

Low pulmonary flow

Presents with cyanosis in infancy.

High pulmonary flow (ventricular septal defect large or PA arising from left ventricle)

Though there is complete intracardiac mixing of desaturated and saturated blood, there may be so much oxygenated blood in the left heart when the pulmonary blood flow is high that the child does not appear cyanosed at all (the patient is usually clubbed).

Clinical examination

General

Cyanosis and clubbing. Dyspnoea if the pulmonary blood flow is high.

Jugular venous pressure

May be elevated. If the ASD is restrictive, the 'a' wave may be palpable in the liver.

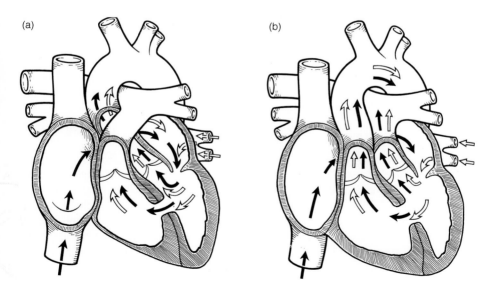

(a)　　　　　　　　　　　　　　　(b)

Fig. 9.32. Tricuspid atresia. (a) With ventriculo-arterial concordance. (b) With ventriculo-arterial discordance.

Cardiac impulse

Prominent apical impulse (LV is volume loaded and supports both the systemic and pulmonary circulations).

Auscultation

Murmur of the VSD.

Electrocardiography

The combination of left axis deviation, RA hypertrophy and LV hypertrophy is characteristic.

Chest radiography

Enlarged RA and LV. The lung fields are oligaemic or plethoric, depending on whether there is restriction to pulmonary flow.

Echocardiography

Establishes the diagnosis.

Cardiac catheterization and angiography

Shows a right to left shunt at atrial level (LA saturation less than pulmonary venous saturation). Before definitive surgery is undertaken, it is important to confirm that the PA pressure and pulmonary vascular resistance are low.

Natural history

Unpalliated, few patients survive infancy.

Surgery

Palliative

A systemic to pulmonary shunt improves the cyanosis in those with a low pulmonary flow. A PA band improves those whose main symptom is breathlessness due to excessive pulmonary flow.

Definitive (Fontan procedure — Fig. 9.33)

Since there is only one normal ventricle and atrioventricular valve, no 'corrective' operation can be offered. The patient can be rendered pink and the complications of paradoxical embolism abolished by a Fontan operation.

The ASD is closed and the RA anastomosed directly to the PA. The connection of the PA to the ventricle is closed. Desaturated blood returning via the cavae is thus carried to the PA. Oxygenated pulmonary venous blood returns to the LA and ventricle and is ejected into the aorta. There is no ventricle serving the pulmonary circulation so that after a Fontan operation the right atrial pressure is chronically elevated by an amount related to the PVR (Fig. 9.33). The operation has applications to many congenital malformations in which there is only one ventricle or only one AV valve.

(a)

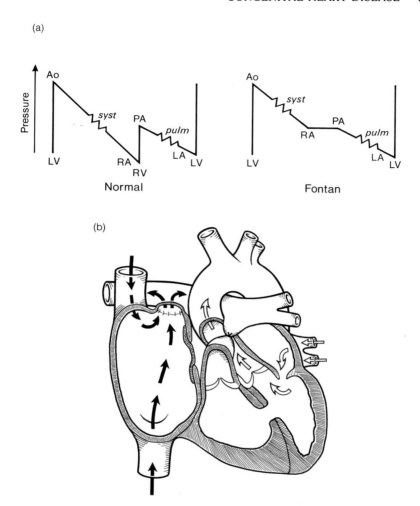

Fig. 9.33. Fontan operation for Tricuspid atresia. (a) Haemodynamics. (b) Surgery.
Ao = aorta.

Mortality and morbidity
Mortality about 30%. The long term sequelae of the high right atrial pressure are
unknown. Atrial arrhythmias may supervene.

Double inlet ventricle
Two AV valves or a 'common' atrioventricular valve emptying into a single
ventricle.
Presentation and natural history depend on associated lesions, principally the
presence of pulmonary stenosis. Palliation in early childhood is directed at
optimizing the pulmonary blood flow. Later, provided the pulmonary vascular
resistance is low, a modified Fontan operation is performed. A few patients are

suitable for a septation operation using a large patch to divide the large ventricle into two, each with an inlet atrioventricular valve. The operative risk is high.

Total anomalous pulmonary venous drainage

Anatomy (Fig. 9.34)

The pulmonary veins collect in a confluence behind the heart and then drain to the RA by one or other of the following anomalous routes:

- *Supracardiac* to the innominate vein or right superior vena cava
- *Cardiac* to the coronary sinus or RA directly
- *Infracardiac* to the portal vein or inferior vena cava

There is always an ASD.

Haemodynamics

Saturated and desaturated blood mix in the RA. Enough blood crosses the ASD to sustain the systemic output but the remainder passes into the RV and is ejected into the PA. Pulmonary blood flow can thus be very high. Sometimes the pulmonary venous return is obstructed somewhere along its abnormal pathway back to the heart, causing pulmonary oedema. If left untreated, pulmonary vascular disease develops secondary to the high pulmonary flow.

Clinical presentation

Symptoms

Usually presents in infancy with cyanosis and breathlessness.

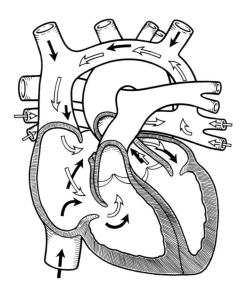

Fig. 9.34. Total anomalous pulmonary venous drainage. Haemodynamics.

Clinical examination
1   *General.* Mild cyanosis, failure to thrive.
2   *Cardiac Impulse.* RV hypertrophy (RV volume overload, later pressure overload if pulmonary vascular disease supervenes).
3   *Auscultation.* As in ASD (p. 171).

Electrocardiogram
Right axis deviation and RV hypertrophy.

Chest radiography
RA, ventricle and PA enlarged. Pulmonary plethora. Pulmonary oedema in obstructed cases. If the drainage is to the innominate (brachiocephalic) vein, the dilated ascending vein joining the pulmonary venous confluence to the innominate vein produces a characteristic shadow — 'cottage loaf' appearance.

Further investigation
Ultrasound is usually sufficient to establish the diagnosis but if cardiac catheterization is undertaken, the site of connection of the anomalous pulmonary veins is marked by a high oxygen saturation. Because of the complete mixing within the RA, the saturations in all the cardiac chambers are similar. The anomalous venous drainage is demonstrated on the venous phase of a PA angiogram.

Prognosis
Untreated, most patients die in infancy.

Surgery
A window is created between the pulmonary venous confluence and the back of the LA. The ASD is closed.

Truncus arteriosus

Anatomy (Fig. 9.35)
Situs solitus, atrioventricular concordance, single outlet heart. There is a large subtruncal VSD so that the common aortic and pulmonary trunk arises from both ventricles.

Haemodynamics
There is complete mixing of blue and red blood in the common trunk. The VSD is unrestrictive, the systolic pressure in the two ventricles and the trunk being the same. The amounts of blood flowing through the systemic and pulmonary circuits is determined by the relative resistances of the systemic and pulmonary beds. At birth, the PVR is high, the pulmonary flow relatively normal and the lesion often unrecognized. Over the next few weeks, the pulmonary resistance falls and the pulmonary flow rises, the child becoming breathless. Unoperated, pulmonary vascular disease progresses quickly, usually becoming irreversible by 18 months of age.

(a)   (b)

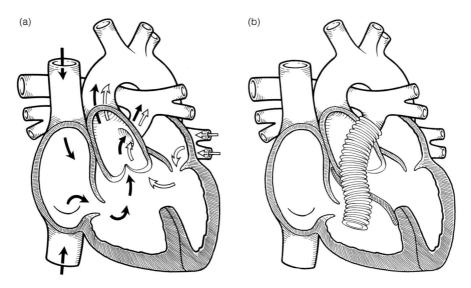

Fig. 9.35. Truncus arteriosus. (a) Haemodynamics. (b) Repair.

Clinical examination

The degree of cyanosis depends on the pulmonary blood flow and hence on the PVR. Cyanosis is mild in the phase of high pulmonary flow and heart failure. The truncal valve opening into the large trunk produces an ejection click. The second heart sound is single. When pulmonary flow is high, there is a mitral flow murmur.

Prognosis

Without surgery, most patients die in infancy. If they survive this phase, they die later of pulmonary vascular disease.

Surgery (Fig. 9.35b)

The VSD is closed so that the LV ejects into the trunk. The PA is detached from the aorta and connected to the RV with a valved extracardiac conduit. The operation is undertaken before six months of age. The mortality is above 50%. Survivors eventually need replacement of the extracardiac conduit which does not grow with the child.

OTHER CONDITIONS

Cor triatriatum

Anatomy and haemodynamics (Fig. 9.36)

A membrane divides the LA in two, typically separating the pulmonary veins from the mitral valve. A hole in the membrane ensures survival but, when this hole is small, there is severe pulmonary venous hypertension.

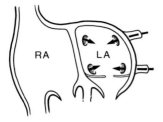

Fig. 9.36. Cor triatriatum.

Clinical presentation
Clinically, the condition simulates mitral stenosis.

Diagnosis
The membrane is well visualized with two-dimensional echocardiography.

Treatment
The membrane is excised on cardiopulmonary bypass.

'Corrected transposition'
Atrioventricular discordance, ventriculo-arterial discordance (the condition has been called isolated ventricular inversion). There are usually associated lesions e.g. VSD, pulmonary stenosis or tricuspid regurgitation.

Anatomy and haemodynamics (Fig. 9.37)
The systemic venous blood returns to the RA and passes through a mitral valve into a LV, from where it is ejected into the PA. Pulmonary venous blood returns to a LA, passes through a tricuspid valve into a RV and is ejected into the aorta. All the red and blue blood is thus delivered to the 'right place' but the function of the ventricles is inverted.

Natural history
May be completely asymptomatic in the absence of associated lesions — patients present with the associated anomalies.

About 1% per year develop complete heart block.

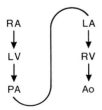

Fig. 9.37. 'Corrected transposition'. Ao = aorta.

Clinical features

These are mainly of the associated abnormalities. However:

Electrocardiography

This typically shows a qR pattern in leads V4R and V1 and absence of the normal q wave in V5 and V6. This is due to the septum being depolarised in the opposite direction to normal, related to the ventricular inversion.

Chest radiography

Typically the aorta lies to the left of the PA, forming the upper left border of the cardiac shadow.

Surgery

This is directed at the associated lesions. Most repairs leave the RV serving the systemic circulation. Late tricuspid regurgitation produces pulmonary oedema. Postoperative heart block is a hazard.

Pulmonary arteriovenous fistula

Anatomy and haemodynamics

May be part of Osler–Weber syndrome (with cutaneous vascular malformations). Pulmonary AV fistulae may be multiple, the shunt causing systemic cyanosis.

Clinical presentation

The patient presents with cyanosis or with paradoxical embolism.

On examination, cyanosis with an otherwise normal cardiovascular examination, no murmur and a normal ECG. Chest radiography sometimes shows a vascular shadow.

Treatment

Embolization of the malformation or resection of the involved lobe of the lung.

Chapter 10
The Lungs in Heart Disease; The Heart in Lung Disease

PULMONARY HYPERTENSION

Normally the pulmonary vascular bed has a very low resistance to flow through it. Moderate increases in pulmonary blood flow can be accommodated without a rise in pulmonary artery (PA) pressure because the pulmonary blood vessels dilate and previously closed channels open. Thus the PA pressure may not be raised even when cardiac output is increased to three times normal with exercise or because of a left to right shunt at atrial level (e.g. atrial septal defect — ASD).

After the first few days of life, the systolic pressure in the pulmonary artery normally falls below 30 mmHg. Pressures higher than this are defined as pulmonary hypertension. PA pressures can equal or exceed systemic levels.

Aetiology and pathology

The PA pressure may be elevated by abnormal haemodynamics but the pulmonary vasculature may accommodate the pulmonary flow passively without elevation of the pulmonary vascular resistance (passive pulmonary hypertension). However the pulmonary vasculature may itself react to vascular stresses, producing changes in the walls and later the intima of its arterioles which raise the pulmonary vascular resistance (reactive pulmonary hypertension).

Passive pulmonary hypertension

Pulmonary venous hypertension (Fig. 10.1a)

Any elevation of pulmonary venous pressure necessarily causes a parallel rise in PA pressure (e.g. associated with mitral valve disease or left ventricular failure). The PA pressure is mildly elevated but the pulmonary vascular resistance is normal.

Obligatory pulmonary hypertension (Fig. 10.1b)

The PA pressure is necessarily elevated in the presence of a large ventricular septal defect (VSD) if there is no right ventricular outflow tract obstruction. If the pulmonary vascular resistance is normal, the pulmonary blood flow (shunt) is high.

Reduction of the pulmonary bed

When two-thirds of the pulmonary bed is obliterated, the PA pressure rises. Causes of loss of pulmonary vascular bed are:

1 Recurrent pulmonary emboli. These are usually of clots from the pelvic or deep leg veins but may be of tumour particles, bilharzia ova or fat globules.

(a)   (b)

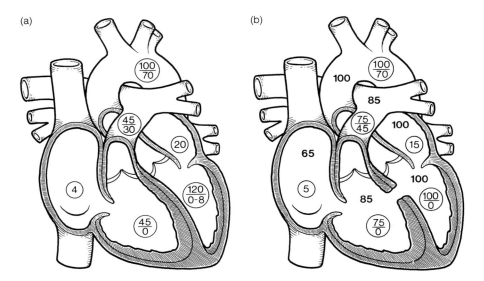

Fig. 10.1. (a) Passive pulmonary hypertension. Mitral stenosis. (b) Obligatory pulmonary hypertension. Large VSD. Oxygen saturation pressures are circled.

2 Pneumonectomy or congenital pulmonary hypoplasia.
3 Widespread destructive lung disease e.g. emphysema, extensive pulmonary fibrosis.

Reactive pulmonary hypertension

Pulmonary vascular changes are usually triggered by vascular stresses imposed on the pulmonary bed by increased pressure or flow from congenital or longstanding acquired heart disease. Early changes such as medial hypertrophy are reversible if the abnormal haemodynamics are corrected but more advanced changes such as intimal proliferation and dilatation of arteries are not, the pulmonary vascular disease becoming 'autonomous'. The pulmonary arterial pressure and pulmonary vascular resistance rise with advancing disease and any response to vasodilator therapy is lost.

Response to pulmonary venous hypertension

Some patients develop pulmonary arteriolar vasoconstriction in response to pulmonary venous hypertension so that the rise in PA pressure is out of proportion to the rise in pulmonary venous pressure and the pulmonary vascular resistance is increased. The mechanism sustaining this reactive pulmonary vasoconstriction is unclear but, when severe, it has a profound influence on the natural history of the disease. This reactive component is more commonly seen with mitral stenosis than with mitral regurgitation or left ventricular failure.

Response to high pulmonary blood flow

Occasionally patients develop a reactive pulmonary hypertension associated with high pulmonary blood flow alone (e.g. in ASD). More commonly a high PA pressure compounds the vascular stress (e.g. pulmonary vascular disease complicates the natural history of VSD more often and earlier than ASD).

Response to hypoxia

Hypoxia is a potent pulmonary vasoconstrictor. This contributes to the pulmonary hypertension of lung disease both in adults (e.g. chronic bronchitis) and children (e.g. bronchopulmonary dysplasia). Reactive pulmonary hypertension from all causes is a more 'aggressive' complication in patients living at high altitude.

Multiple defects

Some congenital defects stress the pulmonary bed by more than one mechanism so that irreversible pulmonary vascular disease is present extremely early (e.g. transposition of the great arteries with an intact atrial septum and large VSD stresses the lungs with a high pulmonary flow and pressure, pulmonary venous hypertension and hypoxia, so that irreversible pulmonary vascular disease is commonly present before the age of 1 year).

Primary pulmonary hypertension

Idiopathic. Usually affects young women or children. The pulmonary arterioles develop intimal changes, some becoming occluded, others dilated and thin walled.

Prognosis

Poor, 50% dead within 5 years of diagnosis. Some respond symptomatically to oral vasodilators e.g. nifedipine. Anticoagulation may prevent thrombosis within the damaged vascular bed. Some patients will become candidates for heart/lung transplantation.

Eisenmenger syndrome

Definition

1 The Eisenmenger complex, as originally described, consists of a large VSD with elevation of the pulmonary vascular resistance above systemic level. Under these conditions, net flow through the defect is from right to left, producing central cyanosis.

2 The definition has widened to include any connection between systemic and pulmonary circuits with pulmonary vascular disease causing reversal of the net flow and cyanosis.

Haemodynamics

Balanced shunt

When the pulmonary and systemic resistances are similar, the direction of overall shunt will fluctuate, reflecting minor changes in systemic or pulmonary vascular resistance. In general, the systemic vascular resistance is more labile, so that falls in systemic resistance — e.g. with exercise — produce right to left shunting.

There are no murmurs caused by the defect because it is large and the overall blood flow across it is small.

Shunt reversal (Fig. 10.2)

The patient becomes chronically cyanosed once the pulmonary resistance consistently exceeds systemic.

Right ventricular failure

The afterload faced by the right heart rises with the pulmonary resistance, with right ventricular failure and low cardiac output eventually appearing. The pulmonary artery and valve ring dilate and the pulmonary valve may become regurgitant. Tricuspid regurgitation may also add a volume load to the failing ventricle.

Clinical presentation

Symptoms

- Dyspnoea
- Cyanosis
- Angina (high myocardial oxygen demand but low oxygen content of blood and low cardiac output).
- Haemoptysis (often pulmonary infarction from intrapulmonary thrombosis)
- Oedema (right heart failure)
- Headache
- Menorrhagia in women (related to polycythaemia)
- Syncope

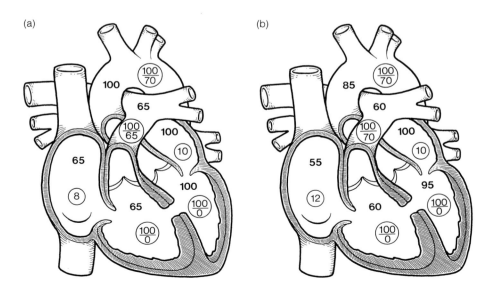

Fig. 10.2. (a) Eisenmenger syndrome. Balanced shunt. (b) Shunt reversal.

Clinical Examination

General

Polycythaemia and central cyanosis, particularly on exercise. If a persistent ductus arteriosus (PDA) is the basis of the Eisenmenger syndrome, the feet will be bluer than the hands (differential cyanosis).

Pulse

Normal or small volume (low cardiac output). Atrial fibrillation may appear late.

Jugular venous pressure

Elevated with large 'a' wave (right ventricle (RV) thick and incompliant).

Precordial impulse

Prominent left parasternal heave from RV hypertrophy. Pulmonary closure may be palpable.

Auscultation (Fig. 10.3)

The defects are large and the flow across them small, so there is no murmur corresponding to the defect itself. The audible signs are thus only those corresponding to the pulmonary hypertension.
- Right atrial fourth heart sound
- Pulmonary ejection click murmur (dilated pulmonary artery)
- Loud pulmonary component to the second heart sound (p. 30)
- Early diastolic murmur of pulmonary regurgitation (late)
- Pansystolic murmur of tricuspid regurgitation when the RV fails

Electrocardiography

P pulmonale (right atrial hypertrophy) with qRs and T wave changes of RV hypertrophy (see Chapter 14, p. 289).

Chest radiography

Large proximal pulmonary arteries (dilated under high pressure) and peripheral 'pruning' (narrow distal vessels). Large right atrium.

Cardiac catheterization

- Pulmonary artery pressure at systemic level.
- Small right to left shunt at the level of the defect.

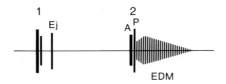

Fig. 10.3. Pulmonary hypertension with secondary pulmonary regurgitation. Heart sounds and murmurs in the pulmonary area.

Angiography is avoided. Radiographic contrast medium promotes systemic vasodilatation and a sudden increase in any right to left shunt.

Differentiation of the site of the defect
By auscultation (Fig. 10.4).

Atrial septal defect
Wide fixed split second heart sound. Severe pulmonary vascular disease is rarely seen before adult life.

Ventricular septal defect
Single second heart sound. Ventricular pressures equalize through the large defect and aortic and pulmonary valves close together.

Persistent ductus arteriosus
The second heart sound moves normally (RV ejection is prolonged by the increased venous return in inspiration, as normal). Differential cyanosis is pathognomonic.

Prognosis
The average age of death is 36 years, earlier in PDA, later in ASD. Because the placental bed lowers systemic vascular resistance, pregnancy is hazardous for patients with Eisenmenger syndrome. Death occurs from:
- *Haemoptysis* (pulmonary infarction or rupture of a bronchial vessel)
- *Arrhythmias,* sometimes related to low cardiac output and myocardial ischaemia, can cause syncope or sudden death
- Right heart failure
- Cerebral abscess and stroke from paradoxical embolism

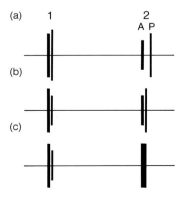

Fig. 10.4. Eisenmenger syndrome. Differentiation of the site of the defect by auscultation in the pulmonary area. (a) ASD. (b) PDA. (c) VSD.

Treatment

No drug is available which reliably lowers the pulmonary vascular resistance without also dropping systemic resistance. Surgical closure of the causative defect is usually fatal and, even if the patients survives, established pulmonary vascular disease progresses and its late consequences are not averted. Heart/lung transplantation may be appropriate.

PULMONARY EMBOLISM AND INFARCTION

Pathogenesis

Pulmonary embolism

Clot, fat or air originating at another site obstructs part or all of the pulmonary arterial tree. Pulmonary infarction does not necessarily occur because bronchial arteries from the systemic circulation maintain viability of lung tissue.

Pulmonary infarction

Necrosis of a wedge of lung tissue related to pulmonary arterial or venous occlusion. Particularly likely to occur in the presence of heart failure.

Pulmonary thrombosis

In situ thrombosis of pulmonary vascular tree.

Pulmonary embolism

A clot arises in legs or pelvic veins or in the right side of the heart (e.g. in atrial fibrillation).

Intravascular clotting is exacerbated by: stasis (bed rest, operation, obesity, heart failure); polycythaemia; dehydration; and malignant disease.

The haemodynamic effects of clot lodging in the lungs depends on the size of the clots and the time course of the vascular occlusion.

Massive pulmonary embolism

A large embolus or multiple smaller emboli block two-thirds of the pulmonary arterial tree precipitating acute right heart failure with a rise in right atrial (RA) pressure and fall in cardiac output.

Clinical presentation

Symptoms:

Syncope; sudden death; central chest pain (inadequate coronary flow, acute increase in RV myocardial oxygen demand); dyspnoea (hypoxia).

Clinical examination

- *General.* Collapsed, peripherally cool and cyanosed, dyspnoeic (low cardiac output)
- *Pulse and blood pressure.* Sinus tachycardia, hypotension

- *Jugular venous pressure*. High, but not excessively as cardiac output poor
- *Cardiac impulse*. Normal, the RV has not had time to hypertrophy
- *Heart sounds*. Pulmonary component of second heart sound loud unless cardiac output is low (pulmonary arterial hypertension) and delayed (long RV ejection time); RV third and fourth heart sounds.

Electrocardiography (*see* Chapter 14, p. 317)

Acute right heart strain: q wave and T inversion in lead III, S wave in lead I; atrial arrhythmias or sinus tachycardia; right bundle branch block; T wave inversion in lead III and anterior chest V1–4.

S–T depression in the left chest leads owing to LV ischaemia secondary to reduced blood flow.

Chest radiography

May be almost normal. Regional diminution of lung markings and enlarged proximal pulmonary arteries may be visible.

Isotope lung scan

Ventilation/perfusion scan shows a perfusion defect.

Cardiac catheterization and angiography

- Low mixed venous oxygen saturation (low cardiac output)
- Moderately elevated pulmonary artery pressure
- Angiography shows site and size of emboli

Prevention

This is more effective than treatment of established major embolism. e.g. early mobilization, elastic stockings and low dose heparin as prophylaxis around the time of elective operations.

If deep venous thrombosis is diagnosed, heparin and subsequently warfarin may prevent embolization of fresh clot.

Treatment

Medical

- Maintain high venous pressure, support myocardium with digoxin or other inotrope, e.g. isoprenaline, dopamine
- Fibrinolysis. Intravenous streptokinase or tissue plasminogen activator (TPA) accelerates natural lysis of clot
- Anticoagulation with heparin and subsequently warfarin to prevent recurrence

Surgical

Condition may warrant pulmonary embolectomy if hypotension persists and the clot is proximal. Embolectomy is ideally performed on cardiopulmonary bypass but in an emergency inflow (caval) occlusion alone can be used.

Mortality

Early mortality of massive pulmonary embolism is high (10% within 10 min, 30% within 1 hour, 60% within a few days). Survivors usually make a complete recovery, though may be at risk of recurrence.

Recurrent pulmonary emboli or thrombo-embolic pulmonary hypertension

Less severe symptoms and signs but the diagnosis suspected with any unexpected attack of dyspnoea. Recurrent emboli may be clinically silent, the patient presenting with the sequelae of widespread pulmonary vascular obstruction indistinguishable from primary pulmonary hypertension.

Clinical presentation

Symptoms

- Dyspnoea, fatigue, syncope on exertion, angina (low cardiac output)
- Ankle swelling, ascites (right heart failure)

Clinical examination

Signs of pulmonary hypertension (RV hypertrophy, loud pulmonary component of second heart sound, raised jugular venous pressure — JVP).

Chest radiography

Large proximal pulmonary artery but ischaemic peripheral lung fields.

Isotope scan

Injection of iodine 131 or chromium 51 will demonstrate patchy perfusion defects.

Prognosis

After onset of symptoms, outlook is poor (> 50% dead after 5 years).

Treatment

- Anticoagulation aimed at preventing further thrombo-embolism
- Digoxin and diuretics when right heart failure is established
- Sometimes plication, ligation or insertion of 'umbrella' in the inferior vena cava is appropriate to prevent further thrombi from reaching the lungs

Fat embolism

Aetiology and pathology

Fat embolism can occur after bone fractures or external cardiac massage. The fat emboli can provoke a florid pulmonary capillary leak, adding to the patient's respiratory distress.

Clinical presentation

- Sudden dyspnoea and chest pain with many crepitations over the lungs (systemic venous fat emboli carried to the lungs)

- Coma or disorientation (cerebral fat embolism)
- Petechial rash (emboli in the skin)
- Haematuria

Treatment

Oxygen and vasopressor drugs.

Air embolism

Aetiology and pathology

Inadvertent injection of air intravenously (15 ml/kg is necessary for the production of symptoms) or opening of a neck or cerebral vein. An air lock is caused in the right heart and obstructs the circulation.

Clinical presentation

Similar to massive pulmonary embolism but sometimes a churning murmur is audible over the right ventricle — produced by the air lock.

Treatment

The patient is nursed with the feet up and the right side up to keep air out of the right ventricular outflow tract.

Foreign body embolism

Occasionally foreign bodies such as dislodged intravenous catheters are carried to the lungs. Some can be removed transvenously with a snare under X-ray control. Others require thoracotomy for removal.

Pulmonary infarction

May follow occlusion of smaller pulmonary arteries. A wedge-shaped infarcted area develops which is often haemorrhagic because of exudation of blood from the bronchial arteries, which remain patent.
Infarction also follows pulmonary venous thrombosis.

Clinical presentation

Symptoms

Pleuritic pain (the wedge-shaped infarct reaches the pleural surface of the lung).
Haemoptysis (bronchial bleed into the infarcted area).

Clinical signs

Often negative but may be: tachypnoea (shallow breathing due to pleuritic pain); pyrexia; pleural rub (inflamed pleura); bloodstained pleural effusion.

Chest radiography

May be negative but may show patchy opacities of infarcted area(s). The diaphragm on the affected side may be raised.

Isotope scan
Demonstrates area of underperfusion.

Treatment
- Pain relief
- Anticoagulation to prevent recurrence

Pulmonary thrombosis

Aetiology and Pathology
Intravascular thrombosis occurs in areas of sluggish flow and is exacerbated if the vascular endothelium is damaged or the patient polycythaemic, e.g. some cyanotic congenital heart disease, Eisenmenger syndrome.

Treatment
Directed where possible at the cause. Polycythaemia may be improved by venesection, retransfusing with the appropriate volume of colloid. Treatment with anticoagulants may be complicated by haemoptysis.

THE HEART IN LUNG DISEASE (Cor pulmonale)
Lung disease may cause secondary heart disease (cor pulmonale) by its effects on the pulmonary vascular bed. An increase in pulmonary vascular resistance leads to pulmonary hypertension, RV hypertrophy and right heart failure.

Pathogenesis
The increase in pulmonary vascular resistance may be mediated by pulmonary arteriolar vasoconstriction (hypoxia and hypercapnia are potent pulmonary vasoconstrictors) or reduction of the total pulmonary bed by destructive lung disease. Lung diseases responsible include:

Diseases of the lower airways and alveoli
Chronic bronchitis and emphysema; pulmonary fibrosis and granulomatous infiltrations; destructive lung diseases — cystic fibrosis, bronchiectasis; and bronchopulmonary dysplasia in preterm babies surviving prolonged artificial ventilation.

Upper airway obstruction (e.g. by huge tonsils in children)

Hypoventilation
Resulting from: thoracic cage deformities — kyphoscoliosis, neuromuscular disorders (polio); and obesity with alveolar hypoventilation.

Clinical presentation (of cor pulmonale secondary to chronic bronchitis and emphysema)

Symptoms
1 *Early*. Cough and expectoration for many years, especially in winter.

2 *Intermediate.* Progressively disabling acute respiratory infections accompanied by dyspnoea and wheeze.

3 *Late.* Dyspnoea on slight exertion with peripheral oedema and central cyanosis. Cardiovascular symptoms are much worse during exacerbations of the bronchitis, because of hypoxia and hypercapnia related to the respiratory failure.

Clinical examination

General

- Laboured breathing using accessory muscles of respiration (obstructive airway disease)
- Central cyanosis (intrapulmonary shunt which is due to perfused but under-ventilated alveoli)
- Mental confusion or disorientation (hypoxia and hypercapnia)
- Warm extremities (peripheral vasodilatation related to hypercapnia)
- Peripheral oedema (salt and water retention which are due in part to RV failure)

Jugular venous pressure
Elevated when there is right heart failure.

Precordial impulse
Overexpanded lungs obscure any evidence of RV hypertrophy.

Auscultation
Faint heart sounds (overexpanded lungs). Loud pulmonary valve closure (raised pulmonary diastolic pressure). Third heart sound from a failing RV.

Lungs
Limited respiratory excursion, hyper-resonant to percussion (overinflated lungs), faint breath sounds, wheeze and prolonged expiration.

Electrocardiography (see Chapter 14, p. 289)
Normal or right atrial and RV hypertrophy.

Chest radiography
1 Evidence of emphysema — localized areas of translucency in the lung fields. Low flat diaphragms lying below the level of the seventh rib anteriorly.
2 Dilatation of the main pulmonary artery and its proximal branches (pulmonary hypertension).
3 The heart shadow is often small (low diaphragm).

Respiratory function tests
1 Forced vital capacity is reduced (high residual volume).
2 Forced expiratory volume in the first second (FEV1) is reduced below normal (obstruction to expiration).

3   Oxygen tension and saturation of the arterial blood are reduced and the carbon dioxide tension increased (respiratory failure).

Treatment

Prevention of chronic bronchitis

Cigarette-smoking plays a large part in the development of chronic bronchitis. Other factors include atmospheric pollution and dusty working environments.

Treatment of cor pulmonale

General

- Progression of the disease becomes slower if the patient stops smoking
- Prompt treatment of acute respiratory tract infections

Treatment of acute exacerbations

1   Antibiotics appropriate to the infecting organism. *Haemophilus influenzae* is often the cause of the exacerbation.

2   Oxygen by Venturi mask which delivers about 40% oxygen and does not exacerbate carbon dioxide retention.

3   Bronchodilators, e.g. ventolin inhaler, aminophylline may be effective intravenously or orally.

4   Physiotherapy to remove infected sputum.

5   Artificial ventilation may be necessary but weaning from ventilation may be prolonged and difficult. Respiratory stimulants may be of value. Sedatives such as morphine are contraindicated as the respiratory depression exacerbates respiratory insufficiency.

Treatment of heart failure

Treatment of the lungs and ensuring adequate oxygenation produces a drop in pulmonary artery pressure. Diuretics for peripheral oedema, digoxin not very effective.

Prognosis is poor once pulmonary vascular resistance is elevated.

Chapter 11
Diseases of the Pericardium; Cardiac Trauma and Tamponade

The fibrous pericardium is a thick unyielding sac which separates the heart from the surrounding organs. It is lined by a serous layer which also covers the surface of the heart (epicardium) and the proximal great vessels. The pericardial 'cavity' is thus a potential space normally containing only a few millilitres of fluid.

ACUTE PERICARDITIS

Definition
Acute inflammation of the pericardium, usually accompanied by a small pericardial effusion.

Aetiology

Infective

Viral (acute benign pericarditis)
Coxsackie virus not uncommon. Occasionally influenza or other viruses. More often the infective agent cannot be identified and a viral origin is assumed.

Tuberculous
Spread into the pericardium from contiguous tuberculous lymph nodes in the mediastinum.

Pyogenic
Following a streptococcal, staphylococcal or haemophilus septicaemia or pneumonia.

Traumatic
Recent cardiac surgery (postpericardiotomy syndrome); injury to thorax.

Systemic disease
Pericarditis is a common complication of rheumatic fever, systemic lupus erythematosus, serum sickness and polyarteritis nodosa.

Neoplastic
Invasion of the pericardium by bronchogenic carcinoma or other neoplasm. A common cause in the elderly.

Metabolic

Pericarditis due to uraemia is a common incidental finding in renal failure. Hypothyroidism is associated with a high cholesterol pericardial effusion which is usually clinically silent.

Myocardial infarction

Local pericarditis over the infarct is present in some patients with myocardial infarction. A generalized pericarditis of immunological origin may occur later (Dressler's syndrome).

Clinical presentation

Symptoms

Malaise and fever are present at the onset of the illness.

Pericardial pain. Typically sharp and aggravated by coughing, inspiration and movement, but otherwise difficult to distinguish from ischaemic pain. The site of the pain is usually central across the chest or upper abdomen, radiating to the shoulders and neck, but may be experienced only in the neck. Pain is often sensitive to position and may be relieved by sitting forwards. Pain eases as an effusion accumulates.

Clinical examination

General

Fever appears at the onset of pericarditis, unlike myocardial infarction.

Jugular venous pressure

May become elevated with the development of a pericardial effusion. Very high with tamponade.

Auscultation

Pericardial friction rub present unless the pericardial effusion is large. The friction rub is a superficial scratch, occurring with movement of the heart in atrial systole, mid-ventricular systole and the rapid filling phase. It may be quite localized or positional. It becomes louder during inspiration.

Electrocardiography

Widespread S–T segment elevation is usually present at the onset, because of epicardial involvement in the inflammatory process (Fig. 14.35). Later the T waves become inverted, an appearance which may persist for months. If an effusion accumulates, all leads generally show a low voltage but there is no alteration of QRS. With acute infarction, the S–T elevation is localized to the site of the infarct and abnormal Q waves may appear.

Chest radiography

The transverse diameter of the heart is seen to vary on serial X-rays with the development and later regression of a pericardial effusion. A pericardial effusion cannot be differentiated from cardiac enlargement from the X-ray alone as neither the configuration of the heart shadow on the X-ray nor the change in shape with varying posture is reliable in this respect.

Small bilateral pleural effusions frequently accompany a pericardial effusion.

Echocardiography

A pericardial effusion is best identified by echocardiography which demonstrates an echo-free space between epicardium and parietal pericardium (see Fig. 2.8). Thick exudate may appear as bright echoes on the pericardium.

Diagnostic aspiration

Rarely needed unless aetiology is in doubt, e.g. tuberculosis.

Biopsy

With bioptome via sheath into aspirated effusion under radiological control or at minithoracotomy. For definitive diagnosis, usually to exclude tuberculosis.

Types of pericarditis

Acute benign pericarditis (viral pericarditis)

Begins with an upper respiratory tract infection in 50% of cases. Malaise, fever, sweating and a dry cough precede the abrupt onset of pericardial pain, which is usually brief but may persist for weeks, with relapses and remissions. Pericarditis may recur weeks or months later, perhaps as an immunological reaction.

The aetiological agent is seldom identified but Coxsackie virus may be isolated from stools and peripheral blood. A rising antibody titre is a more useful test. Pericardial fluid obtained by pericardiocentesis is amber-coloured, contains lymphocytes and the virus may be isolated from it.

Postmyocardial infarction (Dressler's syndrome)

Pericarditis may follow infarction within days or months and appears to be immunological. It is suppressed by steroids but may recur. It has no prognostic significance and resembles viral pericarditis.

Tuberculous pericarditis

Pericardial involvement may occur either as an acute, exudative pericarditis, part of a 'primary response', or with granulomatous involvement. Pericardial fluid may be bloodstained, and contain acid-fast bacilli. Differential diagnosis from recurrent viral pericarditis is not easy; usually the patient is more ill with a fluctuating fever and a larger effusion but diagnosis may only be possible by pericardial biopsy. The pericardium is characteristically thick, oedematous, haemorrhagic and often adherent, with granulomas on histology, in contrast to viral pericarditis in which it is thinner and less adherent. Constriction may occur early when the disease is acute, as in Africans, or years later with calcification of the pericardium.

Pyogenic pericarditis

Usually extreme toxicity with the infecting organism isolated from blood cultures.

Traumatic pericarditis

Fever, malaise, chest pain with a pericardial friction rub and effusion following chest trauma or cardiac surgery within days or weeks. This 'postpericardiotomy syndrome' resembles viral pericarditis in its clinical features and prognosis.

Systemic diseases

Rheumatic fever (p. 64)

Pericarditis may complicate a severe attack of acute rheumatic carditis. The myocardium is usually involved and the valves always are.

Systemic lupus erythematosus

Pericarditis is occasionally the first sign of this disease. Any female patient with signs of acute pericarditis of unknown aetiology should be investigated for evidence of this disease.

Metabolic pericarditis

The occurrence of pericarditis is usually a relatively unimportant complication during the course of chronic renal failure and uraemia and only occasionally results in cardiac tamponade.

Prognosis

Acute benign (viral) pericarditis

This is generally a mild illness with no sequelae. Complications are unusual but include: *cardiac tamponade* (collection of fluid in the pericardial sac embarrassing the circulation by impeding the diastolic filling of the heart); *cardiac arrhythmias*; *recurrent attacks* of pain and pericarditis within the next 2–3 months; and *constrictive pericarditis*.

Other causes of acute pericarditis

The prognosis will depend on the severity and management of the underlying condition.

Treatment

Acute benign (viral) pericarditis (including postpericardiotomy syndrome)

1   Bed rest with mild analgesics (activity aggravates symptoms).

2   High dose aspirin (600 mg 6 hourly), or ibuprofen (200 mg 12 hourly if the patient is anticoagulated after cardiac surgery). Damps down fever and pain by anti-inflammatory and antipyretic actions.

3   Steroids (prednisone 10 mg 6 hourly) relieves fever and pericardial pain but does not shorten the course of the disease or prevent the development of large pericardial effusions. Steroids are reserved for severe cases.

4   Pericardiocentesis with aspiration of pericardial fluid may be useful in diagnosis and necessary in a small proportion of cases where the effusion is causing cardiac tamponade. The pericardium is entered by a needle passed between the xiphisternum and lower costal margin, preferably under radiographic screening control. Extrasystoles on the ECG during pericardiocentesis indicate that the needle is touching the epicardium. Insertion of an intrapericardial plastic cannula with underwater seal drainage is less likely to damage the myocardium as the effusion lessens. Dangers of pericardiocentesis include damage to coronary vessels and intensification of tamponade by bleeding from a punctured ventricle.

5   If pericardiotomy and biopsy via a limited thoracotomy has been necessary for differential diagnosis of recurrent pericarditis, as much pericardium as possible is removed. If only a small window is made in the pericardium, the edges of the incision may adhere to the heart and the effusion recur or constrictive pericarditis ensue later.

Other causes of acute pericarditis

Accurate diagnosis leads to treatment of the underlying condition in addition to symptomatic management as above.

CONSTRICTIVE PERICARDITIS (PICK'S DISEASE)

Definition

Gross fibrosis of the pericardium may follow various types of pericarditis, and restrict diastolic expansion of the ventricles.

Aetiology and pathology

Tuberculosis

Tuberculous pericarditis (either blood-borne or by direct invasion from a tuberculous mediastinal lymph node) used to be by far the most common cause of constrictive pericarditis until the advent of antituberculous chemotherapy, and is still common where tuberculosis is prevalent.

The pericardium becomes grossly thickened, fibrous, calcified and even ossified, and the inflammatory process invades the underlying myocardium which becomes atrophic. The outside of the pericardium is adherent to the lung, and tuberculous pleural thickening often coexists.

Haemorrhagic pericarditis

Fibrosis and constriction occasionally ensue.

Rarer causes

Rheumatoid pericarditis, carcinomatous invasion of the pericardium, radiotherapy of the chest.

'Atypical' constrictive pericarditis

Constrictive pericarditis can occur within a few months of non-specific (viral) pericarditis. The pericardium is less thickened and adherent than in tuberculosis, is seldom calcified, and the underlying myocardium is neither invaded nor atrophic.

Haemodynamics of constrictive pericarditis

Effect on cardiac output

Reduced cardiac output

The rigid, contracted pericardium restricts diastolic filling of the ventricles and so reduces the stroke volume and hence the cardiac output. Cardiac output can only be raised by increasing heart rate, which reduces the diastolic interval and exacerbates the fundamental filling problem.

Both ventricles constricted

Constriction of both ventricles limits right ventricular (RV) ejection and hence return to the left ventricle (LV). LA pressure does not therefore rise to high levels, dyspnoea is not a prominent symptom and paroxysmal nocturnal dyspnoea does not occur in contrast with left ventricular failure.

Pulsus paradoxus (p. 11 and Fig. 1.2)

Effect on venous pressures and pulse

Left and right atrial pressures

Both are equally raised. The wave forms of their pressure pulses are identical, (during diastole blood fills all four chambers of the heart until expansion is terminated by the rigid pericardium).

Kussmaul's sign

Normally the jugular venous pressure (JVP) falls during inspiration because the intrathoracic pressure falls, blood flow into the thorax increases and RV output rises to accommodate it. In constrictive pericarditis the JVP may rise on inspiration, probably because the constricted RV is unable to accept the increased systemic venous return.

y descent and trough (Friedreich's sign)

In classical constrictive pericarditis the dominant wave in the jugular venous pulse is a y descent. As the tricuspid valve opens, blood flows rapidly into the RV and the raised venous pressure drops sharply, only to rise again abruptly when filling ceases as the ventricle is brought up against the rigid pericardium ('square root sign'). (p. 11 and Fig. 1.8e)

Systolic descent (p. 19 and Fig. 1.8d)

Effect on auscultatory signs

Third sound

In classical constrictive pericarditis there is an early high-pitched third sound falling 0.1 s after aortic valve closure. Expansion of the ventricles is terminated sooner than usual by the constricted pericardium, and the atrioventricular (AV) valves and ventricles vibrate to produce an early third sound.

Clinical presentation of classical constrictive pericarditis (Pick's disease)

Symptoms

A previous history of tuberculosis or pericarditis is unusual. Onset of symptoms is insidious. Dyspnoea is slight. Fatigue (fixed low cardiac output), oedema and ascites (raised systemic venous pressure) are the main symptoms.

Clinical examination

Pulse and blood pressure

Pulse small (reduced pulse pressure and cardiac output) and sometimes paradoxical, almost disappearing during inspiration (increased RV filling compressing LV), irregular from atrial fibrillation in a third of cases. Low blood pressure.

Jugular venous pressure

Raised and sometimes rising further on inspiration — Kussmaul sign (RV unable to accept increased flow into thorax). Dominant wave is y descent and trough.

Cardiac impulses

Barely palpable (fibrosis around ventricles and small stroke volume). Systolic retraction at the apex is characteristic.

Auscultation

Early third sound (rapid ventricular filling abruptly halted).

Enlarged liver, ascites and oedema (raised systemic venous pressure)

Electrocardiography

Widespread T inversion (chronic pericarditis).

Chest radiography

Heart size normal or slightly enlarged (thick pericardium). Calcification in pericardium usual but not invariable.

Echocardiography

The rigid, calcified, thickened pericardium is seen.

Cardiac catheterization

Right atrial (RA) and left atrial (LA) pressures are both raised equally at rest with similar wave form and rise together on exercise (both ventricles equally constricted).

Differential diagnosis

Cardiomyopathy

Dyspnoea is greater in cardiomyopathy affecting mainly the LV: heart size is larger (failing ventricle). Echocardiography shows a thin pericardium and a dilated LV with poor ejection fraction. The LA pressure rises significantly higher than the right on exercise (RV function better than left).

Biventricular failure

Indistinguishable as both atrial and end-diastolic pressures rise equally. The greatest difficulty is in differentiating endomyocardial fibrosis when the heart may not be enlarged.

Clinical presentation of atypical (postviral) constrictive pericarditis

Symptoms and signs similar to classical Pick's disease except that it arises relatively soon after viral pericarditis; dominant descent in the jugular venous pressure is systolic (RA fills when blood is ejected from pericardial cavity); different from Pick's disease because the AV ring can move down and allow RA filling; thus no third sound; often no calcium; and pericardiectomy is simpler than in Pick's disease (myocardium not so invaded by calcium) with postoperative course smoother (good myocardium).

Treatment

Only surgical removal of the thickened pericardium is of curative value. Treatment with diuretics further decreases cardiac output.

Indications for surgery

The presence of chronically raised venous pressure which ultimately causes irreversible liver damage.

Technique

Bilateral fourth intercostal space, left thoracotomy or median sternotomy incisions are all used; mobilization and removal of pericardium from ventricles and AV groove. Antituberculous cover is not usually necessary as the tuberculous process is seldom active.

Results

Mortality (10%)
From technical difficulty (calcium and bone invading myocardium) and post-operative cardiac failure and respiratory complications (myocardium affected by disease).

Postoperative function
Higher than normal venous pressure and third sound may persist if the myocardium is badly involved, but symptoms disappear.

Reconstriction
Five to ten per cent (usually due to inadequate first operation).

CARDIAC TRAUMA AND TAMPONADE

Types of cardiac trauma

Blunt chest injury
Deceleration injuries (car and aeroplane accidents); acceleration injuries (pedestrians struck by cars); and crush injuries (e.g. weight falling on chest).

Penetrating chest injury
Stabbing, gunshot wounds, cardiac surgery.

Other causes
Perforation by cardiac catheter, pacemaker or bioptome.

Effects of trauma

Damage to functional components of the heart

Myocardium
Myocardial contusions and lacerations and damage to coronary arteries may lead to infarction.

Ventricular septum
Perforation produces a ventricular septal defect.

Valves
Rupture of valve cusps or papillary muscles may be caused by either blunt or penetrating injury.

Conduction mechanism
Heart block and other arrhythmias result.

Lacerations within the pericardium causing tamponade

Lacerations of ventricles, atria or great vessels allow rapid haemorrhage into the pericardial sac and life-threatening tamponade.

Aortic lacerations outside the pericardium

Aortic lacerations are due to blunt or penetrating injury and may be closed by clot, allowing the patient to reach hospital alive (p. 246).

Cardiac tamponade

Compression of the heart by fluid in the pericardium, which may be blood (trauma, ruptured aneurysms) or inflammatory exudate (any pericarditis).

Haemodynamics of tamponade

1 *Poor ventricular filling.* The presence of fluid in the pericardium prevents adequate filling of the ventricles during diastole. The JVP rises, the blood pressure falls and a reflex tachycardia occurs. Death ensues when the intraperi-cardial pressure reaches about 17 cm of water which may occur acutely with as little as 200 ml of pericardial fluid. In more chronic cases there is time for dilatation of the pericardium allowing large effusions to form.

2 *Systolic descent in JVP* (Fig. 1.8d)

3 *Pulsus paradoxus.* The pulse pressure markedly diminishes during inspiration (p. 11).

Clinical presentation of patient with recent cardiac trauma

Symptoms

History of recent injury.

Clinical examination

General

Evidence of a blunt or penetrating chest injury is usually but not always obtained.

Signs of haemorrhage (if the heart is lacerated)

Pallor; sweating; tachycardia; hypotension; and low JVP.

Signs of tamponade (when bleeding is into pericardium)

Tachycardia, pulsus paradoxus, hypotension, raised JVP with a systolic descent, diminished heart sounds. The diagnosis of tamponade is confirmed by pericardial aspiration.

Arrhythmias

Atrial fibrillation, heart block, ventricular extrasystoles and fibrillation can all result from cardiac injury.

Murmurs of traumatic valve incompetence and septal defects (rare)

Electrocardiography
High-peaked T waves may indicate blood in the pericardium. Changes of myocardial ischaemia and infarction may be seen. Arrhythmias are frequent. A triad virtually diagnostic of pericardial effusion is low voltage, S–T segment elevation and electrical alternans.

Chest radiography
Widening mediastinum on serial films indicates a ruptured aorta or dissecting aneurysm. Haemothorax and fractured ribs are common. CT scan confirms. Wide cardiac silhouette may indicate haemopericardium.

Echocardiography
Pericardial separation from the ventricle is seen in tamponade.

Prognosis
Sixty to seventy per cent of patients with penetrating injuries of the heart die before reaching hospital, but up to 85% of the remainder can be rescued by efficient treatment.

Treatment

Conservative management
Treatment is initially conservative.

Myocardial contusion
As for myocardial infarction (rest, sedation, etc.) Anticoagulants are contra-indicated.

Lacerations inside the pericardium
Tamponade is corrected by pericardial aspiration with a wide-bore needle or, better, plastic cannula inserted under the xiphoid process, accompanied by transfusion to replace blood loss.

Surgery

Indications for operation
1   Persistence or recurrence of signs of tamponade after one pericardial aspiration. The blood in the pericardium is often clotted (the rapid rate of bleeding prevents the defibrinating action of the beating heart) and then cannot be withdrawn through a needle.
2   Increasing widening of the mediastinum or enlarging haemothorax on serial chest X-rays (ruptured aorta).

Technique
Left anterior thoracotomy and suture of lacerations.

Results of treatment

Cardiac lacerations

Conservative management by aspiration has surprisingly been shown to have a better survival rate (up to 85% of those reaching hospital alive) than surgery, but necessarily such a series includes mainly the smaller wounds. Best results are obtained if immediate surgery is available when a single, or at the most two, pericardial aspirations fail to resuscitate the patient.

Aortic lacerations

Thirty per cent of those reaching hospital alive may survive if immediate thoracotomy and suture of the lacerations are performed.

Chapter 12
Diseases of the Thoracic Aorta

ANOMALIES OF THE AORTIC ARCH

Embryology

The six branchial arches each have an artery connecting ventral to dorsal aorta on either side of the foregut (trachea and oesophagus). The first, second and fifth arches disappear. The third arch forms the carotid arteries, the fourth arch the aortic arch and right subclavian artery, and the sixth arch the pulmonary arteries and ductus arteriosus (Fig. 12.1).

Anomalies causing obstruction to trachea and oesophagus

All the following anomalies may exist without causing obstruction. Obstruction occurs when a tight ring is formed around the trachea and oesophagus, or when an anomalous artery kinks the lumen of either.

Right aortic arch (Fig. 12.2a)

A right aortic arch alone causes no obstruction, but forms a ring when associated with a left ductus passing behind the oesophagus to the right arch.

Double aortic arch (Fig. 12.2b)

Both arches persist, one usually smaller than the other.

Aberrant subclavian artery (Fig. 12.2c)

Aberrant innominate artery (Fig. 12.2d)

Treatment is surgical division of one part of the ring, dividing the fascia accompanying it as obstruction may otherwise persist after operation.

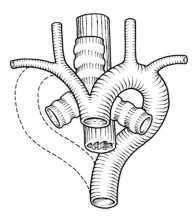

Fig. 12.1. Normal anatomy of great vessels.

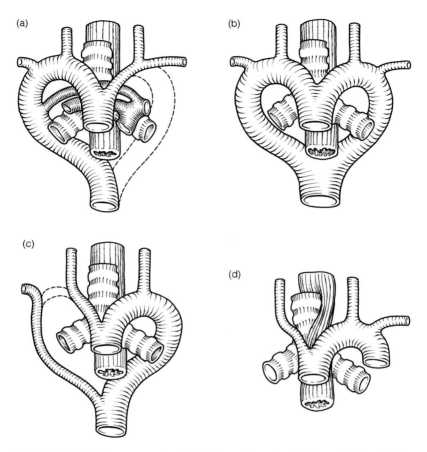

Fig. 12.2. (a) Right aortic arch. (b) Double aortic arch. (c) Aberrant left subclavian artery. (d) Aberrant innominate (brachio-cephalic) artery.

COARCTATION OF THE AORTA

Definition

Coarctation is a congenital narrowing of the aorta. In 98% of cases the coarctation is immediately distal to the origin of the left subclavian artery.

Types

Nomenclature is difficult as no recognized name embodies the essential difference between the two types, a difference that is physiological rather than anatomical:

Descending aorta supplied from the aortic arch (post-ductal, adult)

Blood reaches the lower half of the body through the coarctation and collateral vessels. If a persistent ductus arteriosus is present, blood flows from aorta to pulmonary artery regardless of the position of the ductus in relation to the coarctation. This type may present at any time from infancy to old age.

Descending aorta supplied from the pulmonary artery (preductal, infantile)

The distal aorta below the coarctation is really a continuation of the ductus arteriosus and the lower body receives venous blood from the pulmonary artery, mixed with some arterial blood flowing through the coarctation. Usually presents in infancy because it is often associated with other congenital cardiac anomalies such as a ventricular septal defect (VSD) which maintains a high pressure and oxygen saturation in the pulmonary artery, ductus and lower limbs. Little stimulus to the formation of collateral vessels.

Haemodynamics of the adult type (Fig. 12.3)

The constriction in the aorta results in the following:

Proximal hypertension

The blood pressure in the head and arms above the coarctation is elevated for reasons that are not clear. Neither the mechanical obstruction to blood flow nor the effects of a small pulse pressure on the kidneys offer adequate explanations.

Hypertension gives the left ventricle (LV) an extra work load and the increased cerebral arterial pressure predisposes to cerebral haemorrhage, particularly if there is a congenital berry aneurysm. Very high pressures occur during exertion.

Turbulence at the narrowed segment

Blood forced through the narrowed orifice causes turbulence.

Distal hypotension and delayed femoral pulses

The blood flow to the body beyond the coarctation is maintained by collateral vessels which arise above the coarctation from branches of the subclavian artery and empty into the aorta below the coarctation.

These collateral vessels are large and numerous so that the mean blood pressure distally is often normal but the pulse pressure is reduced and there is a

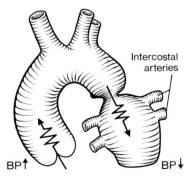

Fig. 12.3. Coarctation ('adult' type). BP = blood pressure.

delay in transmission of the pulse wave to the aorta beyond the coarctation. The first few pairs of aortic intercostal arteries carry the largest flow of blood, which makes them tortuous so that they erode the under surface of the ribs.

Associated abnormalities are a bicuspid aortic valve (60%); aortic stenosis and regurgitation; berry aneurysms on the cerebral arteries; persistent ductus arteriosus; left heart syndrome (hypoplasia of the left heart, congenital mitral stenosis, endocardial fibro-elastosis, aortic stenosis and coarctation of the aorta); and anomalous origin of subclavian arteries below the coarctation.

Clinical presentation of postductal, adult type

Usually presents as a chance finding of hypertension in the arms with a diminished and delayed femoral pulse.

Symptoms

1 Usually none (60%). The diagnosis is made at a routine medical examination.

2 Proximal hypertension may cause dyspnoea on exertion and finally frank LV failure. Cerebral arterial hypertension and cerebral aneurysms may result in cerebrovascular accidents.

3 Turbulence at an associated bicuspid aortic valve or occasionally at the narrowed segment predisposes to infective endarteritis.

4 Intermittent claudication and cold feet are not prominent symptoms because blood flow through collaterals is usually adequate below the coarctation.

Clinical examination

General

Disproportionate build with well-developed shoulders and thin legs (collateral vessels in shoulder muscles).

Pulses and blood pressure

- Brachial, suprasternal and carotid pulsation; increased amplitude with blood pressure raised
- Femoral pulses small (small pulse pressure) and delayed compared with the radial pulses (effect of constriction in the aorta and long course of pulse wave via collateral vessels)
- Palpable collateral arteries felt around the scapulae

Cardiac impulses

LV hypertrophy.

Auscultation

Aortic ejection sound and murmur in 60% (associated bicuspid aortic valve). The 'coarctation murmur' is heard at the back to the left of the vertebral column at the fourth intercostal space (turbulence at the coarctation) and may be equally loud at the front, absent if coarctation is complete.

Electrocardiography

LV hypertrophy.

Chest radiography

1 Disappearance of aortic knuckle owing to dilatation of the left subclavian artery.
2 Rib notching (collateral blood flow along the aortic intercostal arteries). Maximal in the intercostal spaces of the first intercostal arteries arising from the aorta (third, fourth and fifth).
3 Little enlargement of the cardiac shadow (LV hypertrophy rather than dilatation).
4 Computerized tomography (CT) scan shows site of coarctation.

Echocardiography

Shows a bicuspid aortic valve and the site of the coarctation.

Cardiac catheterization and angiography

Not normally necessary because the site and the severity of the coarctation are obvious on clinical grounds: the site by the position of the coarctation murmur in the back and by those ribs showing maximal notching being the ones immediately distal to the narrowing: the severity by radiofemoral diminution and delay, the presence of collateral vessels and the height of the blood pressure in the arms.

Retrograde femoral aortic catheterization, for measurement of the pressure gradient across the coarctation and aortography, is essential when the coarctation is atypical (i.e. minimal diminution and delay of the femoral pulse, suspected abnormal site of the coarctation or anomalous subclavian arteries).

Other types of coarctation

'Preductal', 'infantile' coarctation

Presentation

Commonly associated with other congenital anomalies, long atretic segments of the aorta and poor development of collateral vessels. It presents usually with heart failure in infancy, although some patients survive to older childhood.

Differential diagnosis from 'postductal' 'adult' type

• Feet may be bluer than the hands, though this sign is rarely marked because almost invariably a VSD raises the oxygen content of the blood flowing into the pulmonary artery
• Echo and angiography demonstrate the anatomy

Abdominal and lower thoracic coarctation

Two per cent of all coarctations. The coarctation murmur is low in the thorax or abdomen and on the chest X-ray the aortic knuckle is normal with rib notching affecting the lower ribs only.

Anomalous subclavian arteries

A diminished and delayed pulse in one arm compared with the other indicates a subclavian artery arising below the coarctation. Angiography confirms.

Prognosis

Ninety per cent of patients with coarctation who have not undergone an operation die before the age of 40, most commonly from cardiac failure in infancy. If they survived infancy, their average life expectancy is 33 years. Death due to the coarctation is caused by: *rupture* of the aorta (dissecting aneurysms of proximal aorta) in one-third of cases; *infective endocarditis* (usually on a bicuspid aortic valve) in one-third; or effects of systemic hypertension (*LV failure and cerebral haemorrhage*) in one-third.

Surgical treatment

Indications

All typical coarctations are recommended for surgery on diagnosis because of their poor long-term prognosis. The optimal age for operation is 7–15.

Exceptions

1 Mild coarctations (normal blood pressure and no femoral arterial delay).
2 Infancy, unless cardiac failure is unresponsive to medical treatment. The operative mortality and recurrence rate is high in infancy but the risks are justifiable in the few who do not respond to medical treatment.

Technique (Figs 12.4–12.7)

The aorta is occluded, the coarctation resected and an end-to-end anastomosis performed (Fig. 12.4). If the gap is too large, a crimped woven Dacron graft is inserted to establish continuity (Fig. 12.5) or a lateral patch used after excising the shelf of the coarctation itself (Fig. 12.6). In infants and small children the subclavian artery may be divided and turned down to bridge the opened

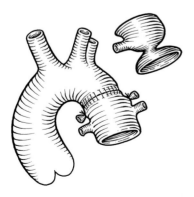

Fig. 12.4. Resection of coarctation and end-to-end anastomosis.

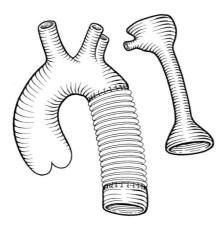

Fig. 12.5. Insertion of prosthetic graft.

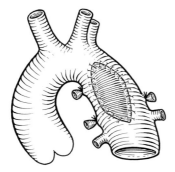

Fig. 12.6. Lateral patch.

coarctation (Fig. 12.7) — recurrence is less likely, but long term results are less satisfactory than end-to-end anastomosis.

Results

Blood pressure reduced, though not always to normal. The incidence of surgical complications varies with the age of the patient (e.g. in infancy operative mortality is 70% under 3 months and recurrence of coarctation 5%).

After infancy, mortality is 2–6% (haemorrhage and infection of the anastomosis). Morbidity is due to hypertensive crises of unknown aetiology, mesenteric arteritis due to the unaccustomed pulse pressure, recurrent nerve palsy. After lateral patch operations, aneurysms may occur at the site of the coarctation 10–15 years later.

Over 40 years of age, operative mortality 10%, almost entirely from haemorrhage but relief of symptoms and reduction of blood pressure are comparable to those under 40.

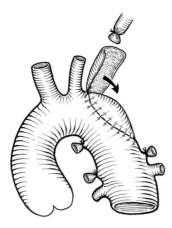

Fig. 12.7. Subclavian patch.

ANEURYSMS OF THE THORACIC AORTA

Definition
A localized dilatation of the aortic wall. Aneurysms may be subdivided for descriptive purposes into saccular, fusiform and dissecting types. Dissections (p. 249) are not localized, nor do they involve the whole aortic wall, so strictly they do not fit the definition.

Strength of normal aortic wall
The aortic wall consists of intima (endothelial lining), media (smooth muscle and elastic tissue) and adventitia (fibrous tissue). Fibrous tissue is the check fibre which resists stretch until the intraluminal pressure reaches 1000 mmHg when the aorta bursts. Sixty per cent of the tensile strength of the aorta lies in the fibrous tissue of the adventitia, the prime function of the media being to supply elasticity rather than strength.

Saccular and fusiform aneurysms

Pathology

Syphilitic
Proximal aorta: round cell infiltration and endarteritis accompanied by necrosis and fibrous tissue replacement. Saccular aneurysms begin at the inflammatory stage if endarteritis and necrosis outstrip fibrous tissue replacement in localized areas (Fig. 12.8).

Arteriosclerotic
Intimal atheromatous plaques involve the media and adventitia secondarily, weakening the aorta and producing fusiform aneurysms, usually of the descending aorta (Fig. 12.9).

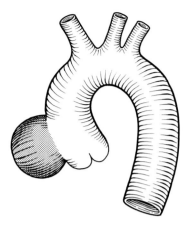

Fig. 12.8. Saccular aneurysm of ascending aorta.

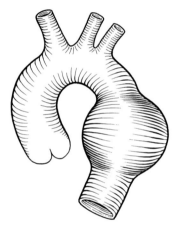

Fig. 12.9. Fusiform aneurysm of descending aorta.

Traumatic (Fig. 12.10)

The thoracic aorta is fixed to other structures at its origin, at the site of the ligamentum arteriosum, and at the diaphragm. Sudden deceleration, as in a car crash, may tear the aorta at these points when the remainder of the aorta is carried forward by the momentum of its contained blood. The aorta tears most often above the aortic valve in the pericardium when death is usually instantaneous from tamponade. Less commonly it tears at the site of insertion of the ligamentum arteriosum, when 10–20% survive with blood contained by surrounding tissues to form an aneurysm.

Other causes

Congenital, mycotic, cystic medionecrosis. The last may produce a markedly dilated ascending aorta and aortic regurgitation ('triple sinus aneurysm', 'aortic annulo-ectasia') with or without a dissection.

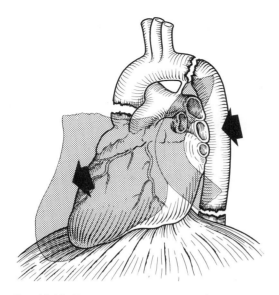

Fig. 12.10. Traumatic rupture sites in thoracic aorta.

Clinical presentation

Symptoms

Often asymptomatic (chance finding on X-ray), pressure on neighbouring structures — e.g. bronchus (pneumonia, wheeze); oesophagus (dysphagia); sternum and vertebrae (pain); and recurrent laryngeal nerve (hoarseness).

Clinical examination

Usually no abnormal signs. Visible pulsation (ascending aorta); tracheal tug (arch pushing down left main bronchus at each pulse beat), and cogwheel breathing (compression of bronchus with each pulse beat).

Chest radiography

Mass associated with aorta on postero-anterior and lateral views; CT scan with contrast shows lesion is vascular. May be confused with uncoiled aorta.

Echocardiography

Dilated aorta.

Angiography

Confirms aortic aneurysm and number of involved branches; contained clot (disparity of lumen with external dimension); and width of neck of sac.

Prognosis

Life expectancy

Fifty per cent die within 5 years from rupture, pressure on surrounding structures, and cardiac failure (from aortic regurgitation in syphilitic aneurysms and from associated coronary disease in arteriosclerotic cases).

Factors carrying a poor prognosis
   Large aneurysm causing symptoms: systemic hypertension.

Treatment

Indications for surgery
   Symptoms; large or enlarging aneurysm; embolism.

Technique

Ascending aortic aneurysm
   Cardiopulmonary bypass with cardioplegic myocardial protection. Excise and patch neck (saccular) or replace aorta (fusiform) (see Fig. 12.16b).

Aortic arch (Fig. 12.11a)
   Cardiopulmonary bypass with profound hypothermic circulatory arrest. Patch neck (saccular) or excise with graft replacement (fusiform) (Fig. 12.11b).

Descending thoracic aorta (Fig. 12.12)
   Bypass the occluded descending aorta with a heparinized plastic tube from the ascending aorta to femoral artery (Gott shunt — see Fig. 12.12a); or perfuse the femoral artery with blood from the left atrium, or from the right atrium via an oxygenator (see Fig. 12.12b).
   Excise aneurysm and replace with a graft.

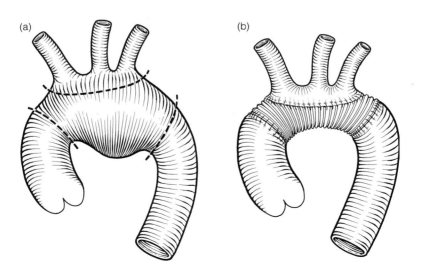

(a)   (b)

Fig. 12.11. (a) Aortic arch aneurysm — resection sites. (b) Resection and graft.

(a)
(b)

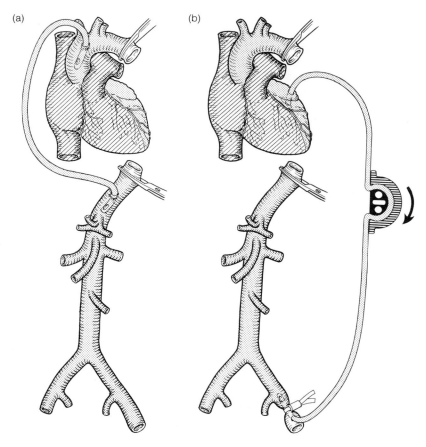

Fig. 12.12. (a). Aortofemoral shunt. (b) Left atriofemoral bypass for descending thoracic aortic aneurysms.

Results

The mortality and morbidity of surgery of aortic aneurysms have been markedly reduced by the use of profound hypothermia, prosthetic grafts which do not leak in spite of heparinization, cardioplegic myocardial protection, and glues for readhering dissections and reducing haemorrhage.

Mortality 10% (haemorrhage, cardiac and renal failure). Increased by old age, hypertension and pre-existing heart disease: paraplegia may occur from a divided spinal artery in descending aortic surgery.

Dissecting aneurysms

Pathology

Definition

The entry into and spread of blood along the media.

Aetiology

A physical change in the media allows its layers to separate easily, usually associated with cystic medial necrosis in which mucopolysaccharide is laid down between degenerating elastic fibres. Its aetiology is unknown but is associated with: Marfan's syndrome (arachnodactyly, dislocation of the lenses, high-arched palate, pigeon chest, increased carrying angle of elbows and muscular hypotonia); coarctation; and pregnancy. Often associated with systemic hypertension.

Pathology

An intimal tear allows blood to enter the media and spread along it, flattening the true lumen, occluding large branches of the aorta and shearing off small ones. The intimal tear may be initiated by a haemorrhage in the media, by an atheromatous plaque or may occur spontaneously.

Types of dissecting aneurysm

- *Type A*. The most common type, beginning in the ascending aorta and either confined to it (Type II DeBakey — Fig. 12.13) or extending round to the descending aorta (Type I DeBakey — Fig. 12.14)
- *Type B* (Type III DeBakey). Dissection begins in the descending aorta and may be confined to it or extend into the abdominal aorta (Fig. 12.15).

Clinical presentation

Symptoms

- Severe tearing pain in chest (ascending aortic dissection), back (descending) or abdomen (abdominal dissection), usually associated with collapse.
- Symptoms of infarction of organs supplied by blocked aortic branches (cerebral, spinal, renal or mesenteric arteries).

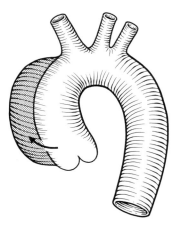

Fig. 12.13. Dissection Type A confined to ascending aorta.

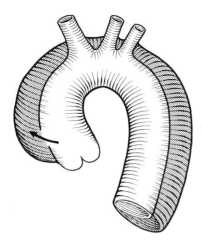

Fig. 12.14. Dissection Type A extending into descending aorta.

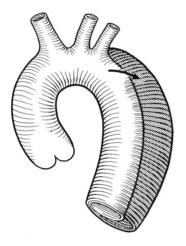

Fig. 12.15. Dissection Type B.

Clinical examination

Shocked patient in severe pain; aortic regurgitation (if dissection has detached an aortic cusp); murmurs in back or abdomen (narrowed lumen); and absent pulses in branches involved by the dissection (particularly femoral).

Electrocardiography

No typical feature. LV hypertrophy (previous systemic hypertension).

Chest radiography

Wide mediastinum: increasing width on serial radiographs is diagnostic. CT or nuclear magnetic resonance (NMR) scan shows the double lumen.

Echocardiography (transoesophageal)
Shows dilated aorta and 'shelf' separating true from false lumen.

Angiography
Confirms diagnosis and extent of aneurysm with site of the intimal tear.

Prognosis

Life expectancy
Twenty per cent die in 24 hours; 50% in 4 days; and 5 year survival rate is 1%.

Cause of death
Rupture; occluded aortic branches; or cardiac failure (aortic regurgitation).

Treatment

Indications

Type A (ascending aorta)
Acute aneurysms are treated surgically because of the risk of aortic regurgitation and blockage of cerebral vessels.

Type B (descending aorta)
Treatment is initially medical, lowering the blood pressure and reducing the rate of rise of pressure in the aorta with β-blocking agents, with surgery recommended if there is continued enlargement or extension.

Technique
Protect brain, spinal cord and myocardium (p. 249). Divide aorta at the level of the intimal tear, oversew the double lumen distally and re-anastomose the aorta, with or without a graft (Fig. 12.16).

Type A aneurysms confined to the ascending aorta are excised (Fig. 12.16a) and the ascending aorta replaced with a prosthetic graft (Fig. 12.16b). If the aortic valve is regurgitant, the prolapsing commissures are resuspended or the valve replaced, inserting the coronary ostia into the graft (Fig. 12.16c).

Type A aneurysms extending into the descending aorta are treated by dividing the ascending aorta, excising the intimal tear (Fig. 12.17a), oversewing the distal false lumen and re-anastomosing the ends to redirect blood into the true lumen (Fig. 12.17b).

Type B aneurysms are treated similarly in the descending aorta.

Results
Mortality 20%; increased by hypertension, cardiac disease, and subsequent extension of the dissection leading to rupture or blockage of vital arteries.

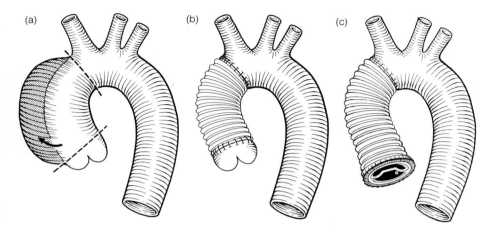

Fig. 12.16. (a) Area of resection for Type A dissection confined to ascending aorta. (b) Ascending aortic prosthetic graft. (c) Aortic valve and ascending aortic prostheses (coronary arteries subsequently attached)

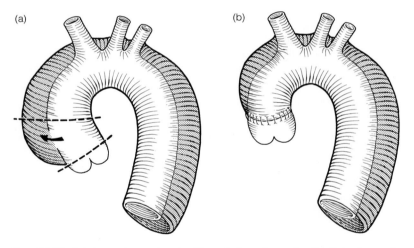

Fig. 12.17. (a) Area of resection for Type A dissection extending into descending aorta. (b) Completed anastomosis redirecting blood to true lumen.

Chapter 13
Surgery in Heart Disease

Low-risk cardiac surgery depends as much on meticulous pre-operative study and medical preparation of the patient, followed by intensive care after surgery, as on technical correction of the defect. A knowledge of the basic principles of cardiac surgery and postoperative management are nowadays necessary for anyone involved in management of cardiac patients.

INDICATIONS FOR SURGERY IN HEART DISEASE

The presence of a technically correctable cardiac lesion is an indication for surgery when:

1 Medical treatment fails to relieve symptoms. The severity of symptoms that demand an operation depends on the risks of the corrective procedure, e.g. mitral valvotomy is recommended for mild symptoms but symptoms have to be more severe before multiple valve replacement is recommended because of the greater operative mortality and long-term complications.

2 The current mortality and morbidity of surgery are less than that of the natural history of the lesion. Even if the patient is asymptomatic, ligation of a persistent ductus arteriosus is performed because the risk of the operation is lower than the risk from infective endarteritis without surgery.

CONTRA-INDICATIONS TO SURGERY

Even though the above indications apply, correction of the defect *alone* is not recommended if the situation is physiologically irrecoverable because of long-standing changes in the heart and circulation:

1 Irreparable damage to the myocardium, e.g. extensive myocardial infarction.

2 Pulmonary vascular resistance at systemic level. Closure of septal defects in the Eisenmenger situation (p. 215) is uniformly fatal.

3 Irreversible damage to other systems e.g. liver, lungs, kidneys. Despite correction of the cardiac lesion, death will occur from hepatic, respiratory and renal failure.

The feasibility of heart, heart and lung, or heart/lung/liver and kidney transplantation means that surgery for defects with myocardial damage or multi-organ involvement is no longer contra-indicated.

PHYSIOLOGICAL DISTURBANCES ASSOCIATED WITH CARDIAC SURGERY

Any operation on the heart produces temporary physiological deterioration during the postoperative period and a cardiac, pulmonary, hepatic and renal reserve is necessary for survival, however well the primary defect has been corrected.

Changes inherent in thoracotomy

A thoracic incision results in pain on breathing which in turn reduces ventilation with the danger of sputum retention, bronchial obstruction and bronchopneumonia. The vital capacity falls and underventilated alveoli cause a respiratory acidosis, ventilation–perfusion mismatch (see below) and a fall in arterial oxygen tension.

Changes inherent in cardiotomy

Opening the pericardium has no sequelae except the occasional postpericardiotomy syndrome (p. 229). An atrial incision carries little inherent morbidity unless it is made too close to the sino-atrial node when arrhythmias may follow.

Right ventriculotomy, e.g. for closure of ventricular septal defects, damages muscle fibres and right bundle branch block develops. Atrial incisions are preferred. Left ventricular (LV) incisions, e.g. for closure of postinfarct ventricular septal defects, are made through old infarcts.

Changes inherent in aortic cross-clamping

Cross-clamping the aorta is often required to obtain a still, bloodless field for accurate surgery but this renders the myocardium ischaemic. Techniques for protection of the myocardium during the period of ischaemia, e.g. cardioplegia, ameliorate later ventricular dysfunction.

Changes inherent in cardiopulmonary bypass

Blood damage

Haemolysis, denaturation of proteins and micro-embolism with particles of fibrin, fat, silicone, aggregated red cells and air bubbles occur with cardiopulmonary bypass, the effects increasing with the duration of bypass and amount of blood sucked from the heart and pericardium. Platelets are reduced in number and clotting factors diluted. Improved oxygenators with inbuilt filters have minimized this problem. Fibrinolysis may be activated. Later a normochromic, normocytic anaemia is common.

Alteration of pulmonary function

Patchy collapse of alveoli and increased stiffness of the lungs, maximal on the second postoperative day, allows shunting of pulmonary arterial blood through underventilated alveoli to the pulmonary veins, so that the arterial blood may become desaturated (ventilation–perfusion mismatch). It is of particular importance in infant lungs and is aggravated by a high left atrial (LA) pressure.

Electrolyte disturbance

Loss of potassium ions in the urine is inevitable during and after cardiopulmonary bypass if a diuresis is produced by a crystalloid prime e.g. Hartmann's solution, for the pump/oxygenator. This may critically lower the level of potassium and cause arrhythmias.

Acid–base changes

With 'normal' flows of oxygenated blood, there is little anoxia of tissues but if the output of the heart/lung machine falls or the blood is underoxygenated, metabolic acidosis occurs which may depress myocardial contractility.

PREPARATION FOR OPERATION

For surgery to have its best chance of success, the patient must reach the operating table with an accurate assessment of the underlying lesion and its complications, and in as good a circulatory condition as possible.

Accurate diagnosis

The site of the lesion, the presence of associated lesions and the severity of complicating factors such as pulmonary hypertension are elucidated before operation because diagnosis on the operating table is difficult, time-consuming and often incomplete, and, in the case of coronary disease, impossible.

General preparation of the patient

Psychological preparation of the patient and relatives is facilitated by explaining the operative and postoperative management, particularly if positive pressure ventilation is likely to be necessary. Anaemia is corrected and other coincidental diseases e.g. diabetes, controlled.

Cardiac failure is corrected or reduced to a minimum by a suitable period of rest, diet and drugs. Electrolyte imbalance is corrected. Bronchospasm, bronchial secretions and infection are controlled by admission to hospital,bronchodilators, antibiotics, physiotherapy and cessation of smoking. Operations performed within 3 weeks of smoking carry an increased morbidity.

GENERAL OPERATIVE TECHNIQUE

Anaesthesia

Anoxia or hypotension are dangerous during anaesthesia, particularly when the pulmonary vascular resistance is raised, after pulmonary embolism or in coronary artery surgery. Anoxia increases pulmonary vascular resistance and potentiates ventricular arrhythmias.

Access to the heart

A median sternotomy can be used for almost any operation, but is especially valuable for operations on the coronary arteries, ascending aorta, pulmonary artery, RV, LV, and LA. A right anterolateral incision in the fourth or fifth intercostal space may be used for cosmetic reasons for access to the right or left atrium or if the patient has had a previous median sternotomy. A similar incision on the left side can be used for a closed mitral valvotomy. A left posterolateral incision is used for access to the descending thoracic aorta and ductus arteriosus.

Access to the defect

Closed heart surgery

Intracardiac operations

A few intracardiac operations can be effectively performed by touch without the surgeon being able to see the lesion. The circulation is maintained by the patient's heart which is obstructed for a few beats during the intracardiac manoeuvre. The advantage of closed heart surgery is that it is cheap and simple, requiring only such equipment as valvotomes and dilators. Its disadvantages are inevitable inaccuracy, a greater chance of thrombo-embolism, and the limited number of lesions correctable by such crude techniques. Defects suitable for closed heart surgery are:

1 Mitral stenosis (dilated through the LV (Fig. 4.15) — rarely in Europe, USA, but frequently in Asia and Africa. Balloon angioplasty possible.
2 Stenosed aortic and pulmonary valves in small children (dilated through left or right ventricles). This operation has largely been replaced by angioplasty.
3 Transposition of the great arteries (Blalock–Hanlon palliation by making an atrial septal defect if balloon atrial septostomy fails).

Extracardiac procedures

1 Palliative operations for congenital heart disease include systemic to pulmonary shunts (Fig. 9.25a) and pulmonary artery banding (Fig. 9.8b).
2 Corrective operations for congenital heart disease include repair of aortic coarctation, ligation of persistent ductus arteriosus and division of vascular rings.
3 Pericardiectomy for constrictive pericarditis.

Open heart surgery

The defect is corrected under direct vision. The heart can be opened and a bloodless field maintained by diverting the venous return to an extra-corporeal cardiopulmonary bypass circuit and occluding the aorta.

Total circulatory arrest may be valuable in infant and aortic arch surgery. By cooling the blood in the extracorporeal circuit, the patient's temperature is reduced to 15–18°C and the pump and oxygenator are switched off. At this temperature the brain will tolerate circulatory arrest for 50–60 min.

CARDIOPULMONARY BYPASS

Technique

The heart and lungs are excluded from the circulation, their function being taken over by a pump and an artificial oxygenator. Venous blood is withdrawn by gravity through catheters in the superior and inferior venae cavae into the oxygenator from which it is pumped back into the ascending aorta — partial bypass (Fig. 13.1). When the cavae are snared tightly around the catheters, all the venous return is diverted into the oxygenator — total bypass (Fig. 13.2). The ascending aorta is clamped below the point of arterial return from the oxygenator. The heart is now dry except for blood from bronchial arteries, which returns via the pulmonary venous system to the left atrium. This is sucked out, defoamed and returned to the oxygenator. After closure of cardiac incisions, the heart is allowed to fill, the aorta is unclamped, air is removed from the cardiac chambers, the heart restarted, and finally the bypass is discontinued.

Myocardial protection

When the aorta is occluded, the heart is rendered ischaemic. The myocardium is protected from ischaemic damage by intermittently releasing the aortic clamp

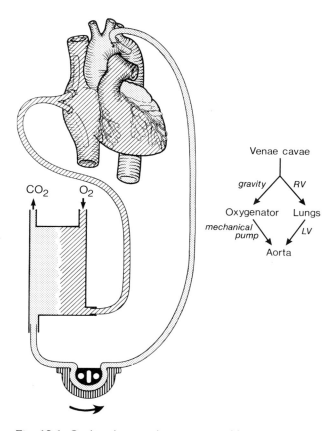

Fig. 13.1. Cardiopulmonary bypass — partial bypass.

to allow coronary perfusion (*intermittent occlusion*) or by infusing a 4°C paralysing protective solution into the coronary arteries via the ascending aorta or, in aortic valve surgery, via separate coronary cannulae (*cold cardioplegia*). The *St. Thomas' cardioplegic solution (Plegisol)*, for instance, has a high potassium and magnesium content with reduced calcium and sodium and a normal pH. With it aortic occlusion is tolerated for 2–3 hours.

Pump oxygenators

The pump used is a roller pump compressing plastic tubing containing blood. Venous blood is oxygenated by bubbling oxygen through it, defoaming the froth over silicone (*bubble oxygenators*) or keeping blood separate from oxygen by gas permeable membranes (*membrane oxygenators*).

POSTOPERATIVE MANAGEMENT

The object of postoperative management is the maintenance of a cardiac output that is adequate for tissue perfusion.

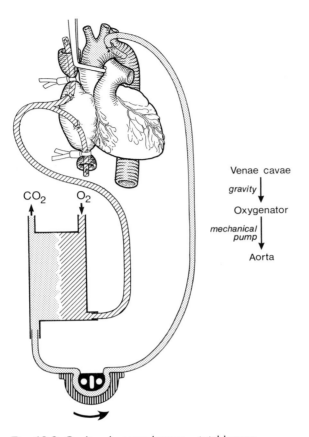

Venae cavae

gravity ↓

Oxygenator

mechanical pump ↓

Aorta

Fig. 13.2. Cardiopulmonary bypass — total bypass.

Cardiac output

The cardiac output is assessed either directly, e.g. by thermodilution methods, or indirectly from evidence of perfusion of brain (cerebral function), kidneys (hourly urine output > 0.5 ml/kg/h) and feet (warm, filled veins, palpable arterial pulses).

The cardiac output is a function of the stroke volume and the heart rate. The stroke volume is adjusted by altering the filling pressure and myocardial contractility. The heart rate is maintained with drugs or a pacemaker. If the cardiac output remains low, the afterload on the LV may be reduced with vasodilators and the effects of poor tissue perfusion are minimized by reducing the body's oxygen consumption.

Stroke volume

Filling pressure of ventricles (preload)

The filling pressure (atrial pressure) of the ventricle most under stress, e.g. LV in aortic, mitral and coronary disease, right ventricle in Tetralogy of Fallot, is raised by transfusion until the cardiac output is judged to be adequate. Further transfusion only causes pulmonary venous congestion (stiff lungs, falling Po_2) and systemic venous congestion (rising haemocrit, PCV). An LA pressure of 25 mmHg (15 mmHg from sternal angle) is the maximum which can be sustained without pulmonary oedema. Capillary leakage occurs at lower atrial pressures in infants or if the albumin level is low.

Myocardial contractility

If the cardiac output is still inadequate with optimal filling pressures, myocardial contractility can be improved by an inotrope, e.g. dopamine, isoprenaline (Isuprel), adrenaline, calcium. Metabolic acidosis, which depresses contractility, is corrected with sodium bicarbonate. Arterial blood oxygenation is maintained by keeping the lungs clear of secretions and atelectasis, and avoiding excessively high LA pressures.

Heart rate

The heart rate is kept near 100/min with isoprenaline or an atrial pacemaker (temporary pacing wires are implanted at surgery). Arrhythmia is dealt with by drugs or DC shock if interfering with function.

Reduce afterload

The peripheral resistance (afterload) is reduced with vasodilators such as sodium nitroprusside or nitroglycerine.

Prevent effects of reduced cardiac output on other organs

1 Maintain urine output — e.g. frusemide. The kidneys tolerate ischaemia better if they are producing urine.

2 Reduce oxygen consumption of body — sedate patient, use intermittent positive pressure ventilation, prevent hyperpyrexia, if necessary use muscle relaxants.

POSTOPERATIVE COMPLICATIONS OF CARDIAC SURGERY

Low cardiac output

Restlessness, cold venoconstricted extremities, peripheral cyanosis, sinus tachycardia, falling urinary output, low oxygen saturation from increased tissue extraction, and metabolic acidosis suggest that the cardiac output is low. Different causes of low cardiac output have characteristic diagnostic features.

Haemorrhage

Haemorrhage is due to inadequate surgical haemostasis or a decreased capacity of the blood to coagulate. In addition to the signs of a low cardiac output, the patient is pale and sweating, breathing rapidly, with a low venous pressure. Treatment involves transfusion of blood and correction of the cause of the haemorrhage by re-exploration of the patient for proper haemostasis or by infusion of appropriate clotting factors.

Tamponade

Tamponade is due to haemorrhage into the pericardium preventing filling of the ventricles. A low cardiac output picture is associated with pulsus paradoxus and a raised jugular venous pressure with a dominant early systolic descent. It is treated by immediate thoracotomy.

Cardiac failure

Cardiac failure may be due to myocardial damage at surgery or persistence or recurrence of defects. Severe ventricular dysfunction causes a low cardiac output, a raised jugular venous pressure, a third sound on auscultation and perhaps basal pulmonary crepitations. It is treated by adjusting the filling pressure of the ventricles (Frank Starling's law), inotropes (to improve contractility), vasodilators (to reduce afterload) and removal of the work of respiration by intermittent positive pressure ventilation. Pulmonary oedema is reduced by diuretics and a positive end-expiratory pressure on the ventilator.

If these measures fail, left ventricular dysfunction may be relieved with an intra-aortic balloon pump (IABP) inserted via the femoral artery into the descending aorta. The balloon is inflated during systole and deflated during diastole, improving blood pressure and coronary blood flow. Long-term bypass with an atraumatic pump and membrane oxygenator can be used if IABP fails.

Implantation of an artificial mechanical heart can be used as a last resort, replacing it with a transplanted donor heart if necessary.

Pulmonary hypertension

Cardiopulmonary bypass often raises further the pulmonary vascular resistance in patients with pre-operative pulmonary hypertension. Postoperative RV failure complicates the repair of some congenital cardiac defects. Most vasodilators are not 'selective' for the pulmonary circulation but tolazoline and prostacyclin are used, together with an inotrope to support the right ventricle.

Arrhythmias

Tachycardias arising from either atria or ventricles can compromise cardiac output and may require drug treatment, e.g. digoxin, verapamil, or cardioversion. Severe bradycardias are best treated with atrial or ventricular pacing via temporary epicardial wires placed at the time of surgery.

Renal failure

Oliguria following cardiac surgery is usually due to acute tubular necrosis caused by a low renal blood flow and pulse pressure. It is recognized by the passage of < 400 ml per day of poorly concentrated urine in spite of large doses of frusemide (up to 500 mg). The blood urea and serum potassium rise. Treatment involves restriction of fluid intake to 400 ml daily and reduction of the serum potassium level with ion exchange resins. Peritoneal or haemodialysis is used if conservative measures fail.

Hepatic failure

Jaundice is not uncommon after cardiac surgery, but hepatic failure is usually the late result of a low cardiac output and is often accompanied by renal failure.

Cerebral damage

Cerebral damage is due to anoxia or embolism of air, thrombus, calcium, fat or silicone and may be complicated by cerebral oedema. Cerebral damage is treated by maintaining a normal blood pressure, reducing carbon dioxide tension to around 30 mmHg with positive pressure ventilation, avoiding hyperpyrexia, and giving steroids (e.g. dexamethazone).

Respiratory failure

Respiratory complications are common after cardiopulmonary bypass which increases lung water, promoting patchy atelectasis and hence ventilation/perfusion mismatch and hypoxia. Diuretics and optimizing cardiac output improves lung compliance. Chest wall pain is controlled to enable effective physiotherapy and avoidance of hypoventilation.

VARIATIONS WITH SPECIFIC OPERATIONS

Valve surgery

Valve replacement

Preparation for surgery

Discontinue digoxin and warfarin 48 hours and diuretics 24 hours before surgery (to maintain potassium levels and avoid digitalis toxicity).

Technique

Cardiopulmonary bypass, aortic occlusion, cold cardioplegic myocardial protection, avoid air embolism.

Complications of artificial cardiac valves

NB   Cardiac valve disease is replaced with 'prosthetic valve disease'.
• *Thrombosis*. Causes valve obstruction or embolism
• *Valve failure*. Mechanical breakage (prosthesis) or tissue calcification and cusp rupture (bioprostheses)
• *Infective endocarditis*. From turbulence and prosthetic material
• *Paravalvular leak*. Technical error or due to poor tissues, e.g. calcium, active infective endocarditis
• *Obstructive gradients*. Too small a valve; occlusive ball or disc necessarily partially obstructs lumen; or tissue ingrowth of pannus onto valve ring
• Haemolysis and, rarely, jaundice

Choice of artificial cardiac valve for valve replacement

Basically this is a decision between the risks of prosthetic valve thrombosis and embolism with the necessary anticoagulation and the probability of tissue valve (bioprosthesis) deterioration.

Prosthesis

There are two types of valve:

1   Ball valve, e.g. Starr cage and silastic ball (Fig. 4.5a & b). Historically this is the most durable valve (25 years) but it is less satisfactory haemodynamically, particularly in the small ventricle and aorta.

2   Disc valve, e.g. single disc (e.g. Bjork-Shiley (Fig. 4.16)) or double disc (e.g. St. Jude). Haemodynamically better with lower embolic rate than Starr valve.

Advantages and disadvantages of a prosthesis. Potentially lasts a lifetime but lifelong anticoagulation is necessary with the risk of anticoagulant related haemorrhage; there is still a risk of valve thrombosis and embolism; it is noisy; and if it fails, it fails acutely.

Specific indications for use of a prosthesis. Child (with aspirin antiplatelet therapy or warfarin); young male adult (for its long-term function).

Bioprosthesis (tissue graft, xenograft)

Types. Porcine valve (e.g. Carpentier–Edwards; Hancock) (Fig. 4.5c) or bovine pericardium (e.g. Ionescu–Shiley) mounted on a frame and sewing ring.

Advantages and disadvantages. It is quiet; has a lower embolic rate than a prosthesis so no anticoagulants are necessary if patient is in sinus rhythm; and when it fails, it fails slowly. However, there is a sharp increase in cusp deterioration after 6 years; and it calcifies rapidly in children.

Specific indications for a bioprosthesis. Avoidance of anticoagulation, e.g. female of childbearing age: elderly over 70; patient with bleeding tendency, e.g. ulcers.

Free aortic allograft (homograft)
Preserved human aortic valve inserted without a frame.

Advantages and disadvantages. It is cheap and has the advantages of bioprostheses but it also has their disadvantages, plus it is more difficult to procure, store and insert; and the aortic wall component calcifies.

Specific indications for a homograft. Widely used as an extracardiac conduit to connect right ventricle to pulmonary artery in patients with pulmonary atresia; for cheapness in less developed countries.

Valve repair (valvoplasty)

Mitral valve

Ruptured chordae (Fig. 4.18)
- Excise redundant segment and suture edges of cusp (Fig. 4.20a)
- Support valve ring with, e.g. Carpentier–Edwards ring (Fig. 4.20b)

Rheumatic stenosis and regurgitation
- Divide fused commissures
- Mobilize posterior leaflet by dividing secondary chordae
- Adjust length of chordae
- Narrow valve ring to fit size of cusp

Tricuspid valve
- Dilated tricuspid ring — DeVega valvoplasty; double circumferential Teflon-supported suture narrows ring (Fig. 4.21)
- Organic stenosis — bicuspidize and Carpentier ring

Valvotomy

Mitral
- Closed valvotomy; in less developed countries with high rheumatic fever incidence (Fig. 4.15)
- Open valvotomy; as part of valve repair

Aortic (Fig. 4.4) **and pulmonary** (Fig. 13.3)
If balloon angioplasty fails in young patients.

Subvalve aortic stenosis
Excise stenotic ring: resect hypertrophic septal muscle (Fig. 6.6).

Supravalvar aortic stenosis
Longitudinal incision and patch (Fig. 4.6).

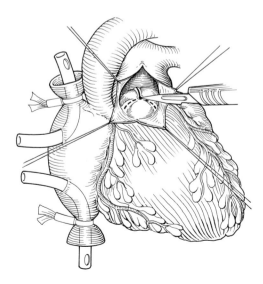

Fig. 13.3. Open pulmonary valvotomy.

Coronary artery surgery

Preparation for surgery

Beta-blocking drugs and calcium antagonists are continued up until surgery to minimize arrhythmias during induction of anaesthesia, aided by adequate premedication and a quiet anaesthetic room.

Myocardial protection

Opinions differ as to whether intermittent aortic occlusion (aortic cross-clamping for 10–15 min at a time) or cold cardioplegia is preferable. The majority of units worldwide prefer cardioplegia because of its better overall results and greater safety margin.

Technique

Coronary artery bypass grafts

Saphenous vein bypass of all significant coronary occlusions with the left internal mammary artery used for the left anterior descending coronary artery. (Fig. 5.1). The right internal mammary may be used for right or circumflex branches.

Ventricular aneurysms

Excise and suture; Teflon felt support if edges are friable (Fig. 5.2b).

Repair of congenital heart disease

Preparation for surgery

Time spent on explanations and reassurance of child and parents avoids the operation becoming a frightening experience.

Procedure

Cardiopulmonary bypass, profound hypothermia in infants, cold cardioplegia. Avoid damage to conducting system. Measure pressures postoperatively and check for residual intracardiac shunts.

Thoracic aneurysms

A temporary shunt has to be set up around the segment of aorta being resected. For details, see Chapter 12.

Cardiac transplantation

Cardiac transplantation is used in patients with irreparably damaged myocardium (e.g. extensive myocardial infarction, cardiomyopathy) and heart and lung transplantation for irreparably damaged lungs (e.g. Eisenmenger's syndrome).

Technique

The heart from a brain-dead donor is perfused with a cold preservative solution, removed, transported rapidly and re-implanted into the recipient on cardiopul-monary bypass with atrial, aortic and pulmonary arterial anastomoses. If heart and lungs are transplanted, the anastomoses are right atrial, aortic and tracheal.

Postoperative management

1   *Antirejection regime*, e.g. cyclosporine A, azothiaprine, steroids; rejection monitored by serial transvenous RV biopsies and reduced voltage on ECG.

2   *Treatment of rejection.*

(a) Acute rejection — increase antirejection regime.

(b) Chronic rejection similar to accelerated coronary artery disease but without angina (due to cardiac denervation) may require retransplant with a second donor heart.

Results

- *Survival.* One year 80%, 5 years 60%
- *Quality of life.* Greatly improved

Chapter 14
Electrocardiography

Electrocardiography is the technique of recording the electrical activity of the heart from the surface of the body. The conventional 12-lead ECG recording consists of three bipolar limb leads (I, II and III), three unipolar limb leads (aVR, aVL and aVF) and six unipolar precordial leads (V1 to V6). The unipolar leads are termed 'voltage' leads since the connections are so arranged that they effectively measure the voltage at one recording position — right arm, left arm, foot (left leg), or precordial location — compared with a reference voltage which is the sum of voltage recordings from around the heart and is close to zero. These 'voltage' leads are termed 'V' leads. In the case of the unipolar limb leads the voltages are augmented automatically to produce larger deflections and hence the augmented lead VR is referred to as 'aVR', VL as 'aVL' and VF as 'aVF'.

The bipolar leads I, II and III assess the voltage differences between two limb electrodes. Lead I is the result of connecting the left arm (LA) to the positive terminal and the right arm (RA) to the negative terminal. Similarly lead II connects RA to the positive and F (the 'foot' lead, i.e. the left leg) to the negative terminal. Lead III connects F to the positive and RA to the negative terminal. The limb leads (which are remote from the heart) are arranged in the frontal plane of the body and the precordial leads (which are close to the heart, and therefore usually of higher, voltage) are in the horizontal plane (Fig. 14.1).

THE NORMAL ELECTROCARDIOGRAM

The basic electrocardiographic wave form

The basic ECG wave form consists of three recognizable deflections, labelled 'P', 'QRS' and 'T' (Fig. 14.2). The most obvious deflection is usually the QRS complex which has the highest frequency components (i.e. is sharp and spiky). *The QRS complex is the surface electrocardiographic manifestation of ventricular myocardial depolarization.* After each QRS complex there is a rounded wave called the *T wave which is the surface electrocardiographic manifestation of ventricular myocardial repolarization.* The gap between the end of the QRS complex and the beginning of the T wave is the *S–T segment which is also part of the repolarization process.* A small, brief, rounded wave *(the P wave)* precedes each QRS complex and is *the surface electrocardiographic manifestation of atrial myocardial depolarization.* Atrial myocardial *repolarization* follows each atrial myocardial depolarization producing a small (often difficult to see) wave called the Ta wave. This inconspicuous wave is often obscured by the much larger QRS complex which tends to occur about the same time (Fig. 14.3). The Ta wave usually increases in magnitude during sinus tachycardia (Fig. 14.4).

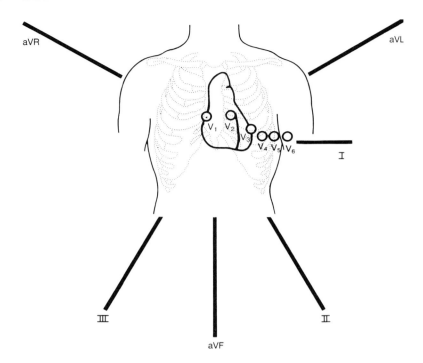

Fig. 14.1. Arrangement of the 12 conventional ECG recording leads. The limb leads are remote from the heart and are arranged in a frontal plane. The precordial leads are close to the heart and are arranged in the horizontal plane.

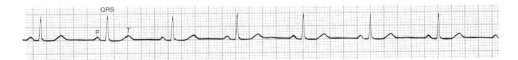

Fig. 14.2. The normal ECG.

This prominent Ta wave is often mistaken for ischaemia S–T segment depression during an exercise stress test (see Fig. 2.1). The main distinguishing point is that the Ta wave begins *before* the QRS complex although it is more obvious following the QRS complex. In most ECG's a small, very low voltage deflection (the U wave) occurs at the end of the T wave and appears to be attached to it and is part of the repolarization process.

The normal rhythm of the heart

The rhythm of the heart is the ordered sequence of depolarization of the myocardium. Rhythm analysis involves the analysis of P waves (atrial myocardial depolarization) and QRS complexes (ventricular myocardial depolarization) with respect to time, to each other and to space (i.e. the timing sequence and orientation of the waves). Figure 14.2 shows an example of sinus rhythm. The P, QRS and T waves follow each other in ordered, regular sequence.

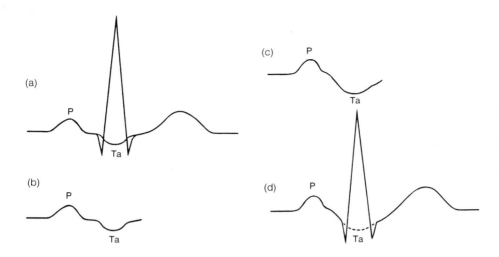

Fig. 14.3. S–T depression in a normal subject due to prominent Ta wave. (a) Atrial depolarization (P wave) and repolarization (Ta wave). (b) The normal 'atrial ECG'. (QRS removed for clarity.) (c) A prominent Ta wave. (d) Prominent Ta wave which is, as usual, partly obscured by the QRS complex. At first sight there is S–T segment depression. More careful inspection reveals that the depression begins before the QRS complex. It therefore cannot be S–T depression. It is a prominent Ta wave.

The pacemaker and conducting tissue (Fig. 14.5)

Normal atrial and ventricular myocardium are incapable of spontaneous depolarization, and myocardial depolarization is induced by specific cells within the heart (the pacemaker and conducting tissue) which have the property of *rhythmicity* i.e. unless they are prematurely activated or modulated by some other cell or agent they self-activate at regular intervals.

The sino-atrial node is a macroscopically visible structure lying within the subendocardial surface of the right atrium, close to the mouth of the superior vena cava. The *atrioventricular (AV) node* is also macroscopic and situated subendocardially in the right atrium close to the tricuspid valve orifice. From the inferior extremity of the AV node, fibres (bundle of His) pass down to the upper part of the interventricular septum. At its lowest point the His bundle divides into *right and left bundle branches* which ultimately spread into a fine arborization, *the Purkinje network*, which spreads over the subendocardial surface of each ventricle. All parts of the atrial myocardium are in electrical continuity with all other parts of atrial myocardium and all parts of the ventricular myocardium are in electrical continuity with all other parts of that myocardium. However, the atrial myocardium is separated from the ventricular myocardium by the non-conducting fibrous AV annulus. This annulus effectively prevents any electrical continuity between atrial and ventricular myocardium. It is pierced by the bundle of His which, under normal circumstances, provides the only electrical continuity between atrial and ventricular myocardium.

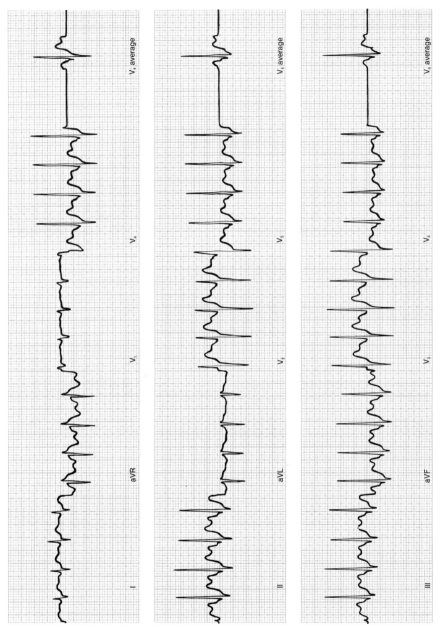

Fig. 14.4. Exercise ECG in a normal subject. Apparent S–T depression which is due to prominent Ta wave. Note that the S–T depression is upsloping (horizontal in ischaemia) and accompanied by P–R depression.

Polarization and depolarization

The cells within the heart (both the myocardial tissue and pacemaker tissue) have complex semi-permeable membranes. In the resting state each cell is *polarized*, the inside having a greater negative charge than the outside, and this state is known as *polarization*. When a cell (myocardium or pacemaker tissue) is activated, the inside of the cell becomes transiently more positive than the outside. This state is known as *depolarization* and is always followed by repolarization. The voltage–time diagram which describes the process of depolarization (which is spontaneous for the active pacemaker cells of the heart and has to be induced for myocardium) is called the *action potential*. The resting, polarized voltage of myocardium is called the *resting membrane potential*. Figure 14.6 shows a typical action potential for a myocardial cell (a) and for a pacemaker cell (b). Note that the absence of a true resting membrane potential for the pacemaker cell gives it the intrinsic property of rhythmicity.

Refractory period

Once a cell (myocardial or pacemaker tissue) is depolarized (i.e. after the upstroke of an action potential) the cell becomes insensitive to further stimulation until the repolarization process is substantially or totally complete. The non-responsive period is called the *refractory period*. The *absolute refractory period*, during which no further response is possible, however great the applied stimulus, lasts from the upstroke of the action potential to the mid-point of the downstroke. The final part of the downstroke of the action potential (extending to the point at which the resting membrane potential is fully restored) is called the *relative refractory period*. During this period a further depolarization can be induced if the applied stimulus is significantly more

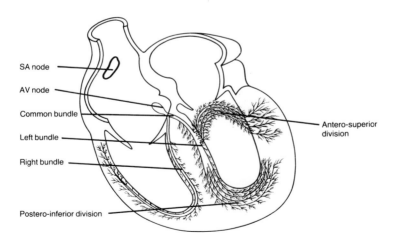

Fig. 14.5. The anatomy of the pacemaking and conduction tissues. The sino-atrial node and the AV node (AV junction) lie in the right atrium. The common bundle (bundle of His) perforates the central fibrous body to reach the interventricular septum, where if divides into the right and left bundle branches. From these the Prukinje network arises.

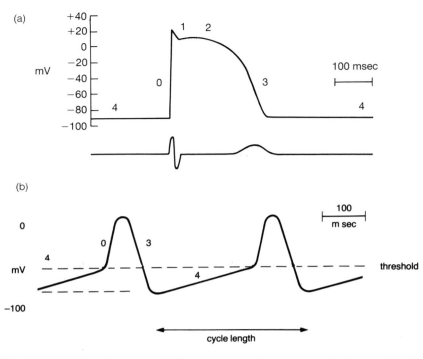

Fig. 14.6. (a) The action potential. The resting membrane potential is about − 90 mV. The onset of depolarization (Phase 0) does not occur spontaneously but must be induced. This induced depolarization (which gives rise to a 'partial reverse polarization' with the inside of the cell transiently becoming somewhat positive with respect to the outside) is inevitably followed spontaneously by the slow and complex process of repolarization (Phases 1, 2 and 3) before the resting potential (Phase 4) is restored. (b) The action potential of a pacemaker cell. Once the threshold level is reached spontaneous depolarization (Phase 0) occurs and an action potential is produced. Phases 1 and 2 (as seen in the myocardial cells) are not apparent but Phase 3 repolarization follows, restoring the maximum (most negative) diastolic potential from which the sloping Phase 4 again ensues giving rise to a further spontaneous action potential. The pacemaker cells thus have the property of rhythmicity or automaticity. The reciprocal of the time interval between identical points in consecutive cycles (i.e. the reciprocal of the cycle length) gives the discharge rate of the pacemaker.

powerful than the minimum required to evoke the initial depolarization of a fully repolarized membrane. Although the rhythm of the heart is determined by depolarization of, and conduction through, the pacemaker and conducting tissue, depolarization of this tissue does not generate sufficient voltage to be detected at the body surface. There are, therefore, no waves on the surface ECG corresponding to depolarization of the pacemaker and conducting tissue. The rhythm of the heart is therefore assessed electrocardiographically from the induced depolarization of the myocardial tissue which produces the P waves and the QRS complexes. The time relations of the action potential of a ventricular myocardial cell and the induced changes on the surface ECG are shown in Fig. 14.6a. Note that ventricular repolarization begins at the height of the action potential which is actually during the terminal part of the QRS complex. The S–T segment is therefore as much part of the repolarization process as the T wave.

The orientation of the 12 electrocardiogram leads

The orientation of the six limb leads with reference to the heart is shown in Fig. 14.7a. Note that all six of these leads are situated in the frontal planes. Leads II, aVF and III 'look at' the inferior aspect of the heart and best show the changes of inferior infarction. Leads aVF and I look at the anterolateral aspect of the heart and best show the changes of anterolateral infarction.

The electrical axis of the heart (the mean frontal plane QRS axis)

These terms (which are used interchangeably) refer to the general (predominant) direction of ventricular depolarization in the frontal plane. Thus the axis is closest to that frontal plane lead with the tallest QRS complex and is at right angles to the smallest QRS complex. The axis position is identified using the hexaxial reference system (Fig. 14.7b) in which lead I is arbitrarily assigned the value 0°. The general direction of ventricular depolarization in the frontal plane is typically towards lead II (+ 60°) but can lie anywhere between aVL (– 30°) and aVF (+ 90°), travelling clockwise. When the axis is in the region of aVL and I (tallest QRS complexes in these leads) the heart is said to be *horizontal*. When the axis is in the region of F and II (tallest QRS complexes in these leads) the heart is said to be *vertical*. With a typical normal axis of 60° there are upright QRS complexes in lead II and to a lesser extent aVF and smaller QRS complexes

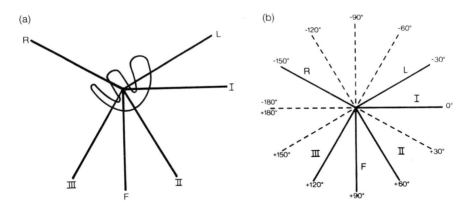

Fig. 14.7. (a) The orientation of the six limb leads around the heart. Note that the distribution of the limb leads around the heart is uneven. Leads L and I look at the anterolateral aspect of the heart. Leads II, F and III look at the inferior aspect of the heart. Lead R looks into the cavity of the ventricles. (b) In this system the six leads are each produced through the origin. The resulting six lines (each line shown half continuous, half interrupted) divide the circle into 12 angles each of 30° and this reference plane is used to define the direction of the axis. Each end of the six lines is labelled in degrees. Lead I is arbitrarily chose as the reference zero. Moving clockwise from lead I the lines are labelled in 30° increments until + 180° is reached. Moving counter-clockwise from lead I the points are labelled – 30°, – 60°, etc.

in III and aVL. Lead aVR 'looks into' the cavity of the heart (Fig. 14.7a). Depolarization of the ventricle is from endocardium (where the Purkinje tissue is) to epicardium, so a cavity lead shows depolarization going away from it and therefore has a negative QRS deflection.

A knowledge of the axis is helpful in understanding the variation in appearances in the limb leads between different subjects with similar (normal or abnormal) precordial ECG appearances. Thus, for example, in a patient with left ventricular hypertrophy (LVH), if the heart is horizontal (axis in the region of $-30°$ to $0°$) appearances similar to those in V5 and V6 will be seen in aVL and I, whereas if the heart is vertical (axis $+60°$ to $+90°$) appearances similar to those in V5 and V6 will be seen in II and aVF.

Determination of the axis is important in the diagnosis of (1) right ventricular hypertrophy (RVH); and (2) left anterior hemiblock (LAH). For diagnosis of RVH, abnormal right axis deviation must be present (i.e. the axis must be more positive than $+90°$ — dominantly positive QRS in aVF and $r < S$ in lead I). For the diagnosis of LAH, abnormal left axis deviation must be present (i.e. an axis more negative then $-30°$ with a dominantly positive deflection in aVL and $r < S$ in II).

The orientation of the precordial leads (V1 to V6) around the heart is shown in Fig. 14.8. The precordial leads are all in the horizontal plane and are situated close to (and are dominantly affected by) local areas of the right or left ventricular myocardium. In general, V1 and V2 face the right ventricular myocardium, V3 and V4 the interventricular septum and V5 and V6 the left ventricular myocardium.

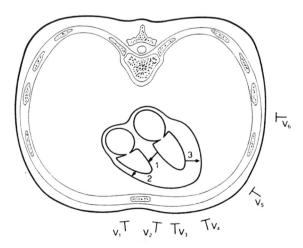

Fig. 14.8. The orientation of the precordial leads with respect to the heart. Horizontal cross-section through the thorax at ventricular level. Phase 1 = depolarization of the interventricular septum. Phase 2 = depolarization of the right ventricular free wall. Phase 3 = depolarization of the left ventricular free wall.

QRS wave form nomenclature

All sharp, pointed deflections resulting from electrical activation of the ventricles are called 'QRS complexes'. Such complexes may start with a positive or negative deflection and may have one, two, three or even more recognizable deflections within them. The presence and relative size of the several possible components of the QRS complex are indicated by a convention using combinations of the letters QRS (Fig. 14.9).

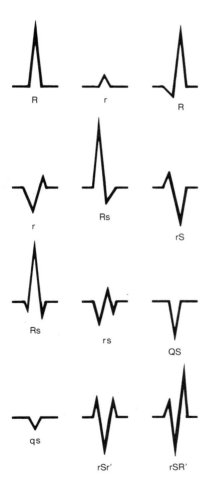

Fig. 14.9. Nomenclature of QRS (also see text). r or R = first positive (up-going) wave; r′ or R′ = a second positive wave; q or Q = negative wave before an r or R wave; s or S = negative wave (i.e. one descending below the baseline) following an r or R wave; qs or QS = entirely negative wave. Large deflections are labelled with an appropriate upper-case letter, and small deflections with an appropriate lower-case letter.

The form of right-sided (V1 and V2) and left-sided (V5 and V6) precordial QRS complexes

Ventricular activation begins on the left side of the interventricular septum (Fig. 14.8) and spreads from left to right within the septum and later from endocardium to epicardium in the free walls of the two ventricles. The ventricular myocardial depolarization can therefore be divided into phase I (depolarization of the interventricular septum), phase II (depolarization of the right ventricular free wall) and phase III (depolarization of the left ventricular free wall). Phase I occurs initially. Phases II and III are, in normal circumstances, virtually simultaneous. Consideration of the sequence of ventricular myocardial depolarization and of the orientation of the recording leads in relation to the heart helps one to understand the typical morphology of a right ventricular and of a left ventricular QRS complex. The typical QRS configuration in V1 and V2 is, therefore, an rS complex (Fig. 14.10a) and in V6 a qR complex (Fig. 14.10b). The important general features about the normal precordial QRS complexes (Fig. 14.11) are as follows:

1   V1 typically has an rS configuration.

2   V6 typically has a qR configuration.

3   In general the size of the initial positive wave increases progressively from V1 to V6. It is quite normal, however, for the R wave in V6 to be smaller than that in V5 and it is also normal for the R wave in V5 to be smaller than that in V4, provided that the R wave in V6 was also smaller than that in V5. (This is because V5 and V6 are progressively further away from the heart (see Fig. 14.8).)

4   The size of the negative wave (S wave) in V2 is usually greater than in V1. The size of this negative wave then progressively falls as one moves from the right to the left precordial leads.

5   The direction of the initial part of the QRS is upwards in V1, V2 and V3 but downwards in V4 to V6. That is, V1–V3 usually show initial r waves and V4–V6 show initial q waves. The potential variations in the shape of the QRS complexes in the precordial leads are shown in Fig. 14.12.

Two additional possible normal variations in the precordial QRS complexes should be noted. V1 may show a QS complex instead of an rS complex and V6 may show an R wave, qRs or Rs complex (Fig. 14.13). The second variation concerns the concept of clockwise and counterclockwise cardiac rotation (Fig. 14.14) which affects the *transition zone* demarcating right ventricular and left ventricular precordial QRS complexes indicated as the vertical dotted line in Fig. 14.12.

Precordial QRS dimensions

The following criteria define normality of the precordial QRS complexes:

• The total QRS duration should not exceed 0.10 s (two and a half small squares)

• At least one R wave should exceed 8 mm (assuming a standard ECG calibration)

• The tallest R wave should not exceed 27 mm

• The deepest S wave should not exceed 30 mm

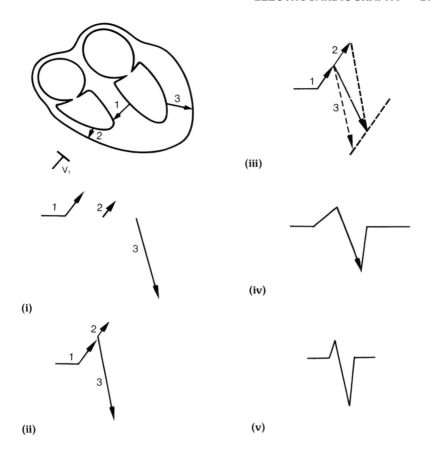

Fig. 14.10 (a). The phases of depolarization. The interventricular septum is depolarized first. Depolarization of the right and left ventricular free walls then follows. Thus phase 1 activation occurs initially, alone, and Phase 2 and 3 activation occur simultaneously after Phase 1. (i) Three phases of depolarization are shown in V1. Phases 1 and 2 give positive and Phase 3 negative deflections in V1. The relative magnitudes of their resulting deflections are represented by the length of the arrows. Phase 3 produces the largest effect because of the dominance of the left ventricle in terms of mass and therefore, of electrical activation. (ii) Phase 1 occurs initially alone. Phase 2 and 3 follow, together. (iii) The resultant of Phases 2 and 3 acting simultaneously is determined by constructing the parallelogram of vectors. (iv) When the recorded deflection is over, the pen returns to the baseline. (v) The magnitude of the Phase 1 wave was exaggerated in (i) to (iv) for clarity. The deflections were also spread out for the same reason. The typical QRS deflection in V1 has a small initial positive wave followed by a larger negative wave.

- The sum of the tallest R in the precordial leads and the deepest S in the precordial leads should not exceed 40 mm
- The ventricular activation time should not exceed 0.04 s (onset of q to peak of R in a lead with a qR complex)
- Any q wave seen should not have a depth exceeding one-quarter the height of the ensuing R wave or a duration exceeding 0.04 s

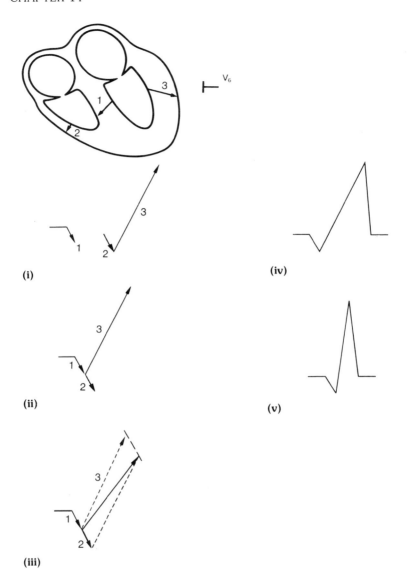

Fig. 14.10 (b). Using the same approach, the typical QRS deflection in V6 can be predicted. (i) Three phases of depolarization are shown. Phases 1 and 2 give negative and Phase 3 positive deflections in V6. Phase 3 gives a larger deflection (positively) in V6 than it gave (negatively) in V1 since the left-ventricular free wall is closer to V6 than to V1. Conversely Phases 1 and 2 give smaller deflections in V6 than they did in V1. (ii) Phase 1 occurs initially, alone, then 2 and 3 follow together. (iii) The resultant of Phases 2 and 3 acting simultaneously may be determined by constructing a parallelogram of forces. (iv) When the recorded deflection is over, the pen returns to the baseline. (v) In (i) to (iv) the deflections were spread out for greater clarity. Here it is shown in its normal perspective. The typical QRS deflection in V6 has a small initial negative wave followed by a large positive wave.

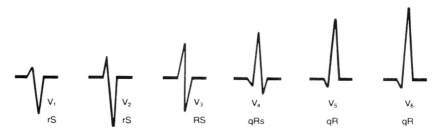

Fig. 14.11. Typical normal precordial QRS morphology.

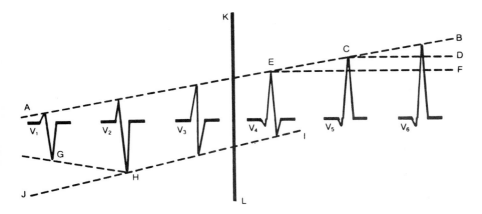

Fig. 14.12. Line AB illustrates that the R wave in each precordial lead is larger than in the lead preceding it in the series from V1 to V6. However, it is quite normal for the R wave in V6 to be smaller than that in V5 (line CD). It is also normal for the R wave in V6 to be smaller than that in V5 (line EF). The size of the S wave diminishes progressively across the precordial leads and may ultimately disappear altogether (line JI). The size of the S wave in V2 is often greater than that in V1 (line GH). Leads before the line KL have an initial deflection which is positive (an r wave). Leads after line KL have an initial negative deflection (a q wave). The position of KL varies.

Precordial T wave polarity and size

The criteria for the normal T waves are less precise than those for the QRS complexes:

• the T wave in V1 may be upright, flat or inverted but if upright in earlier records it should still be upright

• the T wave in V2 may be upright, flat or inverted but if upright in earlier records or simultaneously upright in V1 it must be upright in V2

• T waves from V3 to V6 must be upright

In general in left chest leads the taller the R wave the taller the T wave should be, but over the right ventricle tall T waves relative to the R wave heights are often seen in V2 and V3.

The precordial S–T segments

The S–T segments of the precordial leads must not deviate from the isoelectric line (time interval between the end of the T wave and the beginning of the P

(a)

(b)

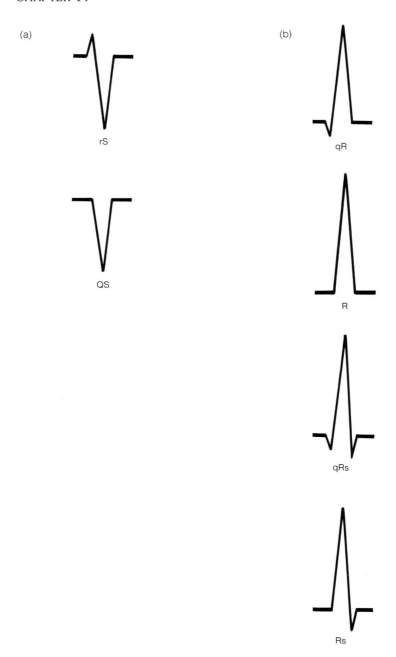

Fig. 14.13. Variations in possible QRS wavefrom in V1 (a) and V6 (b).

wave) by ± 1 mm. During sinus tachycardia there may be little or no isoelectric line visible and assessment of minor degrees of S–T segment shift may therefore be difficult or impossible. The S–T segment tends to appear more discreet in V5

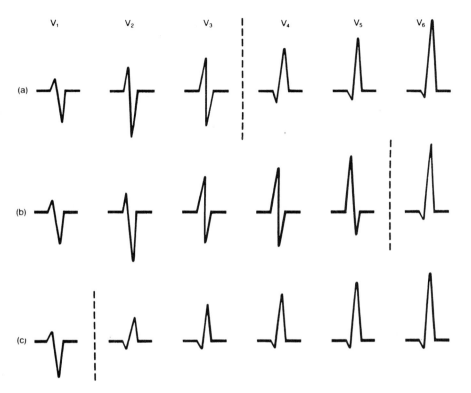

Fig. 14.14. The typical precordial QRS complexes of the intermediate position and of clockwise and counterclockwise rotation. (a) Intermediate position. Transition zone between V3 and V4. (b) Clockwise rotation. Transition zone between V5 and V6 (if appearance of q wave is taken as criterion) or between V4 and V5 (if dominant positive deflection is taken as criterion). (c) Counterclockwise rotation. Transition zone between V1 and V2.

and V6 than it does in V2 and V3 and minor degrees of S–T segment elevation in these latter two leads should be interpreted with great caution. It should be remembered that the S–T segment is just as much part of the repolarization process as is the T wave and there is no intrinsic reason why it should always be recognizable as a discreet entity.

Limb lead QRS complexes

The criteria required to assess normality or otherwise of the limb lead QRS complexes are relatively few. They are as follows:
- A q wave in aVL, I, II or aVF should not equal or exceed 0.04 s in duration
- A q wave in aVL, I, II or aVF should not have a depth > one-quarter of the height of the ensuing R wave
- The mean frontal plane QRS axis should not lie outside the range – 30° to + 90°
- The r wave in aVL should not exceed 13 mm and that in aVF should not exceed 20 mm

- Q waves which are visible only in aVR or lead III are of no significance
- Q waves which are > 0.04 s in duration or > one-quarter the height of the ensuing R wave are permissible in lead aVL if the heart is vertical i.e. has a mean frontal plane QRS axis of + 60° or more positive.

Limb lead T waves

In general the T waves and the QRS complexes in the limb leads should be concordant, i.e. when the QRS is clearly positive the T waves should be positive and when the QRS is clearly negative the T waves should be negative. This rule allows an approximate general assessment of the T waves in the limb leads, but does not define the borderline cases and there are problems in deciding the significance of, for example, shallow T wave inversion in the presence of a small positive QRS complex. The way to get round such difficulties is to work out the mean frontal plane T wave axis, which should not differ from the QRS axis by > ±45°.

Limb lead S–T segments

The rule for the S–T segment in the limb leads is exactly the same as for that in the precordial leads. A normal S–T segment in the limb leads must not deviate from the isoelectric line by > 1 mm (above or below).

The P waves

During normal sinus rhythm atrial myocardial depolarization is initiated from the sino-atrial node. In the frontal plane atrial myocardial depolarization therefore travels predominantly from right to left and from above downwards and gives rise to positive deflections in lead II (and to a lesser extent in lead I and in the foot lead). Right atrial depolarization tends to give deflection towards the right precordial leads and left atrial depolarization deflection away from the right precordial leads and the resulting P wave in V1 may therefore be biphasic (Fig. 14.15).

The P waves are most effectively assessed using lead II and V1 and the rules for normality or otherwise of the P waves are as follows:

1   The P waves should not exceed 0.12 s duration in lead II.
2   The P waves should not exceed 2.5 mm in height in lead II.
3   Any negative component of the P wave in V1 should not have a greater area than the initial positive component.

THE ABNORMAL ELECTROCARDIOGRAM

Intraventricular conduction disturbances

When the normal sequence of conduction of a depolarization wave is disturbed after it has descended beyond the bifurcation of the bundle of His, the following intraventricular disturbances are recognizable on the 12 lead ECG:

- Right bundle branch block (RBBB) — partial or complete, permanent or intermittent
- Left bundle branch block (LBBB) — partial or complete, permanent or intermittent

(a)

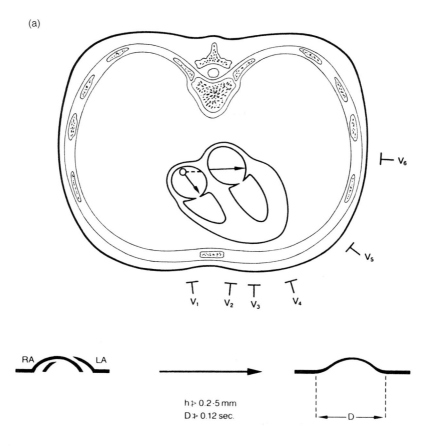

h ⊁ 0.2·5 mm
D ⊁ 0.12 sec.

Fig. 14.15 (a). The origin of the P wave is V1. Atrial depolarization starts at the sino-atrial node and spreads simultaneously in all directions through the myocardium of the right atrium. That direction of spread of depolarization within the right atrium which produces the longest available pathway is the effective, predominant direction of depolarization of the right atrium and this determines the direction of the right atrial P wave vector. The first part of the left atrium to be depolarized is that part lying on the shortest route from the sino-atrial node. From this point depolarization spreads in all directions through the left atrial myocardium. That direction of spread of depolarization within the left atrium which provides the longest available pathway is the effective, predominant direction of depolarization of the left atrium and this determines the direction of the left atrial P wave vector.

- Left anterior hemiblock (LAH) — also known as left superior interventricular block
- Left posterior hemiblock (LPH) — also known as left inferior intraventricular block
- Right bundle branch block plus LAH
- Right bundle branch block plus LPH
- Diffuse intraventricular block

Only RBBB and LBBB will be considered here.

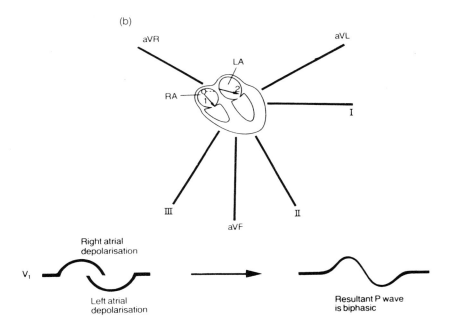

Fig 14.15 (b). The origin of the P wave in lead II. Atrial depolarization begins in the sino-atrial node and spreads in all directions across the right atrial myocardium. The longest available direction determines the direction in which most right atrial myocardium is available for depolarization and therefore the direction in which the right atrial component of the P wave is best seen. Left atrial depolarization begins at that point which is on the shortest depolarization route from the sino-atrial node. The longest available direction within the left atrium then determines the predominant left atrial depolarization pathway. The right and left atrial depolarization waves are therefore both positive in lead II, the right atrial wave beginning before but overlapping with the left.

Right bundle branch block (Fig. 14.16)

Complete failure of conduction in the right bundle branch causes delayed depolarization of the free wall of the right ventricle without a change in the timing or direction of depolarization in the interventricular septum or in the left ventricular free wall. The delay in depolarization of the free wall of the right ventricle gives rise to a late secondary broad R wave in the right precordial leads and a corresponding late secondary broad S wave in the left precordial leads. The R wave in the right precordial lead and the S wave in the left precordial leads are typically broad and slurred. The criteria for the presence of right bundle branch block are as follows:

In relation to a supraventricularly initiated beat: (1) the total QRS duration is 0.12 s or more; and (2) a secondary R wave [R′ wave] is seen in V1. Both criteria must be fulfilled before there is RBBB. The QRS complex in V1 may be rsr′, rSr′, rsR′, rSR′, Rsr′, RSr′, RsR′ or RSR′ or M shaped. These criteria are the only ones *necessary* for the diagnosis of RBBB but, additional secondary changes frequently occur. These are not in, themselves, part of the diagnostic requirement but, when present, should not lead to the conclusion that there is

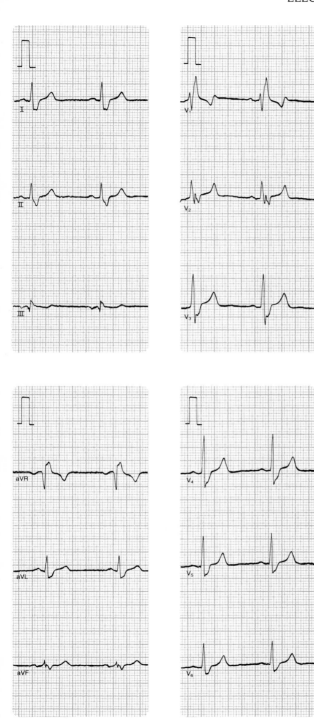

Fig. 14.16. Right bundle branch block. The rhythm is sinus. The total QRS duration is abnormally long (0.16 s — most easily seen in the first QRS in V1 or the second QRS in 1). V1 has a large secondary R wave (i.e. it has an rSR′ complex). The combination of prolongation of the total QRS duration with a secondary R wave in V1 is diagnostic. There is a broad, slurred S wave in V6 (the equivalent of the broad, slurred R wave in V1).

an additional abnormality. The secondary changes include (a) the presence of deep, slurred S waves in lead I, aVL and V4–V6 and (b) S–T segment depression and/or T wave inversion from V1 to V3.

Left bundle branch block (Fig. 14.17)

Left bundle branch block produces more widespread electrocardiographic changes than RBBB. Depolarization of the free wall of the left ventricle is delayed and, in addition, there is reversal of the direction of septal depolarization resulting in reversal of the initial part of each QRS and major alteration of the QRS wave form. Secondary S–T segment and T wave changes occur as a result of the primary QRS abnormality.

The diagnostic criteria for LBBB (all three of which must apply simultaneously) are as follows:

- The total QRS duration is 0.12 s or more
- No initial Q wave is seen in V5, V6, lead I or aVL
- No secondary R wave is seen in V1 to indicate the presence of RBBB

The last criterion is necessary to avoid confusion in cases in which there is simultaneously RBBB and extreme clockwise cardiac rotation. The former feature would give rise to an RSr′ in V1 and an increase in the total QRS duration and the latter would give rise to absence of an initial Q wave in V5, V6, lead I and aVL. As with the RBBB secondary changes also inevitably occur but are not part of the diagnostic process. These include secondary S–T segment depression and T wave inversion most typically in leads I, aVL, V4–V6, broad QS complexes in V1–V3, notching of the R waves in the mid-precordial leads (to give M-shaped complexes) and broad R waves in leads I, aVL and V4–V6.

Ventricular and atrial hypertrophy

Left ventricular hypertrophy (Fig. 14.18)

The increased bulk of the hypertrophied left ventricular myocardium increases the voltage induced during depolarization of the free wall of the left ventricle, giving rise to taller R waves in the left precordial leads and deeper S waves in the right precordial leads. Since the left ventricular free wall thickness is usually increased, the depolarization process takes longer to travel from endocardium to epicardium causing a prolongation of the ventricular activation time (the time interval between onset of the q wave and the peak of the R wave in any lead facing the left ventricle and showing a qR type of QRS complex). Secondary changes in repolarization occur, with S–T segment depression and T wave inversion. S–T, T changes are always non-specific in appearance and their cause can only be inferred from any primary depolarization changes which are present or from the overall clinical picture. Left ventricular hypertrophy is not an 'all-or-none' diagnosis (like LBBB and RBBB) but is a graded diagnosis. The greater the number of criteria fulfilled the more likely it is that the condition exists. The recognized criteria for LVH are as follows:

- R in V4, V5 or V6 exceeds 27 mm
- S in V1, V2 or V3 exceeds 30 mm
- R in V4, V5 or V6 plus S in V1, V2 or V3 exceeds 40 mm
- R in aVL exceeds 13 mm

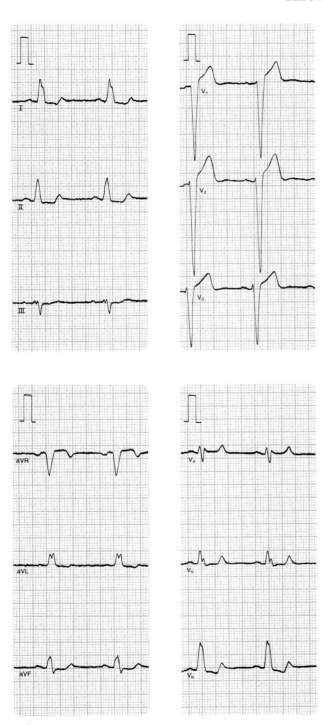

Fig. 14.17. Left bundle branch block. The rhythm is sinus. The total QRS duration is abnormally long (0.14 s — most easily seen in the first QRS complex in V6). Deep S waves (in this case with a small initial r wave) are seen in V1. There is no secondary R wave in V1 to indicate RBBB. There is no initial (septal) q wave in V6 or in leads further to the left than V6 (i.e. 1 and aVL). In the absence of RBBB this combination of absent left-sided q waves and abnormally long total QRS duration is indicative of LBBB. S–T segment depression (which is secondary to the QRS abnormality) is seen in V6, I, II and aVL. The frontal plane QRS axis is within the normal range of + 15°. The heart is horizontal and because of this the appearances in left ventricular leads (typically V6) are transmitted to leads I and aVL (i.e. to those frontal plane leads which lie closest to the direction of the frontal plane axis).

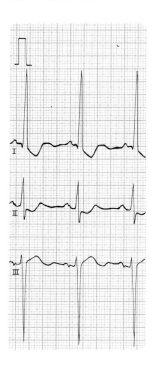

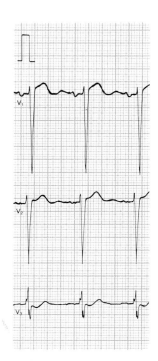

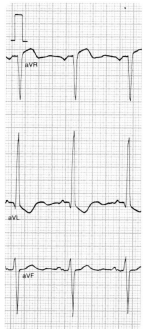

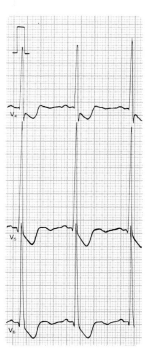

Fig. 14.18. Left ventricular hypertrophy. The rhythm is sinus. The axis is towards the left end of the normal range (−15°) i.e. the heart is horizontal. R wave height in V5 and V6 is abnormal (the peak R wave height in V5 is 41 mm). The S wave depth in V1 is abnormal (31 mm). The ventricular activation time in V5 and V6 is prolonged (0.06 s). There is S–T segment depression and T wave inversion in the left precordial leads. Since the heart is horizontal the changes seen in the left precordial leads are also shown in I and aVL. There is also evidence of LAH.

- R in aVF exceeds 20 mm
- Ventricular activation time exceeds 0.04 s
- S–T segment depression, T wave flattening or T wave inversion in leads facing the left ventricle (V4, V5 or V6, lead I and aVL when the heart is horizontal and leads II and aVF when the heart is vertical)

It should be noted, however, that the thickness of the chest wall greatly affects the height and depth (voltage) of the QRS deflections and these figures may be greatly exceeded in unusually thin but healthy subjects.

Systolic and diastolic left ventricular overload patterns

In the presence of systolic overload of the left ventricle (e.g. in the presence of systemic hypertension or aortic stenosis) S–T to T changes tend to be prominent whereas in the presence of diastolic overload of the left ventricle (for example in the presence of aortic or mitral incompetence) S–T to T changes tend to be minimal or absent and QRS voltage changes are prominent.

Right ventricular hypertrophy (Figs. 14.19, 14.20, and 14.22)*

The increased bulk of the right ventricle results in higher voltages during right ventricular depolarization giving rise to an increase in the size of the positive deflection in the right precordial leads and secondary S–T and T wave changes. Since the left ventricle no longer dominates the electrocardiographic appearances, the electrical axis of the heart moves towards the right. The diagnostic criteria for RVH are therefore:

- R wave in V1 ⩾ the S wave (i.e. an R complex, an Rs, an RR′, a qR or a qRS) together with
- A mean frontal plane QRS axis more positive than $+90°$

Both these criteria must be present for a diagnosis of RVH. A dominant R wave in V1 can also occur in true posterior infarction, in ventricular pre-excitation and in the Duchenne type of muscular dystrophy. As with LVH, secondary S–T to T changes may be present with S–T segment depression and flattening or inversion of the T waves but in the case of RVH these are seen in the right precordial leads.

Left atrial hypertrophy (Fig. 14.21)

The P wave is best seen in lead II and in V1 (Fig. 14.15). The normal P wave in lead II consists of a smooth rounded positive deflection. In the presence of left atrial enlargement the terminal part of the P wave becomes taller and the P wave becomes broader. Since the two parts of the P wave are no longer equal there is often a recognizable notch in the mid portion of the P wave and broad bifid P waves in lead II are characteristic of LAH. The P wave in V1 consists of an initial positive and a later negative component. The negative component is produced by left atrial depolarization, and increases in size with LAH.

The criteria for LAH are as follows:

- The P is notched and exceeds 0.12 s in duration in lead II (and possibly also in leads I, aVF and aVL), or

---

* In childhood the left ventricle is normally much less dominant than in the adult ECG and the normal electrocardiogram in childhood frequently shows a QRS axis more positive than $+90°$ together with T wave inversion in the right precordial leads.

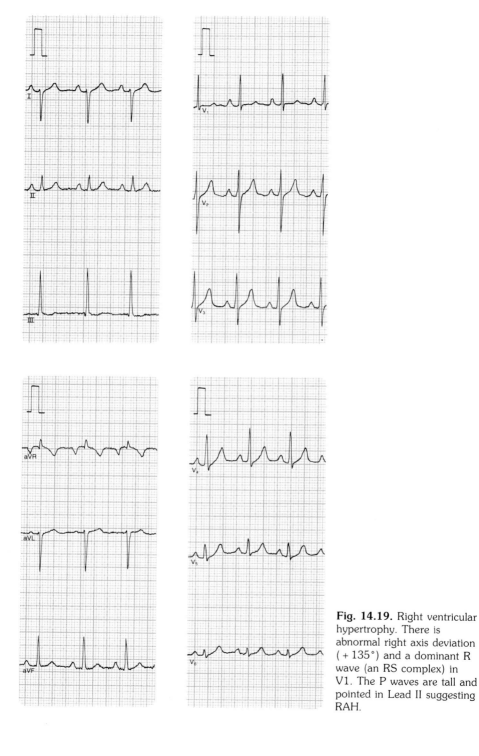

Fig. 14.19. Right ventricular hypertrophy. There is abnormal right axis deviation (+135°) and a dominant R wave (an RS complex) in V1. The P waves are tall and pointed in Lead II suggesting RAH.

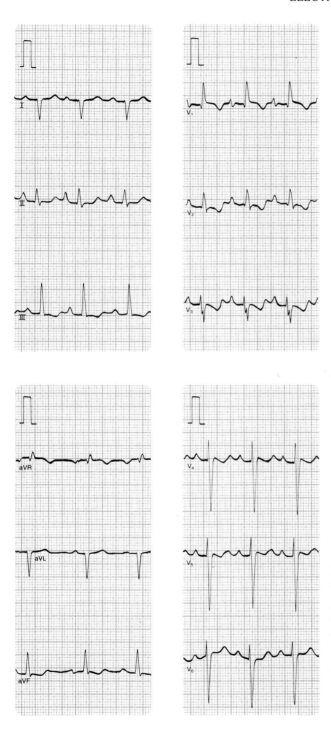

Fig. 14.20. Right ventricular hypertrophy. There is abnormal right axis deviation (+135°) and a dominant R wave (qR complex) in V1. There is a clockwise cardiac rotation and a deep S wave in V6. There is S–T segment depression from V1 to V4. The P waves are tall and pointed in Lead II, indicating RAH. The P–R interval is prolonged at 0.22 s.

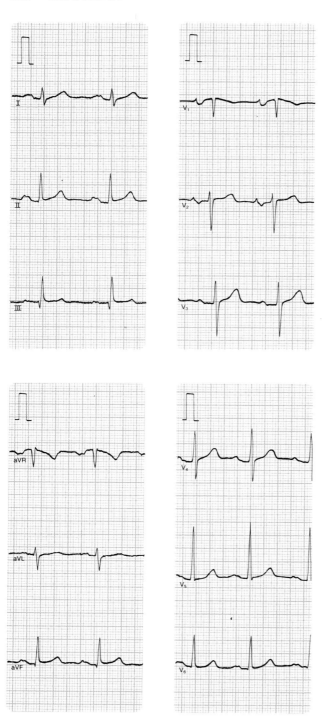

Fig. 14.21. Left atrial hypertrophy. The P waves in lead II are bifid and the phase duration is prolonged at 0.15 s. The P waves in V1 are biphasic with a small brief (and rather sharp looking) initial positive component followed by a deeper and very much broader negative component. The area of the negative component exceeds that of the positive component.

- The P wave in V1 has a dominant negative component (i.e. the area of the negative component exceeds the area of the positive component which precedes it).

Right atrial hypertrophy (Figs. 14.20 and 14.22)

The right atrial component of the P wave increases in height and in duration. The increase in duration is not apparent in the 12 lead ECG since depolarization of the left atrium continues after that of the right, but the increased voltage gives tall (3 mm or more) P waves in lead II.

ISCHAEMIC HEART DISEASE

The electrocardiogram is used most frequently in the detection and evaluation of ischaemic heart disease, but provides no direct information about the state of the coronary arteries. Relatively crude inferences can be made about the coronary arteries if the degree of regional myocardial ischaemia induced by the presence of coronary stenoses is sufficient, either at rest or on exercise, to produce recognizable alterations in myocardial depolarization or repolarization. About half the patients who present with unequivocal angina pectoris have, when first seen, normal *resting* 12 lead ECGs. In the other half the commonest abnormality to find in the presence of ischaemic heart disease is evidence of a previous myocardial infarction. The second commonest abnormalities are minor degrees of S–T segment depression, T wave flattening or T wave inversion. These changes, though non-specific, may be highly *significant* in the clinical context.

When electrocardiographic changes are seen in relation to ischaemic heart disease the range of possible changes is enormous. Since ischaemia can involve any part of the myocardium and/or the conducting tissue, changes can be seen in the P waves, the QRS complexes, the S–T segments or the T waves and almost any arrhythmia or conduction disturbance can be induced. However, the majority of cases in which the ECG shows evidence of ischaemic heart disease can be classified as examples of myocardial ischaemia, myocardial injury or myocardial infarction.

The electrocardiogram in myocardial ischaemia (Figs 2.1, 14.23 and 14.24)

Myocardial ischaemia may give rise to the following electrocardiographic changes:
- Symmetrical T wave inversion
- Deep but asymmetrical T wave inversion
- Horizontal S–T segment depression with or without T wave inversion
- Abnormally tall T waves
- Minor non-specific S–T, T wave changes

The changes in the ECG induced by exertional ischaemia are described in Chapter 2 (p. 39) and are illustrated in Fig. 2.1. They must be differentiated from physiological S–T depression (see Figs. 14.3 and 14.4).

Myocardial injury

Myocardial injury produces changes in the S–T segment of the electrocardiogram. When the injury is confined to or predominantly involves the subendocar-

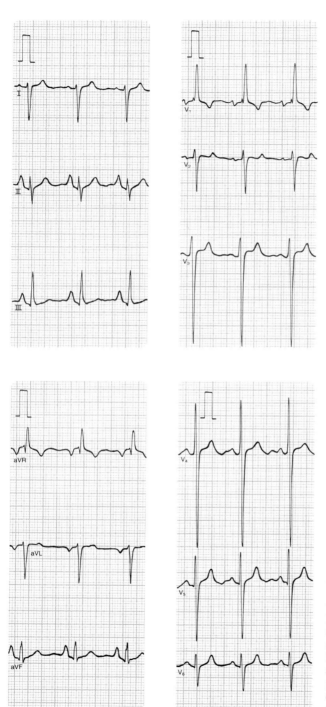

Fig. 14.22. Right atrial hypertrophy accompanying RVH. There is an abnormal degree of right axis deviation (+165°) and a dominant R wave in V1. There is thus RVH. The P waves are tall and pointed in lead II and are > 3 mm. There is thus RAH which frequently accompanies RVH. The pronounced clockwise cardiac rotation is part of the RVH.

dium, S–T segment depression is typically produced. The presence of horizontal (i.e. neither downsloping or upsloping) S–T segment depression suggests subendocardial ischaemia or infarction. It is usually not possible to distinguish between these two possibilities but if the S–T segment depression is persistent (i.e. does not clear within days), infarction is more likely than ischaemia as a cause, particularly if there is clinical or enzyme evidence of infarction. Transient myocardial ischaemia (Fig. 2.1) is most commonly in the subendocardium which is the area most vulnerable to ischaemia. Subendocardial ischaemia is most frequently shown as S–T segment depression.

Subepicardial ischaemia (Fig. 14.24)

This is much less common than subendocardial ischaemia. When episodes of angina pectoris are associated with S–T segment elevation (indicative of subepicardial injury) rather than S–T segment depression (indicative of subendocardial injury) the terms 'Prinzmetal's angina', 'atypical angina' or 'variant angina' have been applied. Both spontaneous and exercise-induced subepicardial ischaemic (i.e. episodes of ischaemic with S–T segment elevation) are very much less common than angina with S–T segment depression (subendocardial ischaemia).

Myocardial injury in the early phase of myocardial infarction

During the electrocardiographic evolution of myocardial infarction evidence of myocardial injury occurs early. This is usually manifested as S–T segment elevation (Fig. 14.24) resulting from injury to the subepicardium. Often the injury is transmural and both the subepicardium and subendocardium are involved but the electrical potential generated in the subepicardium is much greater than that in the subendocardium, so that the ECG changes of transmural injury are similar to those of subepicardial injury. When the S–T segment elevation occurs as a result of an acute coronary occlusion there is usually a steady progression through the sequential changes of myocardial infarction (see below). Occasionally, however, there may initially be evidence of S–T segment elevation with reversion to normal within 24 hours. In such a situation there is likely to be a critical stenosis in the artery supplying the underlying myocardium and the subsequent redevelopment of the injury pattern with progression to the full pattern of infarction remains a distinct possibility.

Myocardial infarction

The term 'myocardial infarction' implies necrosis of a portion of heart muscle as a result of occlusion of its coronary artery. It is most commonly due to thrombus, but may occasionally result from an embolus or spasm. Typically there are changes in the S–T segments, T wave and QRS complexes. It is only the QRS changes which are diagnostic of myocardial infarction.

The QRS changes of myocardial infarction

Two QRS abnormalities may be indicative of myocardial infarction. These are:
- Localised, inappropriately low, R wave voltage
- Abnormal Q waves

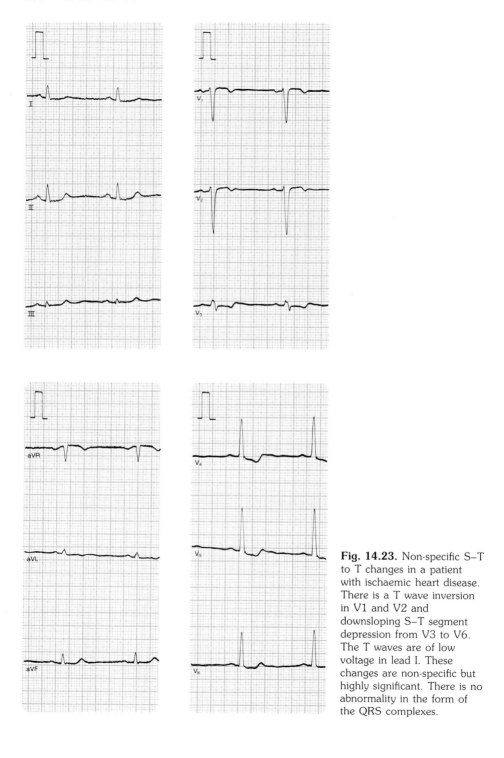

Fig. 14.23. Non-specific S–T to T changes in a patient with ischaemic heart disease. There is a T wave inversion in V1 and V2 and downsloping S–T segment depression from V3 to V6. The T waves are of low voltage in lead I. These changes are non-specific but highly significant. There is no abnormality in the form of the QRS complexes.

Whilst these two changes may seem very dissimilar they are part of the same process. The development of a negative wave (a Q wave) and the reduction in size of the positive wave are the result of loss of positivity from necrosis of myocardium. The QRS changes of infarction are thus related to reduction in the amount of (and in the case of transmural infarction total absence of) viable myocardium beneath the exploring electrode. In the case of the precordial leads the size of the positive wave in each lead is related to the thickness of viable myocardium underlying that electrode and normally this thickness (and R wave voltage) increases progressively from right to left in the precordial series (Fig. 14.25a).

Loss of R wave voltage

If infarction involves only part of the thickness of the myocardial wall the QRS complexes recorded from the area of the infarction will show a reduction on R wave voltage (Fig. 14.25b).

Loss of R wave height can only be judged to be present if either a previous record is available showing a significantly greater R wave height in the appropriate leads before the infarction occurred, or the leads involved are two or more of the leads V2–V5 so that a normal R wave is seen on each side of the lead (V1 and V6) and interpolation between V1 and V6 permits estimation of the approximate size of the anticipated normal R wave (Fig. 14.25b).

Abnormal Q waves and QS complexes

When infarction involves the full thickness of the myocardium ('transmural' infarction — i.e. from endocardium to epicardium) there will be *total* loss of R waves in leads overlying the infarcted zone (Fig. 14.25c), i.e. the waves will be entirely negative (QS complexes). These negative waves are the result of depolarization of the posterior wall of the ventricle travelling from endocardium to epicardium (and therefore away from the precordial leads). These depolar-

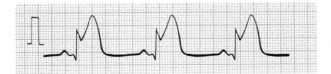

Fig. 14.24. Subepicardial ischaemia or injury and the S–T segment changes of infarction. The rhythm is sinus. The rate is relatively slow. Because of the slow rate a clear iso-electric line is visible between the end of each T wave and the beginning of each P wave. The S–T segment is clearly elevated some 5 mm above the iso-electric line. Note that in the presence of tachycardia, there may be no interval between the end of the T wave and the beginning of the next P wave and no iso-electric line would be visible. In that event, S–T segment elevation may only be regarded as significant if it is striking. Furthermore, minor degrees of apparent S–T segment elevation may be present in leads in which the S–T segment merges imperceptibly into the T wave. This is often the case in normal records in the right precordial leads. One should be very cautious about regarding minor degrees of S–T segment shift in V1 and V2 as being significant. In addition 1–2 mm of S–T elevation may be seen in dominant R pattern leads in some normal subjects (and also in pericarditis — Fig. 14.35).

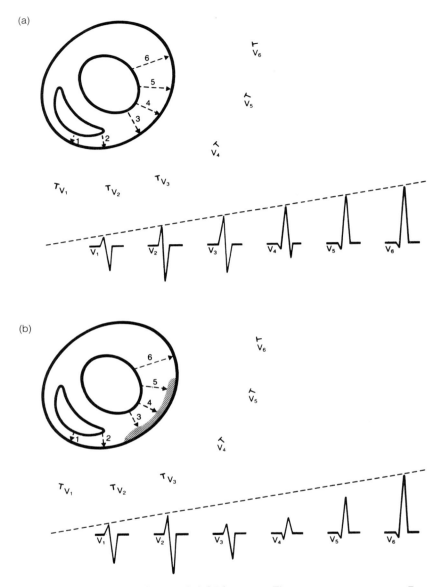

Fig. 14.25. (a) The normal precordial QRS pattern. The progressive increase in R wave height from right (V1) to left (V6) in the precordial series reflects the progressive increase in muscle depth (interrupted arrows) underlying the electrode since depolarization spreads from endocardium to epicardium. (b) Anterior myocardial infarction: changes in QRS. The height of the R wave in each lead is related to the thickness of viable myocardium underlying the lead. With infarction of part of the wall thickness underlying leads V3 to V5 there is loss of R wave height in these leads. (c) Full thickness anterior myocardial infarction: changes in QRS. Depolarization of the free wall of the right and left ventricles takes place normally from endocardium to epicardium in areas underlying V1, V2 and V6. However, leads V3, V4 and V5 are not influenced at all by the subadjacent myocardium, which is electrically inert. These three leads reflect instead the depolarization of the interventricular septum and the posterior wall of the ventricle (continuous arrows). This depolarization also travels from endocardium to

(c)

(d)

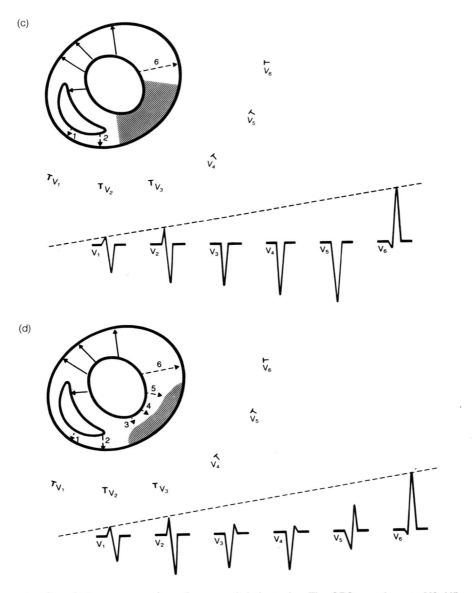

epicardium, but moves away from the precordial electrodes. The QRS complexes in V3–V5 thus show entirely negative complexes (i.e. QS complexes). (d) Myocardial infarction: changes in QRS. Depolarization of the free wall of the left ventricle takes place normally from endocardium to epicardium in areas underlying electrodes V1, V2 and V6. However, infarction has occurred in a substantial part of the left ventricular wall thickness in areas underlying electrodes V3, V4 and V5. As a result of this the R wave voltage is substantially diminished in these leads. The size of the residual R waves in leads V3–V5 is related to the thickness of remaining viable myocardium (interrupted arrows 3, 4 and 5). The situation differs from that shown in (b) only in degree, i.e. in the extent of the wall thickness involved in infarction. In this case most of the wall thickness is involved and the thickness of the remaining viable myocardium is insufficient to overcome the effects of the posterior left ventricular wall depolarization passing away from the precordial leads giving rise to deep, broad Q waves.

ization waves from the posterior wall of the heart are normally obscured by the dominant depolarization of the anterior wall of the ventricle which lies much closer to the precordial leads. When infarction involves less than the full thickness of the myocardium, but still involves a major part of the wall thickness, less severe changes occur in which the R waves, whilst appreciably reduced in size, are still present and there are abnormal Q waves. The finding of abnormal Q waves (defined later) and reduced R wave voltage is the commonest electrocardiographic appearance in established infarction (Fig. 14.25d).

The four possible QRS changes which may indicate the presence of myocardial infarction are therefore as follows:
- Reduced R wave voltage (where it can confidently be ascertained that this has occurred)
- Abnormal Q waves without any conclusive evidence of R wave reduction
- Abnormal Q waves with evidence of reduced R wave voltage
- Abnormal QS complexes

Normal and abnormal Q waves

The first part of each QRS complex is produced by depolarization of the upper part of the interventricular septum and all leads recording from the left side of the interventricular septum will normally show small q waves (Fig. 14.12). These q waves will be seen from V4 to V6 when the heart is intermediate in position, but may be present from V2 to V6 if there is extreme counterclockwise cardiac rotation.

In the limb leads septal q waves will be seen in those leads which show a left ventricular configuration. When the heart is horizontal normal qR complexes will be seen in leads I and aVL. When the heart is vertical normal qR complexes will be seen in leads II and aVF.

A normal q wave is not > one-quarter of the height of the ensuing R wave *and* is < 0.04 s in duration. Normal QS complexes occur in those leads that look into the cavity of the myocardium. aVR is usually a cavity lead and therefore very frequently shows a QS complex (alternatively it may show a rS). Lead III is a cavity lead when the heart is horizontal, lead aVL is a cavity lead when the heart is vertical and lead V1 is a cavity lead when there is pronounced clockwise cardiac rotation. QS complexes may therefore be found normally in aVR, and in aVL if the heart is vertical, in III if the heart is horizontal, and in V1 with clockwise rotation.

Abnormal Q waves have a depth > 25% of the height of the ensuing R wave, or a duration $\geq$ 0.04 s.

The electrocardiographic criteria for the diagnosis of myocardial infarction from the QRS complexes may be summarized as follows:
- Reduction in R wave height (from a normal level assessed either by a previous record ante-dating the infarction or by interpolation of the precordial leads)
- The occurrence of QS complexes in V1 (except in the presence of pronounced clockwise cardiac rotation), V2, V3, V4, V5, V6, I, II, aVF, and aVL (in the case of the latter excepting those situations where the heart is vertical), or
- Abnormally deep q (or Q) waves in V1, V2, V3, V4, V5, V6, lead I, lead II,

aVF and aVL (except that abnormally deep Q waves (QS complexes) may be seen in V1 in clockwise cardiac rotation and in aVL in vertical hearts)
• Abnormally wide q (or Q) waves in V1, V2, V3, V4, V5, V6, lead I, lead II, aVF, and aVL (except that QS complexes may be seen in V1 in clockwise cardiac rotation and in aVL in vertical hearts)

The S–T segment changes of infarction

In the early stages of infarction S–T segment elevation usually occurs and may occasionally be dramatic in degree (Fig. 14.24). The injury state which accounts for this change is an unstable one and in the majority of cases evolutionary changes of infarction subsequently follow. Abnormal S–T segment elevation of this type usually occurs in leads facing an area of transmural infarction. Leads looking at the heart from the opposite aspect will usually show 'reciprocal' S–T segment depression at a time when there is 'primary' S–T segment elevation in the leads related to the infarction. The precordial leads and lead I and aVL on the one hand and the inferior limb leads (II, III, and aVF) on the other hand are mutually reciprocal in this respect.

The T wave changes of infarction

A whole variety of non-specific T wave changes may occur in association with myocardial infarction. These include flattening of the T waves, inversion of the T waves and abnormally tall T waves. Widespread deep symmetrical T wave inversion, whilst still, strictly speaking a non-specific change, suggests subendocardial infarction.

The sequential changes of myocardial infarction

Although any or all of the changes described above may occur in myocardial infarction, a common, typical *sequence* of changes is recognized and is shown in Fig. 14.26.

The location of changes in myocardial infarction

Primary electrocardiographic changes of the type described will occur in leads overlying the infarct.

Anterior infarction (Figs 14.27 and 14.28)

The 'anterior' leads are the precordial leads (V1–V6) and lead I and aVL. If the infarction pattern involves V1–V3 the term 'anteroseptal' is used. If the pattern involves V4, V5, V6, I and aVL the term 'anterolateral' is used. If the pattern involves V1–V6 and I and aVL the term 'extensive anterior' is used. If the pattern involves some of the group V1–V3 plus some of the group V4–V6 the term 'anterior' is used. Changes confined to aVL (but possibly also present in left-sided precordial leads taken one or more interspaces higher than the conventional positions) indicate 'high lateral' infarction.

Inferior infarction (Figs 14.29 and 14.30)

Typically inferior myocardial infarction shows primary changes in leads II, III and aVF. Not infrequently the infarct also involves the apex of the ventricle in which case the term 'apical' or 'infero-lateral' is used and in this situation changes are

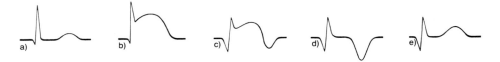

Fig. 14.26. The sequence of changes in acute myocardial infarction. (a) Shows the control, normal appearances in a lead, which by the QRS morphology, lies over the left ventricle. (b) Within hours of the clinical onset of infarction there is S–T segment elevation. At this stage no QRS changes or T wave changes have occurred. Although such a pattern is frequently spoken of, loosely, as showing 'acute infarction', no definitive evidence of infarction is shown. There is evidence of myocardial damage. This is an unstable situation. In the vast majority of cases evolutionary changes of infarction follow. Occasionally the record returns to normal. (c) Within days the R wave voltage has fallen and abnormal Q waves (in this case both in duration and in depth relative to the R wave height) have appeared. These changes are sufficient to prove the occurrence of infarction. In addition T wave inversion has appeared. The S–T elevation is less pronounced than in (b). (d) Within one or more weeks the S–T segment changes revert completely to normal. The R wave voltage remains reduced and the abnormal Q waves persist. Deep symmetrical T wave inversion may develop at this stage. In some patients this pattern remains permanently, in others it progresses to the appearances shown in (e). (e) Months after the clinical infarction the T waves may gradually return to normal. The abnormal Q waves and reduced R wave voltage persist.

expected in leads II, III, aVF, V5 and V6. QS waves or T inversion confined to lead III may however be simply due to a horizontal electrical position of the heart (axis more negative than $+3°$).

Subendocardial infarction

This typically gives rise to widespread S–T segment depression or widespread T wave inversion.

Posterior infarction

This is a relatively uncommon infarct pattern in which changes which might be *anticipated* in true posterior leads can be estimated from reciprocal changes anteriorly in V1 and V2 with abnormally tall and broad R waves, loss of S wave depth and S–T segment depression (Fig. 14.28).

Reciprocal changes of acute myocardial infarction

Leads V1–V6, I and aVL on the one hand and leads II, III and aVF on the other hand are mutually reciprocal. Whenever primary S–T segment elevation is seen in one of these two groups of leads there is usually simultaneous reciprocal S–T segment depression in the other group. When the primary S–T segment changes revert, the reciprocal S–T segment changes also clear. Thus during acute inferior myocardial infarction S–T segment elevation is to be anticipated in leads II, III and the foot lead and reciprocal S–T segment depression in some of the precordial leads. Likewise in acute anterior myocardial infarction primary S–T segment elevation is to be anticipated in the mid-precordial leads and reciprocal S–T segment depression in the inferior limb leads.

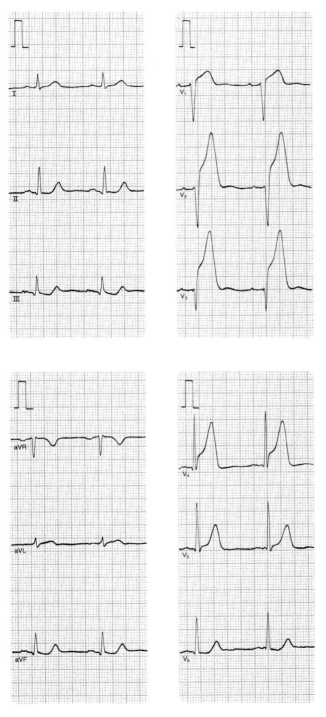

Fig. 14.27. Acute anterior myocardial infarction. There is S–T segment elevation from V1 to V4 and loss of R wave height in V2 and V3. The changes are those of acute anteroseptal infarction. There is reciprocal S–T segment depression in leads II, III and aVF.

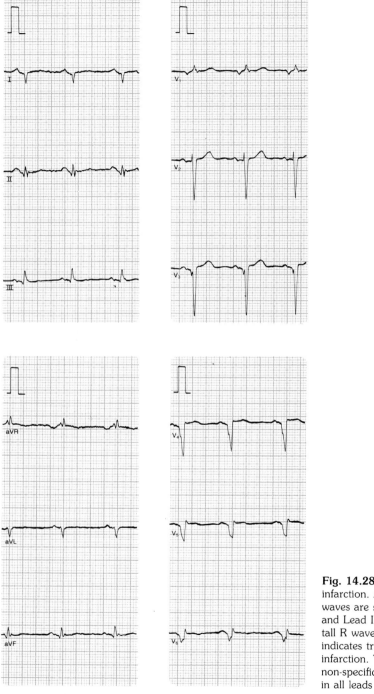

Fig. 14.28. Old anterior infarction. Abnormal Q waves are seen in V3–V6 and Lead I. The abnormally tall R wave in V1 probably indicates true posterior infarction. There are non-specific S–T, T changes in all leads except V2.

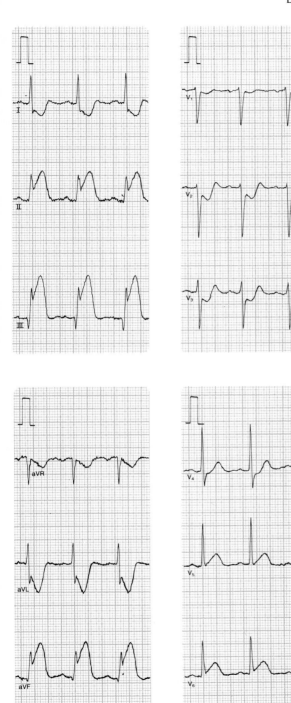

Fig. 14.29. Acute inferolateral myocardial damage. There is striking S–T segment elevation in II, III and aVF and minimal S–T elevation in V5 and V6. These changes indicate inferolateral (i.e. 'apical') myocardial damage. The S–T elevation in the inferior leads is convex upwards. This shape is typical of ischaemic damage. The S–T segment depression in I, aVL and V1–V3 is reciprocal to the primary S–T elevation. There is no QRS evidence of infarction.

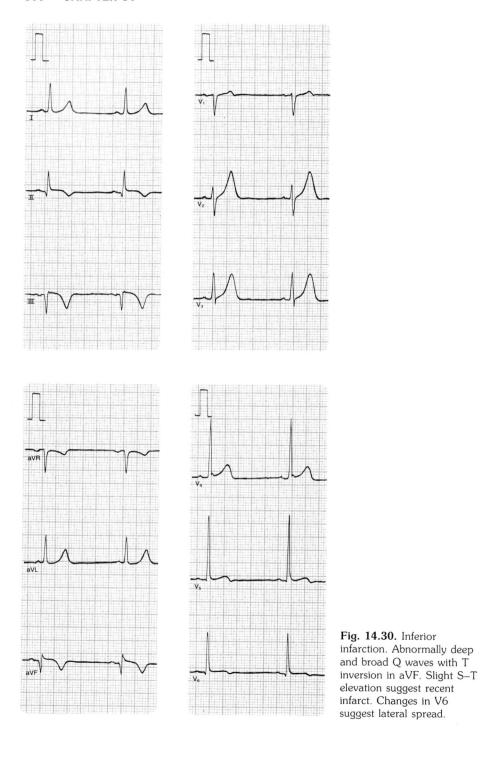

Fig. 14.30. Inferior infarction. Abnormally deep and broad Q waves with T inversion in aVF. Slight S–T elevation suggest recent infarct. Changes in V6 suggest lateral spread.

MISCELLANEOUS ABNORMALITIES

Within this section a variety of subjects will be covered which do not easily fit into major diagnostic categories and in addition the electrocardiographic features of certain relatively common cardiac syndromes will be discussed.

Space constraints preclude the inclusion of a comprehensive coverage of miscellaneous abnormalities. Therefore, with the exception of ventricular pre-excitation, these topics will be covered only in a brief summary.

Ventricular pre-excitation (Figs 14.31, 14.32, 14.33 and p. 150)

This abnormality occurs in approximately 1/1000 of the normal population. The ECG changes result from the fact that the ventricular myocardium receives the depolarization wave early from the abnormal (anomalous), 'accessory' pathway which links atrial and ventricular myocardium in such a way as to bypass the slowly conducting AV node. A variety of anatomical substrates permit ventricular pre-excitation. These include: AV connections (often referred to as Kent bundles and these may be left-sided, right-sided or septal), atrio-Hisian bypass tracts (which connect the atrial myocardium with the bundle of His or the bundle branches), nodo-ventricular fibres (which connect the AV node to the ventricular myocardium) and fasciculoventricular fibres (which pass from the His bundle to the ventricular myocardium). The commonest variety is the AV bypass tract which results in shortening of the P–R interval. The bypass tract inserts into ventricular myocardium away from the His bundle resulting in an abnormal shape and duration of the QRS complex. The initial part of the QRS is slurred and this represents depolarization induced via the bypass tract. The addition of this slow slurred part of ventricular depolarization to the beginning of the QRS complex causes abnormal widening. The combination of the electrocardiographic features of ventricular pre-excitation induced by AV bypass tracts and clinical episodes of paroxysmal tachycardia constitutes the Wolff–Parkinson–White (WPW) syndrome.

The diagnostic criteria of the Wolff–Parkinson–White type of ventricular pre-excitation are as follows:

- A P–R interval < 0.12 s in the presence of sinus rhythm, together with
- An abnormally wide QRS complex of > 0.10 s, together with
- The presence of initial (first 0.03–0.05) slurring of the QRS complex

All three criteria must be fulfilled for a diagnosis of pre-excitation of the Wolff–Parkinson–White type.

Subjects with AV nodal bypass are capable of having paroxysmal re-entrant AV tachycardia. The abnormal QRS complex resulting from ventricular pre-excitation can easily be confused with right or left bundle branch block (Fig. 14.32), RVH or LVH, or myocardial infarction (Fig. 14.33). Since the initial part of each QRS complex may be changed radically by the presence of pre-excitation the normal criteria for the QRS complexes cannot be applied once the presence of ventricular pre-excitation has been recognized.

Another relatively common form of ventricular pre-excitation occurs when there are atrio-Hisian bypass tracts. The AV node is bypassed but the ventricular myocardium receives its depolarization normally from the terminal part of the His bundle. This results in a short P–R interval without a delta wave and without

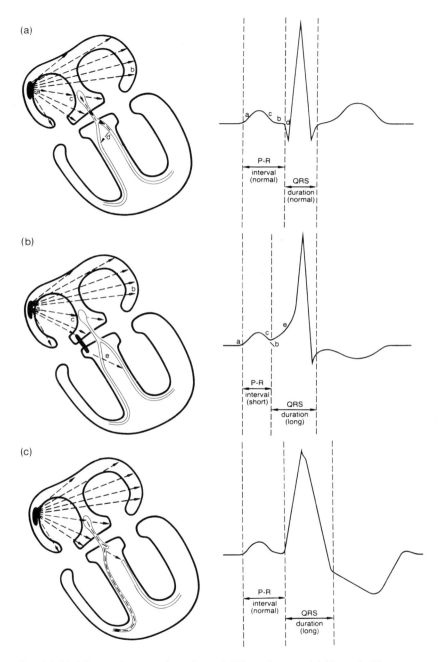

Fig. 14.31. The mechanism of accelerated AV conduction. (a) Normal AV conduction: The P wave is normal; The P–R interval is normal; The QRS is normal; and the S–T segment and T waves are normal. (b) Ventricular pre-excitation. The P wave is normal; the P–R interval is short; The QRS is abnormal in shape and duration; and the S–T segment and T waves are secondarily abnormal. (c) Left bundle branch block: the P wave is normal; the P–R interval is normal; the QRS is abnormal in shape and duration; and the S–T segment and T waves are secondarily abnormal.

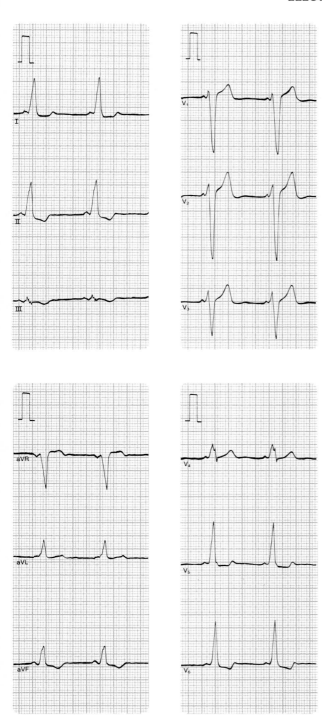

Fig. 14.32. Ventricular pre-excitation. The P–R interval is short at 0.06 s (V2). The total QRS duration is long at 0.18 s. The initial slurring of the QRS complex is seen clearly in I, V2, V3 and V4. Note the similarity in the QRS appearance to LBBB (see Fig. 14.17).

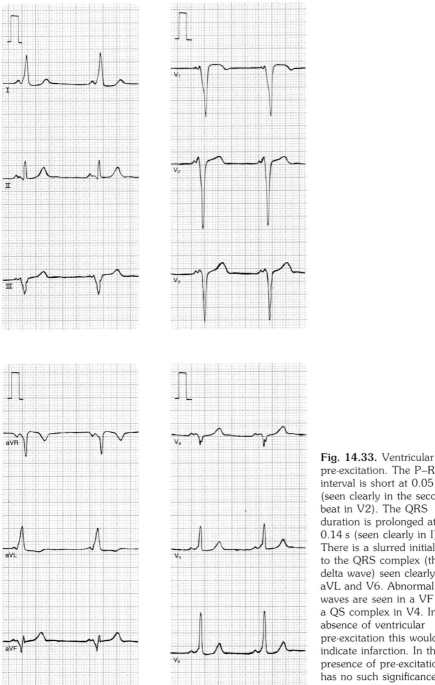

Fig. 14.33. Ventricular pre-excitation. The P–R interval is short at 0.05 s (seen clearly in the second beat in V2). The QRS duration is prolonged at 0.14 s (seen clearly in I). There is a slurred initial part to the QRS complex (the delta wave) seen clearly in I, aVL and V6. Abnormal Q waves are seen in a VF and a QS complex in V4. In the absence of ventricular pre-excitation this would indicate infarction. In the presence of pre-excitation it has no such significance (compare Fig. 14.28).

broadening of the QRS complex (Fig. 14.34). The combination of this type of ventricular pre-excitation with episodes of paroxysmal tachycardia is called the Lown–Ganong–Levine syndrome.

Pericarditis (Fig. 14.35)

Acute pericarditis gives rise to transient, *generalized* S–T segment elevation (except in the case of cavity leads which show S–T segment depression), thought to be due to inflammation of the myocardium in the subepicardial region (adjacent to the inflamed pericardium). The only other common cause of S–T segment elevation is acute myocardial ischaemic damage which gives rise to localized changes.

In chronic pericarditis there are no specific features, just widespread non-specific S–T, T changes. There may be S–T segment depression, low-voltage T waves, T wave inversion and sometimes generalized low voltage of the QRS complexes.

Pericardial effusion

Pericardial effusion does not give rise to specific electrocardiographic changes. There may be generalized reduction in the voltages (of P waves, QRS complexes and T waves, both in limb and chest leads) because of the interposition of pericardial fluid between the voltage generated in the myocardium and that recorded at the body surface. In addition, there may be non-specific S–T, T changes.

Digitalis effect (Fig. 14.36)

Digitalis preparations frequently cause repolarization changes in the ECG (changes in the S–T segment, T wave and U wave) and these changes are known as the 'digitalis effect'. This is typically a downsloping S–T segment depression often associated with T wave flattening. In addition, digitalis may cause a wide variety of cardiac arrhythmias, all of which are indicative of *digitalis toxicity*. The most important arrhythmias associated with digitalis toxicity are ventricular ectopic beats, ventricular coupling, atrial tachycardia with 2 : 1 (or more) AV block, various degrees of heart block, sinus arrest, sino-atrial block and ventricular tachycardia.

Hyperkalaemia

Hyperkalaemia produces changes in the electrocardiogram with a direct but imprecise correlation between the degree of increase in the serum potassium level and the resulting ECG change. The changes are non-specific and may be seen in myocardial damage arising from other causes, e.g. infarction or the action of drugs. P waves, QRS complexes, S–T segments and T waves may be affected in hyperkalaemia and ultimately the cardiac rhythm becomes abnormal. The typical progressive changes of hyperkalaemia are the development of tall pointed narrow T waves, a reduction in the P wave height and the R wave height with widening of the QRS complexes and elevation or depression of the S–T segments. Left anterior hemiblock and first degree heart block may develop. Subsequently more advanced intraventricular blocks occur with very wide QRS complexes, bundle branch block or complete heart block. There may be multiple

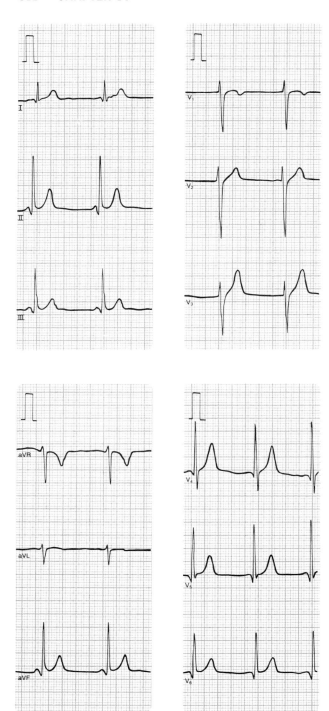

Fig. 14.34.
Lown–Ganong–Levine
syndrome. The basic rhythm
is of sinus origin. The P–R
interval is abnormally short
at 0.08 s. The QRS
complexes are normal. The P
waves are hardly visible in
the precordial leads. This
indicates that the P wave
vector is directed superiorly
and inferiorly and therefore
has no major component in
the horizontal plane.

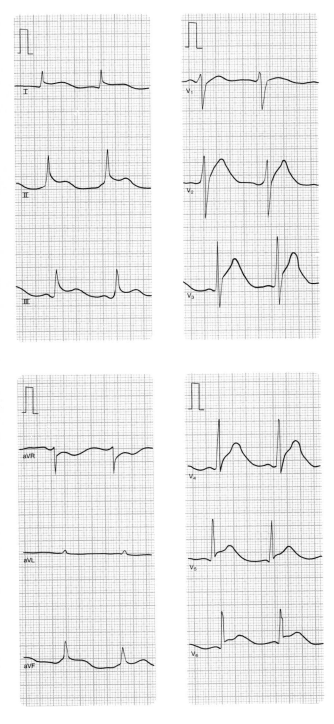

Fig. 14.35. Acute pericarditis. Widespread S–T elevation.

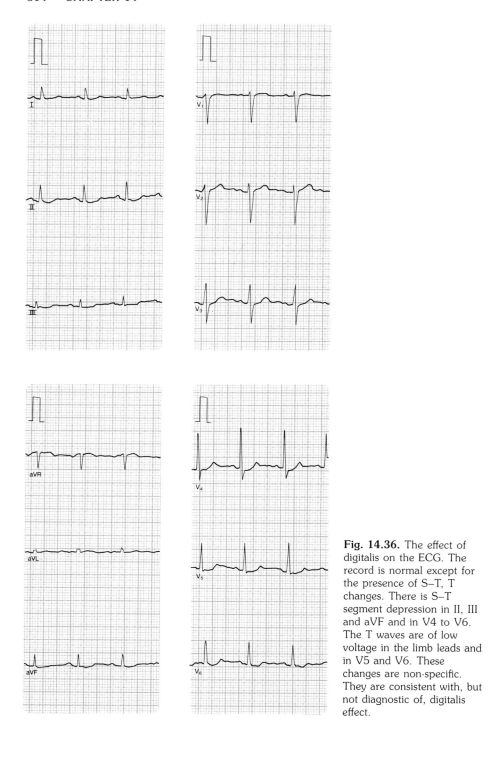

Fig. 14.36. The effect of digitalis on the ECG. The record is normal except for the presence of S–T, T changes. There is S–T segment depression in II, III and aVF and in V4 to V6. The T waves are of low voltage in the limb leads and in V5 and V6. These changes are non-specific. They are consistent with, but not diagnostic of, digitalis effect.

ectopic beats, disappearance of P waves, and very broad bizarre QRS complexes. Finally, there may be ventricular tachycardia, ventricular fibrillation or ventricular asystole.

Hypokalaemia

The important changes of hypokalaemia:
1   S–T segment depression, decreased amplitude of the T waves and increased U wave height (all non-specific changes).
2   The development of cardiac arrhythmias.
3   Prolongation of the QRS duration and increase in P wave amplitude and duration.
The correlation between the serum potassium level and the ECG changes of hypokalaemia is poor.

Hypercalcaemia

In this condition there is a reduction in the Q–T interval approximately proportional to the increase in the serum concentration of ionic calcium. The T wave duration appears unaffected, the reduction being primarily in the duration of the S–T segment itself. At very high levels of serum calcium this relationship breaks down because of progressive T wave prolongation which offsets the effect of reducing S–T segment duration of the total Q–T interval. No appreciable changes occur in the P, QRS or T morphology.

Patients with hypercalcaemia have an increased sensitivity to digitalis, the injudicious use of which may (in hypocalcaemic patients) cause sinus arrest, sino-atrial block, AV ectopic beats, ventricular tachycardia or ventricular fibrillation. Furthermore occasional fatalities have been reported following the intravenous administration of calcium to a fully digitalized patient.

Hypocalcaemia

The main electrocardiographic change in hypocalcaemia is prolongation of the Q–T interval which is due predominantly to an increase in the S–T segment duration. The T wave itself is not significantly changed. The ECG changes of hypocalcaemia appear to be of little or no clinical significance. Hypocalcaemia does not usually predispose to arrhythmias.

Hypothyroidism

When severe or prolonged, generalized electrocardiographic changes frequently occur and are thought to be the result of interstitial myocardial oedema and perhaps of a pericardial effusion.

The main changes are as follows:
• Sinus bradycardia
• Low voltages of the P waves, QRS complexes and T waves
• Slight S–T segment depression
• Prolongation of the P–R interval
• AV conduction disturbances
• Prominent Q waves
• Prolongation of the Q–T interval

Hyperthyroidism

Sinus tachycardia is the most common finding but atrial tachycardia, atrial fibrillation or atrial flutter may also occur.

Hypothermia

In this condition there is sinus bradycardia with prolongation of the P–R and Q–T intervals. Below 25° an extra deflection, the 'J wave' may occur at the end of the QRS complex and just overlapping the beginning of the S–T segment. It is usually upright in the leads facing the left ventricle, increases in size as the temperature falls and is often mistakenly interpreted as prolongation of the QRS duration. The broad second part of the QRS complex (which in V1 may superficially resemble RBBB) is also known as the 'camel hump sign' and it is accompanied by S–T depression and low voltage T waves or T wave inversion. Atrial fibrillation may develop. The Q–T interval may be prolonged.

Electrocardiographic changes in acute disorders of the central nervous system

More than 50% of patients with subarachnoid or intracranial haemorrhage develop transient ECG changes as follows:

- Deep T wave inversion
- Abnormally tall T waves
- Prominent U waves
- S–T segment elevation or depression
- Prolongation of the Q–T interval
- Arrhythmias (sinus tachycardia, sinus bradycardia, nodal rhythm, atrial fibrillation and ventricular tachycardia)

Myocarditis

Transient myocarditis is very common in systemic virus infections and in acute rheumatic fever. In the majority of cases of viral myocarditis the electrocardiogram shows non-specific flattening of the T waves, minimal S–T segment depression and the occurrence of frequent atrial or ventricular premature beats. Occasionally abnormal Q waves simulating those found in myocardial infarction may occur. In acute rheumatic myocarditis the commonest abnormality is prolongation of the P–R interval but second degree heart block (type I) may occur and there may be minor non-specific S–T, T changes.

Cardiomyopathy

In congestive cardiomyopathy there may be abnormalities of the P waves, QRS complexes, S–T segments and T waves and of the cardiac rhythm — almost any electrocardiographic abnormality may occur. The appearances may simulate LVH or RVH, LBBB or RBBB, LAH or LPH or myocardial infarction. The single most characteristic aspect of the electrocardiogram in cardiomyopathy is evidence of involvement of all four chambers (e.g. LVH plus RBBB plus ectopic beats arising in the left atrium). In hypertrophic cardiomyopathy the changes are much more dramatic (see Chapter 6 and Fig. 6.5).

Cor pulmonale

There are no diagnostic features but the common findings are a combination of abnormal right axis deviation and clockwise cardiac rotation in the absence of definitive evidence of RVH. There may, in addition, be evidence of RAH and non-specific S–T, T changes.

Pulmonary embolism

The ECG is widely thought to be helpful in the investigation of the diagnosis of pulmonary embolism but this is actually very far from the truth. Changes which are thought to suggest this condition include the development of large S waves in lead I, large Q waves in lead III, and T wave inversion in lead III (the so-called $S_1Q_3T_3$ syndrome), abnormal right axis deviation, transient RBBB and T wave inversion in the right precordial leads. Often no electrocardiographic changes occur or there may simply be non-specific T wave changes which may be found in any of the precordial leads. Occasionally there may be atrial fibrillation or atrial tachycardia.

Mitral valve prolapse

Common findings in this condition include flattening or inversion of the T waves in leads II, III and aVF, sometimes accompanied by slight S–T segment depression; they may wrongly be interpreted as evidence of inferior myocardial ischaemia. Occasionally prominent U waves may be visible. The Q–T interval may be prolonged. Ventricular pre-excitation is found more commonly in subjects with mitral valve prolapse than in those without. Supraventricular tachycardia, atrial fibrillation and atrial flutter may also occur.

Heredofamilial neuromyopathic disorders

Three major heredity and familial neuromyopathic disorders are often accompanied by electrocardiographic abnormalities. These are the progressive muscular dystrophies, dystrophia myotonica and Friedreich's ataxia. The electrocardiographic findings in all of these conditions include sinus tachycardia, atrial or ventricular ectopic beats, atrial flutter, atrial tachycardia, atrial fibrillation, paroxysmal ventricular tachycardia, RBBB or LBBB and various degrees of heart block. (In addition the Duchenne type of progressive muscular dystrophy frequently has an abnormal R : S ratio in V1 — (i.e. the R wave is dominant in V1). There may also be prominent Q waves in the limb leads or in the left precordial leads and these may simulate infarction.

Dressler's syndrome (the postmyocardial infarction syndrome)

Pleuropericarditis may occur within the first 12 weeks following acute myocardial infarction. The electrocardiogram shows the typical diffuse S–T segment elevation as in pericarditis from any cause. In subsequent weeks there may be flattening of the T waves and minor S–T, T changes.

Haemochromatosis

There may be generalized low voltages of the QRS complexes and T waves and possibly also T wave inversion. Ventricular and supraventricular ectopic beats and tachycardia may occur and there may be RBBB or LBBB and first-, second- or third-degree heart block.

Amyloidosis

Not infrequently associated with cardiac involvement, there may be left axis deviation, LBBB or RBBB or complete heart block. A common finding is absence of the initial R wave from V1 to V3 (simulating anteroseptal infarction).

Dextrocardia

In the presence of cardiac disease, the ECG should be normal, apart from left–right inversion.

Technical dextrocardia

This occurs as a result of the inadvertent interchange of the right and left arm connections during the recording. The appearances of the limb leads are identical with those of dextrocardia but the chest leads are normal.

Chapter 15
Cardiac Emergencies

CARDIAC ARREST

Definition
Cardiac arrest is best defined as the cessation of an effective circulation due to:
1 Cardiac asystole.
2 Ventricular fibrillation (VF) — more than 90% of cases.
3 Grossly inadequate cardiac output (extreme bradycardia or tachycardia, or feeble myocardial contractions).

Aetiology
Multiple factors often present:

Myocardial anoxia

Local. Coronary occlusion produces local anoxia of an area of myocardium surrounded by other areas which are properly oxygenated, a situation of electrical instability which readily precipitates ventricular fibrillation.

General. Any anoxic episode (anaesthesia with underventilation, airway obstruction etc.).

Myocardial disease. End-stage dilated cardiomyopathy and hypertrophic cardiomyopathy.

Disease of the conducting tissue, especially bilateral bundle branch fibrosis (Stokes–Adams attacks, pp. 158–163).

Reflex. Particularly vagal reflexes from tracheal stimulation (intubation, inhaled vomit, tracheotomy) or traction on viscera at operation under light anaesthesia.

Drugs and electrolytes
1 Overdose of cardiac drugs — digitalis, quinidine, procainamide.
2 Anaesthetic drugs — chloroform, cyclopropane, halothane, cocaine.
3 Electrolytes — high or low levels of potassium, high levels of calcium.

Other causes
Electrocution, drowning, air embolism.

Diagnosis of cardiac arrest

Sudden collapse accompanied by:

1 Unconsciousness.

2 Apnoea.

3 Absent pulses. Absent carotid pulsation is the best sign as the more peripheral vessels may be impalpable in any low cardiac output state.

4 Dilating pupils. The pupils start to dilate 30–45 s after circulatory arrest.

No further time is wasted in refinements of diagnosis such as electrocardiography, although this may be available if the patient is already connected to an ECG oscilloscope. Treatment is begun at once, as irreversible changes occur in the brain within 4 min.

Treatment of cardiac arrest

Treatment may be divided into three stages: provision of an artificial circulation of oxygenated blood; restoration of a normal beat; and aftercare and treatment of complications.

Provision of an artificial circulation of oxygenated blood

Such provision entails external cardiac massage and artificial ventilation.

External cardiac massage

The patient is laid flat on a firm surface (floor or board) and the lower half of the sternum firmly but quickly depressed by the palms of the hands 3–5 cm in an adult (less for children) 60–80 times a minute.

The heart is compressed between the sternum and the vertebral column and its contained blood ejected into the pulmonary artery and aorta. Pressure is only applied over the lower half of the sternum because force applied elsewhere fractures ribs or damages the liver and spleen. Efficient cardiac compression results in a pulse being felt in a major artery and the return of circulation to the brain results in the pupils shrinking to a normal size.

Artificial ventilation

The upper airway is cleared, the head extended and the jaw pulled forward. Ventilation can be performed by:

1 Mouth-to-mouth breathing.

2 Brook airway — similar to mouth to mouth breathing but using an airway for better fit.

3 Ambu bag — a self-inflating bag and facemask allowing ventilation without a gas supply.

4 Endotracheal tube.

Adequate ventilation is assessed by expansion of the chest with each inflation and by the patient's colour becoming pink.

Restoration of normal beat

Effective massage and ventilation alone may restart the heart and in any case are continued until a normal beat is restored.

Determination of rhythm

An electrocardiograph is connected to the patient to diagnose whether the arrest is due to asystole (pacing then indicated), VF or other rhythm disturbances. If not available, regard as VF.

Electrical defibrillation (see also p. 322)

Ventricular fibrillation is restored to normal rhythm by a shock from a DC defibrillator. One electrode is placed on the chest in the region of the cardiac apex and the other below the angle of the left scapula. A shock of 200 J is usually sufficient to halt VF, but may be repeated with 360 J.

Injection of drugs

Sodium bicarbonate is given after prolonged arrest to counteract metabolic acidosis (check blood gases). Adrenaline (10 ml of 1 : 10 000) and calcium chloride (10 ml of 2% hydrated solution) increase the tone of the heart. Vasopressor drugs sustain the blood pressure once the heart has restarted. Lignocaine 1% and potassium chloride (40 mEq) depress myocardial irritability if relapse into ventricular fibrillation occurs. Atropine (2 mg) is given for bradycardia or asystole.

The drugs may be given into distended jugular veins, into an intravenous infusion or as an endotracheal aerosol.

Aftercare and treatment of complications

Aftercare

1 Monitor pulse and blood pressure.
2 Oxygen by facemask.
3 Oscilloscope for cardiac rhythm.
4 Nasogastric tube to prevent inhalation of vomit.
5 Urinary catheter to recognize oliguria early and to treat it with dopamine (up to 300 µg/min) and frusemide.

Treatment of complications

Renal failure

Acute tubular necrosis may occur and is treated with ion exchange resins dialysis, or haemofiltration.

Cerebral damage

Severe cerebral damage requires steroid therapy (e.g. dexamethasone for 8 days).

Respiratory failure

Assessed from arterial blood gas analysis. Mechanical ventilation is used until spontaneous respiration is again adequate.

EXTERNAL DIRECT CURRENT CARDIOVERSION

An effective and safe method for the termination of many cardiac arrhythmias (see pages 119, 120, 154, 156). A high voltage of short duration is passed through the chest and this depolarizes the heart, momentarily abolishing all electrical activity. Sinus rhythm is usually re-established as rhythmical electrical activity recommences.

Technique

1 Patient anaesthetized with thiopentone or diazepam.
2 Large electrodes placed on the skin overlying the heart, either at apex and base, or front and back of the chest.
3 One shock given at the peak of the R wave of the electrocardiogram (the shock is not given on the ascending limb of the T wave since this is the vulnerable period of the cardiac cycle and ventricular fibrillation can result. The apparatus automatically gives the shock at a predetermined point on the patient's electrocardiogram). No timing is required for VF.
4 A shock of 40–360 J is necessary, depending on the nature of the arrhythmia and the build of the patient.
5 Usually digitalis is discontinued 36 h prior to the shock as the technique is dangerous in the presence of excess digitalis.
6 Anticoagulants are advisable for embolic risk patients.

CARDIAC TRAUMA AND TAMPONADE

See Chapter 11 page 234.

MASSIVE PULMONARY EMBOLISM

See Chapter 10 page 219.

CARDIOGENIC SHOCK

Myocardial infarction

See page 118.

Dissection of aorta

See page 251.

PAROXYSMAL VENTRICULAR TACHYCARDIA (rarely supra-ventricular)

See page 155.

Index